Hair Disorders: Current Concepts in Pathophysiology, Diagnosis and Management

Editor

JERRY SHAPIRO

DERMATOLOGIC CLINICS

www.derm.theclinics.com

Consulting Editor
BRUCE H. THIERS

January 2013 • Volume 31 • Number 1

ELSEVIER

1600 John F. Kennedy Boulevard • Suite 1800 • Philadelphia, PA 19103-2899

http://www.theclinics.com

DERMATOLOGIC CLINICS Volume 31, Number 1
January 2013 ISSN 0733-8635, ISBN-13: 978-1-4557-7081-6

Editor: Stephanie Donley

Dermatologic Clinics (ISSN 0733-8635) is published quarterly by Elsevier Inc., 360 Park Avenue South, New York, NY 10010-1710. Months of publication are January, April, July, and October. Business and editorial offices: 1600 John F. Kennedy Blvd., Suite 1800, Philadelphia, PA 19103-2899. Customer service office: 11830 Westline Drive, St. Louis, MO 63146. Periodicals postage paid at New York, NY, and additional mailing offices. Subscription prices are USD 346.00 per year for US individuals, USD 512.00 per year for US institutions, USD 404.00 per year for Canadian individuals, USD 613.00 per year for Canadian institutions, USD 473.00 per year for international individuals, USD 613.00 per year for international institutions, USD 161.00 per year for US students/residents, and USD 233.00 per year for Canadian and international students/residents. International air speed delivery is included in all *Clinics* subscription prices. All prices are subject to change without notice. **POSTMASTER:** Send address changes to *Dermatologic Clinics*, Elsevier Health Sciences Division, Subscription Customer Service, 3251 Riverport Lane, Maryland Heights, MO 63043. **Customer Service: 1-800-654-2452 (U.S. and Canada); 314-447-8871 (outside U.S. and Canada). Fax: 314-447-8029. E-mail: journalscustomerservice-usa@elsevier.com (for print support); journalsonlinesupport-usa@elsevier.com (for online support).**

Reprints. For copies of 100 or more, of articles in this publication, please contact the Commercial Reprints Department, Elsevier Inc., 360 Park Avenue South, New York, New York 10010-1710. Tel.: (212) 633-3813; Fax: (212) 462-1935; Email: reprints@elsevier.com.

The *Dermatologic Clinics* is covered in *MEDLINE/PubMed (Index Medicus), Current Contents/Clinical Medicine, Excerpta Medica, Chemical Abstracts,* and *ISI/BIOMED.*

Printed and bound by CPI Group (UK) Ltd, Croydon, CR0 4YY

Transferred to digital print 2012

Contributors

CONSULTING EDITOR

BRUCE H. THIERS, MD
Professor and Chairman, Department of
Dermatology and Dermatologic Surgery,
Medical University of South Carolina,
Charleston, South Carolina

GUEST EDITOR

JERRY SHAPIRO, MD
Hair and Scalp Disorders, Clinical Professor,
University of British Columbia; Department of
Dermatology and Skin Science, Vancouver,
Canada; Adjunct Professor, Department of
Dermatology, New York University Langone
Medical Center, New York City, New York

AUTHORS

ABDULLAH ALKHALIFAH, MD
Riyadh Military Hospital, Riyadh, Saudi Arabia

**NATASHA ATANASKOVA MESINKOVSKA,
MD, PhD**
Department of Dermatology, Dermatology and
Plastic Surgery Institute, Cleveland Clinic,
Cleveland, Ohio

NUSRAT BANKA, MD
Department of Dermatology and Skin Science,
University of British Columbia, Vancouver,
British Columbia, Canada

WILMA F. BERGFELD, MD
Department of Dermatology, Dermatology and
Plastic Surgery Institute, Cleveland Clinic,
Cleveland, Ohio

ULRIKE BLUME-PEYTAVI, MD
Professor, Department of Dermatology and
Allergy, Clinical Research Center for Hair and
Skin Science, Charité–Universitätsmedizin
Berlin, Berlin, Germany

TRISIA BREITKOPF, MSc
Department of Dermatology and Skin Science;
Vancouver Coastal Health Research Institute,
The University of British Columbia, Vancouver,
British Columbia, Canada

M.J. KRISTINE BUNAGAN, MD
Department of Dermatology and Skin Science,
University of British Columbia, Vancouver,
British Columbia, Canada

RITA M. CABRAL, PhD
Postdoctoral Research Fellow, Department of
Dermatology, Russ Berrie Medical Science
Pavilion, Columbia University, New York,
New York

JOHN M. CHILDS, MD
Department of Pathology, Walter Reed
National Military Medical Center, Bethesda,
Maryland

ANGELA M. CHRISTIANO, PhD
Richard and Mildred Rhodebeck Professor of
Dermatology and Professor of Genetics and
Development, Departments of Dermatology,
Genetics and Development, Russ Berrie
Medical Science Pavilion, Columbia University,
New York, New York

RAPHAEL CLYNES, MD, PhD
Associate Professor in Pathology, Medicine
and Dermatology, Departments of
Dermatology, Medicine, and Pathology, Russ
Berrie Medical Science Pavilion, Columbia
University, New York, New York

ZOE DIANA DRAELOS, MD
Consulting Professor, Department of
Dermatology, Duke University School of
Medicine, Durham, North Carolina

ANDREAS M. FINNER, MD
Trichomed Clinic for Hair Medicine and Hair
Transplantation, Berlin, Germany

ANDREW G. FRANKS JR, MD
Director, Skin Lupus & Autoimmune
Connective Tissue Disease Center; Professor
of Clinical Dermatology & Medicine
(Rheumatology), New York University School
of Medicine, New York, New York

**SHANNON HARRISON, MBBS, MMed,
FACD**
Honorary Clinical Lecturer, St Vincent's
Hospital, Fitzroy, Melbourne, Victoria, Australia

ALI JABBARI, MD, PhD
Assistant Clinical Professor of Dermatology,
Department of Dermatology, Russ Berrie
Medical Science Pavilion, Columbia University,
New York, New York

ADRIANNA J. JACKSON, MD
Advanced Dermatology, Katy, Texas

SUNIL KALIA, MD, MHSc, FRCPC
Department of Dermatology and Skin Science,
University of British Columbia, and
Photomedicine Institute, Vancouver Coastal
Health, Vancouver, British Columbia, Canada

GIGI LEUNG, BSc
Department of Dermatology and Skin Science;
Vancouver Coastal Health Research Institute,
The University of British Columbia, Vancouver,
British Columbia, Canada

HARVEY LUI, MD, FRCPC
Professor and Chairman, Department of
Dermatology and Skin Science, University of
British Columbia, and Photomedicine Institute,
Vancouver Coastal Health, Vancouver, British
Columbia, Canada

KEVIN J. MCELWEE, PhD
Department of Dermatology and Skin Science;
Vancouver Coastal Health Research Institute,
The University of British Columbia, Vancouver,
British Columbia, Canada

SIAMAK MOGHADAM-KIA, MD
Fellow in Rheumatology, University of
Pittsburgh Medical Center, Pittsburgh,
Pennsylvania

MALGORZATA OLSZEWSKA, MD, PhD
Department of Dermatology, Medical
University of Warsaw, Warsaw, Poland

NINA OTBERG, MD
Head of Hair Clinic, Skin and Laser Center and
Hair Transplant Center, Potsdam, Berlin,
Germany

MANSI PATEL, MBChB
Department of Medicine, St Vincent's Hospital,
University of Melbourne, Fitzroy, Melbourne,
Victoria, Australia

LYNN PETUKHOVA, MS
Biostatistician and Doctoral Candidate,
Departments of Dermatology, and
Epidemiology, Russ Berrie Medical Science
Pavilion, Columbia University, New York,
New York

VERA H. PRICE, MD, FRCPC
Professor, Department of Dermatology,
University of California, San Francisco,
San Francisco, California

ADRIANA RAKOWSKA, MD, PhD
Department of Dermatology, CSK MSWiA,
Warsaw, Poland

LIDIA RUDNICKA, MD, PhD
Department of Dermatology, CSK MSWiA;
Mossakowski Medical Research Centre, Polish
Academy of Sciences; Department of Clinical
Nursing, Faculty of Health Sciences, Medical
University of Warsaw, Warsaw, Poland

JERRY SHAPIRO, MD, FRCPC
Clinical Professor, Department of Dermatology
and Skin Science, University of British
Columbia, Vancouver, British Columbia,
Canada; Department of Dermatology,
New York University, New York City,
New York

RODNEY SINCLAIR, MBBS, MD, PhD, FACD
Director of Dermatology Research, St
Vincent's Hospital, Professor of Dermatology,
University of Melbourne, Fitzroy, Melbourne,
Victoria, Australia

LEONARD C. SPERLING, MD
Department of Dermatology, Uniformed
Services University of the Health Sciences,
Bethesda, Maryland

EDDY WANG, BSc
Department of Dermatology and Skin Science;
Vancouver Coastal Health Research Institute,
The University of British Columbia, Vancouver,
British Columbia, Canada

MEI YU, MD, PhD
Department of Dermatology and Skin Science;
Vancouver Coastal Health Research Institute,
The University of British Columbia, Vancouver,
British Columbia, Canada

SOODABEH ZANDI, MD
Clinical Research Fellow, Department of
Dermatology and Skin Science, University of
British Columbia, Vancouver, British Columbia,
Canada; Associate Professor, Department of
Dermatology, Kerman University of Medical
Sciences, Kerman, Iran

Contents

Preface   xiii

Jerry Shapiro

The Basic Science of Hair Biology: What Are the Causal Mechanisms for the Disordered
Hair Follicle?   1

Trisia Breitkopf, Gigi Leung, Mei Yu, Eddy Wang, and Kevin J. McElwee

> A hair disorder can be difficult to define, but patients are typically motivated to seek treatment when their hair growth patterns are significantly different from their cultural group or when growth patterns change significantly. The causes of hair disorders are many and varied, but fundamentally the disorder is a consequence of aberrant alterations of normal hair biology. The potential trigger factors for hair disorders can be attributed to inflammation, genetics, the environment, or hormones, of which the relative contributions vary for different diagnoses, between individuals, and over time. This article discusses the causal mechanisms for the disordered hair follicle.

How to Diagnose Hair Loss   21

Adrianna J. Jackson and Vera H. Price

> This review presents a systematic approach to the diagnosis of hair loss. An accurate diagnosis is based on history, clinical examination, laboratory tests, and scalp biopsy. Whether the hair loss is a cicatricial or noncicatricial alopecia guides one's history taking. After assessing the patient's global appearance, the hair and scalp are evaluated, aided by a hair pull, hair tug, Hair Card, and hair mount. Scalp biopsies can confirm a diagnosis and are essential in all cases of cicatricial alopecia. In all patients with hair loss a complete blood count, ferritin, thyroid stimulating hormone, and vitamin D 25OH should be ordered.

Trichoscopy: How It May Help the Clinician   29

Lidia Rudnicka, Adriana Rakowska, and Malgorzata Olszewska

> Trichoscopy (or dermoscopy of hair and scalp) is an easy in-office technique that may be performed with a handheld dermoscope or a digital videodermoscopy system. This method is gaining increasing popularity, because it may be applied in differential diagnosis of multiple hair and scalp diseases. The focus of this article is application of trichoscopy in differential diagnosis of the most frequent hair and scalp diseases in dermatologic practice. Trichoscopy of genetic hair shaft abnormalities are briefly addressed. A new classification of perifollicular and interfollicular skin surface abnormalities is proposed.

Histopathology of Scarring and Nonscarring Hair Loss   43

John M. Childs and Leonard C. Sperling

> This article reviews the histologic findings of alopecia, preceded by a brief discussion of biopsy and processing techniques, the normal follicular anatomy and cycle, and expected findings in transverse sections. Subtle histologic abnormalities will be missed unless the normal follicular anatomy and follicular cycle, when viewed in transverse sections, are understood.

How to Diagnose and Treat Medically Women with Excessive Hair   57

Ulrike Blume-Peytavi

Excessive hair growth in women is common and due to a broad spectrum of causes. Management options comprise different pharmaceuticals, epilation methods, and aesthetic approaches. Because excessive hair growth in women may cause psychological and psychosocial problems, a holistic treatment approach, including support and emotional coping strategies, should be recommended. In this article, diagnostic procedures and treatment options for excessive hair growth in female patients are discussed.

Drugs and Hair Loss   67

Mansi Patel, Shannon Harrison, and Rodney Sinclair

Hair loss is a common complaint, both in men and women, and use of prescription medications is widespread. When there is a temporal association between the onset of hair loss and commencement of a medication, the medication is commonly thought to have caused the hair loss. However, hair loss and in particular telogen effluvium may occur in response to a number of triggers including fever, hemorrhage, severe illness, stress, and childbirth, and a thorough exclusion of these potential confounders is necessary before the hair loss can be blamed on the medication. Certain medications are known to cause hair loss by a variety of mechanisms including anagen arrest, telogen effluvium, or accentuation of androgenetic alopecia by androgens.

Autoimmune Disease and Hair Loss   75

Siamak Moghadam-Kia and Andrew G. Franks Jr

Once systemic disease is in remission, it is prudent to recognize the importance of alopecia in the patient's overall sense of well-being and quality-of-life clinical outcome. Scarring alopecia (scalp discoid lupus erythematosus) can be the presenting manifestation of lupus in more than half of affected individuals. Diffuse nonscarring alopecia in lupus is usually responsive to treatment of the systemic disease. Severe, often intractable burning pruritus of the scalp is a frequent complaint in dermatomyositis. Lichen planopilaris may mimic other autoimmune forms of scarring alopecia. Alopecia can also be caused by medications used to treat systemic autoimmune disease and fibromyalgia.

Alopecia Areata Update   93

Abdullah Alkhalifah

Alopecia areata (AA) is a common nonscarring alopecia. It affects 1.7% of the population at some point in their lives. AA is an autoimmune condition characterized by dense peribulbar lymphocytic infiltrate. The exact cause and triggering factors are still unknown. The scalp is the most commonly affected area but any hair-bearing area can be involved. All available treatment options are neither curative nor preventive. This article will discuss updates in AA with focus on etiopathogenesis, clinical presentation, and treatment options and suggest treatment plans based on the age of the patient and extent of the disease.

Genetic Basis of Alopecia Areata: A Roadmap for Translational Research   109

Ali Jabbari, Lynn Petukhova, Rita M. Cabral, Raphael Clynes, and Angela M. Christiano

Alopecia areata (AA) is a recurrent autoimmune type of hair loss that affects about 5.3 million people in the United States alone. Despite being the most prevalent autoimmune disease, the molecular and cellular mechanisms underlying this complex disease are still poorly understood, and rational treatments are lacking. Further efforts are necessary to clearly pinpoint the causes and molecular pathways leading to this disease and to find evidence-based treatments for AA. The authors focus on the central role of genetics for gaining insight into disease pathogenesis and setting the stage for the rational development of novel effective therapeutic approaches.

Hair: What is New in Diagnosis and Management?: Female Pattern Hair Loss Update: Diagnosis and Treatment   119

Natasha Atanaskova Mesinkovska and Wilma F. Bergfeld

Female pattern hair loss (FPHL) is the most common cause of alopecia in women. FPHL is characterized histologically with increased numbers of miniaturized, velluslike hair follicles. The goal of treatment of FPHL is to arrest hair loss progression and stimulate hair regrowth. The treatments for FPHL can be divided into androgen-dependent and androgen-independent. There is an important adjuvant role for nutritional supplements, light therapy, and hair transplants. All treatments work best when initiated early. Combinations of treatments tend to be more efficacious.

Pattern Hair Loss in Men: Diagnosis and Medical Treatment   129

Nusrat Banka, M.J. Kristine Bunagan, and Jerry Shapiro

Androgenetic alopecia is a common cause of hair loss in both men and women. The exact pathogenesis of androgenetic alopecia is not well understood. As the name implies, the role of androgens and genetic susceptibility predisposes to pattern hair loss due to gradual conversion of terminal hair into vellus hair. Male and female pattern hair loss are clinically distinct entities but histologically indistinguishable. The role of sex hormones in females is less understood. This article discusses current understanding of the etiopathogenesis of hair loss in men, diagnostic tests available, and its medical management.

Hair Transplantation Update: Procedural Techniques, Innovations, and Applications   141

M.J. Kristine Bunagan, Nusrat Banka, and Jerry Shapiro

The advances in hair transplantation, particularly the advent of follicular unit transplantation, have greatly elevated the outcome of this procedure. Various modifications to the basic technique as well as innovations focused on the different aspects of the hair transplantation procedure have further enhanced this type of hair restoration surgery. In addition, there is ongoing expansion of the indications and applications of this procedure beyond the usual male pattern hair loss.

Primary Cicatricial Alopecias   155

Nina Otberg

Primary cicatricial alopecias refer to a group of rare, idiopathic, inflammatory scalp disorders that result in permanent hair loss. Primary cicatricial alopecias comprise a diverse group of inflammatory diseases and can be classified via different approaches, such as clinical presentation, histopathologic findings, or both. Primary cicatricial alopecias are rare scalp disorders. Whiting found a prevalence of 7.3% in all patients who sought advice for hair and scalp problems at the Baylor Hair Research and Treatment Center in Dallas between 1989 and 1999.

Nutrition and Hair: Deficiencies and Supplements   167

Andreas M. Finner

> Hair follicle cells have a high turnover. A caloric deprivation or deficiency of several components, such as proteins, minerals, essential fatty acids, and vitamins, caused by inborn errors or reduced uptake, can lead to structural abnormalities, pigmentation changes, or hair loss, although exact data are often lacking. The diagnosis is established through a careful history, clinical examination of hair loss activity, and hair quality and confirmed through targeted laboratory tests. Examples of genetic hair disorders caused by reduced nutritional components are zinc deficiency in acrodermatitis enteropathica and copper deficiency in Menkes kinky hair syndrome.

Shampoos, Conditioners, and Camouflage Techniques   173

Zoe Diana Draelos

> This article examines hair care in persons with hair loss. The use of shampoos, conditioners, and hair styling products to camouflage hair loss is discussed. Because hair is nonliving, medical treatments are limited to only inducing change in the follicles within the scalp skin and do not improve the hair loss actually witnessed by the patient. There is therefore a need to accompany medical treatment of hair loss with cosmetic hair treatment to optimize patient satisfaction.

Long-Term Removal of Unwanted Hair Using Light   179

Soodabeh Zandi and Harvey Lui

> Laser (or light) hair removal, also referred to as *photoepilation*, is the most commonly used laser or light-based cosmetic medical procedure. The extended theory of selective photothermolysis is the basic principle for destruction of hair follicles using light. In this type of laser application the chromophore is follicular melanin. Several types of lasers and light sources have been effective for hair reduction, including the ruby, alexandrite, diode, and neodymium:yttrium-aluminum-garnet lasers and broadband, intense pulsed light sources. This article provides a broad overview of how hair can be removed using light, with an emphasis on practical considerations.

Utilizing Electromagnetic Radiation for Hair Growth: A Critical Review of Phototrichogenesis   193

Sunil Kalia and Harvey Lui

> Hair loss has a high prevalence in the general population and can have significant medical and psychological sequelae. Pattern hair loss and alopecia areata represent the major reasons patients present to dermatologists in relation to hair loss. Because conventional treatment options are generally incompletely effective, novel methods for hair grown induction are being developed. The role of using electromagnetic radiation, including low-level laser therapy for the management of hair loss through phototrichogenesis, is reviewed in this article.

Index   201

DERMATOLOGIC CLINICS

FORTHCOMING ISSUES

April 2013
Pediatric Dermatology
Moise L. Levy, MD, *Guest Editor*

July 2013
Autoinflammatory Disorders
William Abramovits, MD, and
Marcial Oquendo, MD, *Guest Editors*

October 2013
Dermoscopy
Giussepe Argenziano, MD,
Iris Zalaudek, MD, and
Jason Giacomel, MD, *Guest Editors*

RECENT ISSUES

October 2012
Dermatopathology
Tammie Ferringer, MD, *Guest Editor*

July 2012
Melanoma and Pigmented Lesions
Julie E. Russak, MD, and
Darrell S. Rigel, MD, *Guest Editors*

April 2012
Quality of Life Issues in Dermatology
Suephy C. Chen, MD, MS, *Guest Editor*

Preface

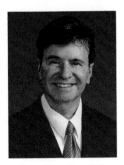

Jerry Shapiro, MD
Guest Editor

Over the past 25 years, I have remarked that the field of hair has continued to gain sizeably more interest now that we have an increasing number of options and accepted approaches to various hair diseases. Twenty-five years ago, there were very few effective treatments to offer patients except the surgical option for pattern hair loss. Patients, knowing there are now more options, are going to dermatologists for treatments. The Internet has made the patient more inquisitive and patients are seeking treatments aggressively. As a result, the dermatologist is now paying far more attention to hair issues than ever before.

There are now symposia at international meetings totally devoted to hair science and disorders. There are also entire international meetings devoted to trichology. The World Congress of Hair Research Societies takes place yearly with an increasing record-breaking attendance of dermatologists and basic science hair researchers convening and sharing their knowledge.

There are now meetings devoted to just specific hair disorders such as alopecia areata and cicatricial alopecia. This was unheard of 25 years ago. At the Society for Investigational Dermatology, the hair presentations have exponentially increased over the past 15 years. With the advancing technology in molecular biology and genetics, the mechanics of the hair follicle are slowly being unravelled.

This issue of *Dermatologic Clinics* includes a "bench-to-bedside" spectrum of hair-related topics: basic science, pathology, pathophysiology, diagnosis, nutrition, endocrine issues, medical treatments, lasers, hair transplantation, and cosmetic camouflage. We hope it will help the dermatologist understand, diagnose, and treat specific hair disorders more effectively.

I am grateful to all the authors for their countless hours in putting together this edition on hair. I also want to thank Bruce Theirs for the opportunity to guest edit this issue as well as Stephanie Donley for her professional editorial assistance.

Jerry Shapiro, MD
Hair and Scalp Disorders
University of British Columbia
Department of Dermatology and Skin Science
Vancouver, Canada

New York University Langone Medical Center
Department of Dermatology
New York City, NY, USA

E-mail address:
jerry.shapiro@vch.ca

Dermatol Clin 31 (2013) xiii
http://dx.doi.org/10.1016/j.det.2012.08.013
0733-8635/13/$ – see front matter © 2013 Elsevier Inc. All rights reserved.

The Basic Science of Hair Biology
What Are the Causal Mechanisms for the Disordered Hair Follicle?

Trisia Breitkopf, MSc[a,b], Gigi Leung, BSc[a,b], Mei Yu, MD, PhD[a,b],
Eddy Wang, BSc[a,b], Kevin J. McElwee, PhD[a,b],*

KEYWORDS

- Hair loss • Hair disorders • Inflammation • Genes • Environment • Hormones

KEY POINTS

- A hair follicle disorder can be defined as when the characteristics of hair growth fall outside the commonly accepted parameters for a particular group, whether identified by gender, age, ethnicity, and/or culture.
- A patient's perception of a hair disorder is determined by differences in "hair coverage" relative to the prior hair growth pattern and/or the growth patterns of others in the patient's cultural group.
- A dermatologist's perception of a hair disorder is determined by objective measurements of hair follicle density per unit area of skin and average terminal hair fiber thickness.

INTRODUCTION: WHAT IS A HAIR FOLLICLE DISORDER?

Hair disorders are not directly life threatening, although they can be a symptom of a more serious condition. A hair disorder may indicate significant threats to life from shedding as a result of toxin exposure, through tumor-secreting hormonal imbalances, to extensive inflammation as occurs with systemic lupus erythematosus. Fundamentally, however, a hair disorder is any condition in which the visible hair coverage over the skin falls outside of normal hair growth parameters. The definition of "normal hair growth" varies with gender, ethnicity, age, and, often, the particular opinion of the individual concerned.

For most people, "normal" scalp hair coverage requires a certain density of terminal hair follicles over the frontal, temporal, auricular, midscalp, vertex, and occipital scalp. Of course, there may be considerable variability in tolerance. The exact geographic limits of terminal scalp hair coverage can differ with ethnicity; the hairline for some East Asian-Indians can be notably more forward on the temples than that for persons of other ethnicities, for example. The nature of the coverage also

Funding sources: McElwee: Canadian Institutes of Health Research (CIHR), Michael Smith Foundation for Health Research (MSFHR), National Alopecia Areata Foundation (NAAF), Canadian Dermatology Foundation (CDF), Replicel Life Sciences. Breitkopf: CIHR Skin Research Training Center (CIHR-SRTC). Wang: CIHR Skin Research Training Center (CIHR-SRTC). Others: None.
Conflict of interest: McElwee is chief scientific officer and shareholder of Replicel Life Sciences Inc. Others: None.
a Department of Dermatology and Skin Science, The University of British Columbia, 835 West Tenth Avenue, Vancouver, British Columbia V5Z 4E8, Canada; b Vancouver Coastal Health Research Institute, The University of British Columbia, 835 West Tenth Avenue, Vancouver, British Columbia V5Z 4E8, Canada
* Corresponding author.
E-mail address: kmcelwee@interchange.ubc.ca

Dermatol Clin 31 (2013) 1–19
http://dx.doi.org/10.1016/j.det.2012.08.006

varies, with a relatively lower density of terminal hair follicles but larger average size of individual hair fibers in persons of Far East Asian ethnicities. Culture also plays a significant role in defining acceptable scalp hair coverage.

There is greater challenge in defining "normal" when it comes to facial hair and body hair. The definition of normal beard growth is highly variable between ethnicities, ranging from mostly full beard growth capacity in Middle East populations to no almost beard growth in Native North Americans. Even within ethnic groups, beard growth capacity can be variable as with North European whites. What is normal also varies with gender; beard growth is normal for men but a disorder when it occurs in women. Terminal, pigmented body hair again varies with ethnicity; Mediterranean people typically have more extensive body hair growth, whereas Far East Asian people may have relatively little body hair. Cultural opinion strongly modifies the definition of normal body hair growth parameters. Concerns related to body hair are mostly limited to those in North America and Far East Asia, although this anxiety is spreading to other ethnic groups. Notably, though, the impact of cultural influence is variable; for example, British and Finnish women regard male body hair growth as desirable, whereas North American women find it unattractive.[1]

Consequently, whether a hair disorder is identified depends in part on the genetic and cultural background of the individual concerned. A hair follicle disorder is probably best defined as when the characteristics of hair growth fall outside the commonly accepted parameters for a particular group, whether defined by gender, age, ethnicity, and/or culture. Rectifying hair disorders, whether perceived or real, has become a global industry. The changeable definition of a hair disorder can also determine whether treatment comes from the cosmetic sector or from medical health care systems. For example, laser hair removal can be regarded as entirely cosmetic, or it may be considered a medical treatment when hypertrichosis can be given a specific diagnostic label. Defining a hair disorder can be challenging.

CONTRIBUTION OF HAIR BIOLOGY TO HAIR DISORDERS
The Patient's Point of View

Whether a patient perceives he or she has a hair disorder is often determined by changes in "hair coverage," usually on the scalp but also on the body. A significant increase or decrease in terminal hair, relative to the prior hair growth pattern or the growth patterns of other people in the same cultural group, can motivate the search for treatment. The definition of hair coverage for a patient is often different from the definition used by dermatologists and other professionals. For a patient, hair coverage is the total amount of hair present, something professionals might describe as total hair mass. A patient's understanding of normal hair coverage typically involves a synthesis of the numbers of hairs, hair thickness, hair length, and hair style.

The Dermatologist's Point of View

For a dermatologist, hair coverage is the combination of hair follicle density per unit area of skin with average hair fiber thickness. A higher density of follicles producing terminal hair fibers gives better coverage; the same density of hair follicles but producing thicker hair fibers also increases coverage. Improvements in both terminal hair density and average hair diameter work synergistically. Hair coverage is a fully quantitative, objective metric that is examined in trichograms, phototrichograms, and, most recently, digital trichogram image techniques.[2] The length of hair is not considered in trichograms, but it can play a role in semiuantitative analyses when global hair coverage is evaluated. Potentially, hair length can interfere with global analysis; an individual with the same hair density and same average hair fiber diameter might seem to have better overall scalp coverage if the hair is allowed to grow.[2] To avoid this issue in clinical trials, participants are usually expected to have their hair cut in a similar style and length before each global evaluation and to avoid styling products. For the dermatologist, then, normal hair coverage is strictly determined by biologic parameters.

Hair Follicle Embryogenesis

The nature of hair follicle formation and growth is described in detail elsewhere.[3] The development and differentiation of hair follicles during embryogenesis is classically divided into 8 stages characterized by distinct morphologies. Extensive research has examined hair follicle embryogenesis and its control, although understanding of the biologic mechanisms involved is quite limited. It is known to require a complex sequence of autocrine, paracrine, and endocrine signals to occur both within and between the epithelium and dermis. How these factors interact with each other, their relative significance, the degree of redundancy in the signaling system, and how these signals determine hair follicle distribution and subsequent growth cycle characteristics are still not well understood.[4] However, it is clear that multiple signaling pathways are required for the correct development and geographic distribution of hair follicle formation through the skin.[5] Consequently, perturbations in hair follicle embryogenesis can produce a hair disorder.[6]

Hair Follicle (Fiber) Density

Outside of experimental induction– or injury-mediated hair follicle formation (neogenesis)[7,8] and cases in which neogenesis may occur naturally in nonhuman species,[9] embryogenesis determines the total number of hair follicles an individual has for the duration of life. Each human typically has 2 million hair follicles across the body.[10] Disorders involving increases in hair follicle number or abnormally increased local density are not found in humans, except perhaps in rare cases involving neogenesis in hyperplastic skin lesions[8] and clustering of follicles in tufted hair folliculitis.[11] However, a failure of embryogenesis can lead to an abnormally low density of hair follicle formation (hypotrichosis), whether in general or in specific body regions. More common is a normal density of hair follicle formation, which is then adversely impacted later in life by an insult yielding a significant reduction in hair follicle number. Plainly, a considerable change in the density of hair follicles per unit area of skin can underlie the development of a hair disorder (**Fig. 1**).

Hair Follicle (Fiber) Size

Hair follicles (fibers) of adults are classified into 3 different groups and size is a key feature that determines their categorization.[3,12] Most human hair follicles produce short, fine, nonpigmented vellus hairs. In contrast, eyebrow, eyelash, and scalp follicles produce much bigger, slowly cycling, usually pigmented terminal hairs from birth. Follicles retain a degree of plasticity with respect to the type of hair produced and they can transform from vellus into terminal hair production, and vice versa. Hair follicles progressing through a transition in size are defined by some as producing intermediate hairs. Essentially, they are neither full terminal hairs nor full vellus hairs and are observed as terminal hair follicles miniaturize or vellus hair follicles enlarge (**Fig. 2**). Hair follicle size, and so the size of the hair fiber the follicle produces, potentially has a great impact on hair coverage (**Fig. 3**). A terminal to vellus scalp hair follicle switch (miniaturization) can be seen with the development of androgenetic alopecia (AGA), chronic alopecia areata (AA), or chronic telogen effluvium (TE), for example. Conversely, a vellus to terminal body hair follicle switch is seen with hirsutism and hypertichoses.

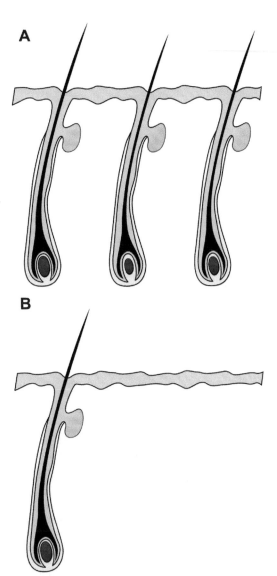

Fig. 1. Changes in hair follicle density elicit a hair disorder. In comparison to normal terminal hair density (*A*), a reduced density of hair follicles, and consequently visible hair fibers, results in reduced hair coverage (*B*).

Hair Fiber Growth Rate

It can be a surprise for patients when they learn that the rate of hair growth does not make a very significant contribution to the development of their hair disorder. In the minds of many, a fast rate of hair growth tends to be associated with hypertrichosis, whereas alopecia is associated with a slow hair growth rate. There is some truth to this relationship; the rate of hair growth does slow in the development of AGA, whereas vellus hair follicles that switch to terminal hair follicles speed up their growth rate. However, compared

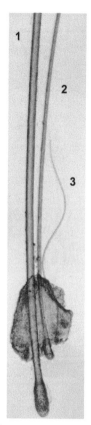

Fig. 2. Hair follicle miniaturization and intermediate hairs. As terminal hair follicles miniaturize they complete a normal hair growth cycle in which a hair fiber of normal thickness is produced (1). In the subsequent growth cycle, a smaller hair follicle produces a finer and sometimes shorter hair fiber (2). The number of cycles needed to fully miniaturize may vary, but in this case the hair follicle entered a third cycle as a fully miniaturized follicle and consequently produced a vellus-like hair fiber (3). Fibers are held together by a sebum plug; taken from an individual with AGA.

with hair follicle size and density, the rate of hair growth provides little toward overall hair coverage as defined in the dermatology clinic. A cluster of hair follicles with slow fiber growth provide the same coverage as a cluster with the same density and size producing hair fiber unusually rapidly; if the patient is willing to wait for the hair to grow. Rate of hair growth is usually only a significant issue when a patient is impatient.

CONTRIBUTION OF THE HAIR CYCLE TO HAIR DISORDERS
Hair Growth Cycle

The nature of hair follicle growth cycles is described in detail elsewhere.[3] There are 3 main phases of the hair follicle cycle: an active growth

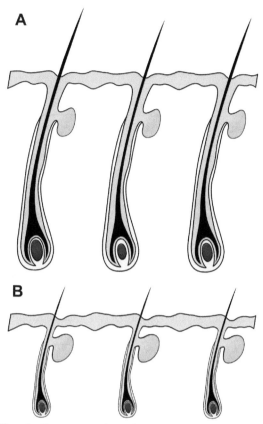

Fig. 3. Changes in hair follicle size elicit a hair disorder. In comparison to normal terminal hair density (A), as terminal hair follicles miniaturize the density of follicles may remain the same (cf **Fig. 1**). However, their reduced size only allows for vellus-like hair fiber production, which fails to provide adequate cosmetic hair coverage (B).

phase called anagen; catagen when the hair follicle regresses; and telogen, when the hair follicle is largely quiescent (**Fig. 4**).[10] How long each phase takes partly depends on the type of hair follicle involved and its geographic location. For someone defined as "normal," roughly 85% of scalp hair follicles are in anagen and 15% are in telogen, although these values can change with ethnicity.[3] Anagen in normal terminal scalp follicles may last from 2 to 6 years, whereas telogen may take about 3 months and catagen about 3 weeks.[3] Potentially, significant changes to the normal hair cycle can elicit a hair disorder.[6]

Hair Follicle Anagen Growth Phase

The duration of anagen is a major determinant of the maximal hair length, along with the rate of hair growth. For example, the anagen phase of eyebrow hair follicles is only 70 days. In addition, the rate of growth is only 0.1 mm/d for eyebrow

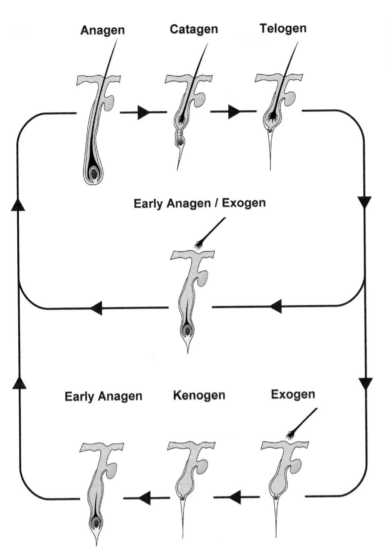

Anagen　　Catagen　　Telogen

Early Anagen / Exogen

Early Anagen　　Kenogen　　Exogen

Fig. 4. Changes in hair growth cycling elicit a hair disorder. As hair follicles progress through a normal cycle, exogen shedding typically occurs close to the time of renewed anagen onset. Consequently, net hair fiber density is maintained. However, in many alopecias, telogen duration increases such that exogen shedding occurs some time before renewed anagen onset. Consequently, hair follicles may remain in telogen without holding a hair fiber, a state termed kenogen.

hair versus around 0.3 mm/d for scalp hair.[3] The net result is a much reduced opportunity for long eyebrow hair to grow. Consequently, eyebrows grow to a certain length and apparently stop, whereas scalp hair can grow much longer. This differential in the time duration of anagen is part of what is known as the hair cycle clock (see later). An increase in the duration of anagen does not alter hair fiber density over the scalp; instead, it determines to what length the hair can grow. A patient tends to value hair length; longer hair can be cosmetically styled to cover areas affected by alopecia, for example.

Hair Follicle Telogen Phase

In and of its self, an increase in the duration of telogen does not alter hair fiber coverage over the scalp. Rather, the longer the time period of telogen, the larger is the window of opportunity for shedding of the telogen club hair to take place. Prolongation of the telogen phase in scalp hair follicles can result in alopecia development as shedding progressively occurs. Telogen hair fibers continue to be shed, but with the failure of the follicles to enter a new anagen phase, new hair fiber is not produced to replace the old shed fibers. This is the most common mechanism by which alopecia may develop, whether describing a distinct alopecic patch or a diffuse thinning. Such a situation can be observed in AGA or TE, for example. Mouse models can provide a demonstration of alopecia development as a result of shedding occurrence before the onset of renewed anagen. Mice with a targeted mutation of the telomerase RNA component have a decreased percentage of hair follicles in anagen, an increased percentage in telogen, and a progressive alopecia as shedding of telogen hair is apparently normal.[13]

Hair Cycle Clock

Under normal physiologic conditions, each hair follicle will continue to cycle throughout life. These cycles are regulated by specific changes in the local signaling milieu, based on changes in expression of hormones, cytokines, and their respective receptors, as well as transcription factors, enzymes, antagonist binding proteins, and epigenetic events.[14] These components may act in endocrine, paracrine, or autocrine manners with positive and negative feedback loops.[15] What determines the clock mechanism and the duration of anagen in individual hair follicles is not known, although many hypotheses have been suggested.[10]

Changes may occur to the hair cycle clock that contribute to the development of alopecias and, to a lesser extent, to hypertrichoses. A prolongation of the anagen growth phase duration (or, alternatively, a delay in the onset of catagen) may be a component of hypertrichosis, yielding excessively long hair. Conversely, a reduction in the anagen growth duration (premature induction of catagen) results in the growth of very short hair fibers as a result of the brief growth phase. This can sometimes be observed in patients with AA, for example. The impact of hair cycle clock changes is most noticeable in animal models. In Angora mice, in which a mutation in *Fgf5* increases the duration of anagen, the fur is up to 50% longer than normal, producing a more fluffy appearance.[16,17] In contrast, truncated anagen growth in mice transgenic for the *Wingless-related MMTV integration site 3 (Wnt3)* yields very short, stubble-like hair growth.[18] A similar density of hair follicles is maintained in both situations.

Hair Follicle Exogen Event

The term "exogen" essentially describes telogen club hair fiber shedding from an individual hair follicle. Previously, hair fiber shedding was believed to be passive, but recent research suggests that shedding is an active and highly controlled process.[19,20] Exogen is a moveable event in the main anagen-catagen-telogen cycle (see **Fig. 4**). The duration of anagen on its own does not alter the density of hair fiber present. Instead, a combination of anagen duration and a lack of exogen shedding allows for increased numbers of hair fibers to be present in the same hair follicle (old telogen club hairs plus new growing anagen hairs). Similarly, an increased duration of telogen alone also does not alter hair fiber coverage. The longer the

time period of telogen, the larger is the window of opportunity for exogen shedding of the telogen club hair to take place. Alternatively, the duration of telogen may be normal but the exogen event is premature, leading to thin hair and alopecia. A good example is the *Msx2* mutant mouse model in which waves of anagen hair growth and telogen rest occur but the exogen event is premature. The result is a mouse with bands of fur apparently migrating over bald skin.[21]

Hair Follicle Kenogen Event

Typically, exogen and shedding of an old hair fiber occur as the follicle is in early anagen actively producing a new hair fiber. However, as noted, exogen can occur when a hair follicle is still in telogen before the onset of renewed anagen (see **Fig. 4**). When this occurs the hair follicle may remain empty of hair fiber for a period of time, in a state termed "kenogen."[22] Not surprisingly then, how long a club hair fiber is retained, and when it is shed in relation to the production of a new hair fiber, helps to determine hair coverage. Kenogen can be observed in healthy scalp skin, but the frequency and duration are significantly greater in individuals with alopecias.[23] With more club hair fibers expelled from hair follicles still in a telogen state, so the numbers of kenogen follicles increase; the net result is bald skin.

Dystrophic Anagen Growth Phase

As noted, kenogen hair follicles devoid of visible hair fiber are most commonly in a prolonged telogen state. However, kenogen hair follicles can also be in an early anagen phase before the emergence of a new hair fiber from the skin surface or in a dystrophic anagen state. A dystrophic anagen state is when the follicle is active but unable to produce a healthy fiber. Such a situation can be observed in anagen effluvium or AA, for example.[24,25] The external insult stops the follicles from successfully forming a recognizable hair fiber.

All of these biologic components can contribute to the development of a hair disorder with different combinations relevant to different disorders.[6]

CAUSAL FACTORS OF HAIR DISORDERS

The authors have attempted to review the basic mechanisms behind hair disorders, but this does not address events that cause a hair disorder to occur. The potential trigger factors for hair disorders are many and varied but can be attributed to one or more categories: inflammation, genetics, the environment, and hormones (**Fig. 5**). In most instances, factors from one of these categories

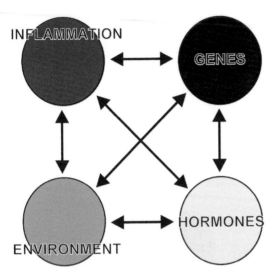

Fig. 5. Potential trigger factors for hair disorders attributed to inflammation, genetics, the environment, and hormones. Factors that elicit or modulate a hair disorder are many and varied but can be categorized as inflammation, genes, environmental, and/or hormones. Disorder-promoting factors may interact and influence each other with the net effect affecting hair follicle biology.

predominate in the development of the hair disorder, but factors in other categories may also contribute (**Fig. 6**). In different individuals with the same condition, the relative contributions of different factors promoting the hair disorder may vary. In addition, the key factors important in promoting the hair disorder may change over time.

INFLAMMATION
Inflammation and Hair Loss

Hair loss promoted by some form of inflammatory insult is not unusual. The inflammation may be specific for the hair follicle or nonspecific. For example, skin inflammation associated with lupus erythematosus may induce a diffuse alopecia in regions of inflamed skin.[26] In this situation, the inflammatory infiltrate is not specifically targeting hair follicles, but because of the general inflammatory effect, hair follicles in the vicinity are adversely affected. Nonspecific inflammation may be a primary promoter of a hair disorder or it may operate in combination with other influential factors. For example, scalp inflammation can be variably associated with AGA. When present, the inflammation may further exacerbate the alopecia.[27] Many forms of nonspecific skin inflammation may promote a degree of alopecia, but in some cases, nonspecific inflammation can also promote hair growth. For example, local injury or irritation can lead to a stimulation of anagen and local increases in terminal hair growth.[28–30] From ancient times, physical and chemical skin irritation techniques have been used to promote hair growth.[31]

Although nonspecific inflammation can promote a hair disorder, inflammatory hair loss disorders can involve an infiltrate targeted to the affected hair follicles. It is worth noting that the target of interest for the inflammatory cells can be exogenous. The hair canal is a known reservoir of bacteria, fungi, viruses, and even parasitic organisms like demodex folliculorum.[32–38] When exogenous stimulators are involved, the inflammatory hair loss condition is usually treatable by removing the antigenic challenge. However, more typically, endogenous hair follicle–specific targets are of interest to inflammatory cells, as occurs with AA or scarring alopecia. These conditions have been studied in some detail, and for both it has been hypothesized that hair follicle–expressed antigens are inappropriately stimulating the immune system.

Hair Follicles and Immune Privilege

Hair follicles, similar to other organs like the testis and the anterior chamber of the eye, are believed to be immune-privileged (IP) sites where immune cell activity is limited.[39,40] IP sites are characterized by downregulation of major histocompatibility complex (MHC)-I complexes, increase in immunosuppressive cytokines, and constitutive expression of cell surface immune regulatory factors such as Fas ligand.[40] Active IP may be especially important during normal hair follicle cycling when apoptosis takes place during the catagen (regressing) phase of the cycle.[41,42] Activation of the immune system by the antigens released from hair follicles during this phase needs to be avoided.[39] The loss of IP is involved in many (auto)-immune diseases such as multiple sclerosis, autoimmune uveitis, fetal rejection, mumps orchitis, and autoimmune chronic active hepatitis.[43] Potentially, when the hair follicle is unable to maintain IP, immune cells are able to infiltrate into the hair follicle and be activated by the hair follicle–specific self-antigens.[42] Activated immune cells express various inflammatory cytokines and proapoptotic molecules that could interfere with hair follicle integrity and may result in hair loss.

AA: An Inflammation-Mediated Hair Loss Disorder

AA is one of the most common forms of autoimmune disease associated with hair follicle.[44] It is characterized by nonscarring, inflammatory patches of hair loss that can progress into alopecia totalis and alopecia universalis.[45] From

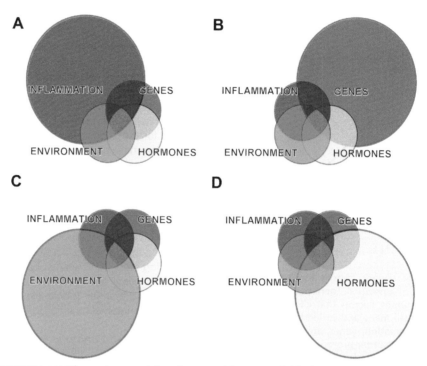

Fig. 6. Inflammatory, genetic, environmental, or hormonal factors variably dominate and interact to affect hair follicle biology. In most instances, factors from one of inflammation, genes, the environment, or hormones predominate in the development of the hair disorder, but factors in other categories may also contribute in a more minor role. Inflammation may dominate in AA or scarring alopecia (*A*); genes may play a principal role in disorders, particularly congenital hypotrichoses and hypertrichoses (*B*); the environment prevails in telogen and anagen effluviums (*C*); but hormones can be the key component for some forms of TE and, of course, in AGA. (*D*) The relative contributions of different factors promoting the hair disorder may vary between different individuals with the same disorder or over time within the same person.

immunohistologic analysis of AA lesions in both humans and rodent models, there is an increase in CD8[+] cytotoxic lymphocytes infiltrating into the hair follicle, whereas CD4[+] cells localize around the hair follicle.[42,46,47] In association with the infiltration is increased expression of MHC class I and II and possibly a loss of IP supporting factors.[48] This could be a sign of collapsed hair follicle IP, allowing lymphocyte infiltration.[42] In response to endogenous inciting antigens,[49–51] the lymphocytes may disrupt the normal hair growth cycle and/or induce apoptosis in the follicular cells via cytokines and other molecules.[41] When depleting CD4[+] or CD8[+] cells in rodent models, there is a significant improvement in AA and hair regrowth.[52,53] Conversely, transfer of AA-activated CD8[+] cells into healthy recipients induces localized AA at site of injection, whereas CD4[+] cells alone eventually promote systemic hair loss, suggesting CD4[+] cells promote AA by "helping" CD8[+] cells.[42,54] The basic inflammatory mechanism of AA has been confirmed by many research groups; however, the exact antigen(s) that trigger the onset of AA are still not yet elucidated.

Role of genetics
Although it is clear that inflammation is the driving force behind the development of AA, genetics also play a role (see **Fig. 6**). It has been found that monozygotic twins have similar times of onset and patterns of AA and some patients have a family history of AA.[45,55–57] These are strong indications that AA is heritable in at least some cases. The genetic composition of a person may affect the expression of self-antigens, which can increase the chance of immune cells targeting and killing hair follicle cells. It has been found that in patients with AA that there is an aberrant expression of specific MHC antigens that likely promote antigen-specific immune cell activation.[58] Mouse and human genomewide screening studies have suggested several more non-HLA gene alleles that may confer AA susceptibility.[44,59]

Role of hormones and the environment
Although genotype may control the relative susceptibility of each individual, environmental inputs are probably important for the onset of AA (see **Fig. 6**).[45] The behavior of hair follicle

immune responses can be modified by environmental factors.[42] In AA, cytomegalovirus has been implicated,[44,60,61] as well as hepatitis B vaccination,[62,63] although conflicting data are presented in different studies. In a mouse model, diet can modify AA susceptibility,[64] and testosterone can increase resistance to AA.[65] Elevated corticotrophin-releasing hormone in AA mice may lead to a dysregulated immune system.[66] The abnormal corticotrophin-releasing hormone and hypothalamic-pituitary-adrenal axis activity in AA could also potentiate an autoimmune response.[67,68] These observations highlight the complexity of AA progression; more than one factor combined with genetic predispositions may be required for the dysregulation of immune response and the onset of hair loss. The development of AA involves input from multiple factors and certain thresholds must be reached before clinically significant changes can be observed.

Cicatricial Alopecia: An Inflammation-Mediated Hair Loss Disorder

Targeted inflammation around the upper, permanent portion of the hair follicle can lead to its destruction, as seen in primary cicatricial (scarring) alopecias.[69] Permanent hair follicle loss results in decreased or completely absent hair follicle density in affected areas. In some scarring alopecias, there is a neutrophil infiltrate, and in others there is a mixed infiltrate of lymphocytes and neutrophils.[70] In the case of lichen planopilaris, Langerhans cells and CD4+ and CD8+ lymphocytes infiltrate the upper permanent follicular epithelium.[69,71,72] Some hypothesize that a loss of IP in the hair follicle bulge region[73] and, therefore, destruction of bulge stem cells are what lead to the permanent hair loss observed in scarring alopecia.[70] Stronger expression of MHC Class I and II and β2-microglobulin are observed in the bulge region of hair follicles in cicatricial alopecia–affected skin compared with uninvolved skin.[74] It is unclear whether the inflammation is the initiating event, causing hair follicle disruption, or a secondary event responding to an unidentified hair follicle abnormality. Additionally, it is unknown whether the inflammatory target antigen is from hair follicle cells or from an external source.

Role of genetics, hormones, and the environment

It is unclear how the different subtypes of primary scarring alopecias are activated and progress, but genetics, hormones, and the environment may play a role in some cases (see **Fig. 6**).[75] A down-regulation of lipid metabolism genes, such as *PPARγ*, have been observed in advance of inflammation suggesting that lipid metabolic issues appear earlier than inflammatory problems in lichen planopilaris.[70] Knockout of PPARγ in bulge cells of mice render them more susceptible to the development of scarring alopecia.[76] Potentially, then, the genetics of lipid metabolism may help determine susceptibility to some forms of scarring alopecia. In lichen planopilaris, postulated stimuli include exposure to quinacrine, vaccinations, or gold.[77] In folliculitis decalvans, *Staphylococcus aureus* infection has been proposed as an antigenic stimulus and antimicrobial treatment can be effective in some cases.[69,77] A case of tick-borne lymphadenopathy was followed by development of cicatricial alopecia.[78] In frontal fibrosing alopecia, estrogens may increase susceptibility to its development.[79] As with AA, scarring alopecias may be inflammatory cell driven, but genetics, hormones, and environmental components may help determine the course of the disease.

GENETICS
Genetics and Hair Loss

Congenital disorders of hair growth are almost always genetic. The environment, hormones, and inflammation may contribute, but the impact of gene-mediated activity predominates (see **Fig. 6**). Fundamentally, a congenital hypertrichosis or congenital alopecia is caused by incorrect or incomplete embryogenic formation of hair follicles. Because hair coverage is defined by hair follicle density, size, and growth cycle, genetic modifications to these parameters can result in congenital hair growth disorders.

Genetics and Hair Follicle Density

The most obvious genetic modification of embryogenesis possible is a reduction in the number of hair follicles formed per unit area of skin. This defect may be localized, as with aplasia cutis congenita or triangular alopecia, when local skin and hair follicles are incompletely formed or follicles fail to achieve terminal size.[80,81] Alternatively, a genetic defect may affect the entire skin and be apparent from birth. As examples, *EDA* gene mutations cause anhidrotic ectodermal dysplasia (ED) and *EDA* receptor gene mutations cause hypohydrotic ED.[82] These syndromes involve a much decreased density of hair follicles, as well as teeth and sweat glands.[83,84] All these epidermal appendages have similar mechanisms of embryogenic development and so can be similarly affected by the same gene mutation.

Genetics and Hair Follicle Growth Cycle

In other genetic hair loss conditions, hair follicle formation may be normal at first, but with time the hair follicles fail to fully regenerate as part of the normal hair growth cycle. In congenital atrichia, the recessive *hairless* (*hr*) gene encodes for a transcription factor that is defective. The hair follicles form and progress through their first full cycle as normal. However, during catagen, the mesenchymal dermal papilla and dermal sheath cells fail to maintain close association with the epithelial cells as the follicle regresses. As the cells separate and can no longer communicate with each other, the follicles fail to regenerate and enter a new anagen phase.[85] Similarly with Marie Unna hereditary hypotrichosis, the hair follicles may initially form and grow hair but fail to survive and successfully enter subsequent hair growth cycles. The late-onset, patterned destruction of hair follicles in Marie Unna hypotrichosis makes this condition unique as a genetic hair loss condition.[86] These and other hair growth disorders involve mutations in genes (usually just one gene) that are functionally significant for cohesive hair follicle structure maintenance throughout the hair growth cycle.

Genetics and Hair Follicle Size

Congenital hypertrichosis is not determined by the number and distribution of hair follicles but instead by whether the hair follicles are terminal or vellus size in a geographic region of skin. Embryos are covered from head to toe by a more or less uniform coat of long fine unpigmented lanugo hair. Shortly before full-term, the scalp hairs progress into terminal hairs while the remaining body hair follicles involute and become vellus hairs.[12] As a result, terminal hair follicle distribution is mostly restricted to the scalp at birth. When terminal hair follicles form beyond these limits on the face and elsewhere in the place of vellus hair follicles, the consequence may be diagnosed as congenital hypertrichosis. Hair growth cycle duration can play a role in some hypertrichoses. In congenital hypertrichosis lanuginosa the duration of anagen is prolonged beyond the norm in vellus hair follicles, the net result being long, fine, unpigmented hair growth.[87] Again, the density of hair follicles has not been altered.

Genetics, the Environment, Hormones, and Inflammation

Of course, genetic hair loss disorders can be modulated and even mediated by factors in the environment, hormonal activity, and inflammatory cell action (see **Fig. 6**). AA may be an inflammatory cell–mediated disease, but the environment and genetics can play a role for at least some patients. Similarly, AGA (see later) has a strong genetic component. Even with TE, generally accepted as a condition that develops in response to environmental insults, genes may play a role in determining an individual's level of susceptibility to the development of hair loss in response to the insult.

ENVIRONMENT
The Environment and Hair Loss

Hair follicle growth and cycling involve the regulation of stem cell quiescence and activation, transit-amplifying cell proliferation, cell-fate choice, cell differentiation, and apoptosis.[88–90] Alteration of any one of these regulatory systems could lead to hair loss. In addition, because hair follicles are receptive to the circadian clock, hair follicle cycling consists of many positive and negative environmental feedback loops.[15] Anything that interrupts the normal hair cycle regulation may cause diffuse hair loss.[14] Hair cycling is sensitive to numerous extrafollicular growth-modulating signals, such as hormones, cytokines, and dietary changes.[14,91–93] In most instances, this modulation of the hair cycle clock leads to TE, either on its own or as part of a larger disorder. When the hair follicle is severely insulted, such as by cytostatic drugs or toxins, the result may be anagen effluvium.

TE: An Environment-Mediated Hair Loss Disorder

TE is probably the most common cause of diffuse hair loss encountered by dermatologists. A wide variety of potential triggers have been implicated including physiologic or emotional stresses, endocrine imbalances, nutritional deficiencies, severe illness, diet deficiencies, and even changes in medication. Clinically, TE shows an abnormality of hair cycling in which anagen hairs are triggered to prematurely stop growing and enter catagen and are then subsequently shed before renewed anagen occurs.[94]

Based on the changes in different phases of follicle cycles, Headington classified TE into 5 functional types. Three types are related to events in anagen and 2 are related to telogen. The types are (1) immediate anagen release; (2) delayed anagen release; (3) short anagen syndrome; (4) immediate telogen release, and (5) delayed telogen release.[94] In immediate anagen release, anagen hairs prematurely enter telogen and hair loss starts to be lost 3 to 5 weeks from the inciting factor. This is a very common form of TE that typically occurs after a physiologic stress such as episodes of high fever and severe illness and with drug-induced hair loss.[94] In fever, the pyrogens, basically circulating cytokines, drive the hair follicle keratinocytes into apoptosis, initiating catagen with following telogen.[95,96] Released cytokines, such as interferons α and γ, have also been shown to inhibit keratinocyte proliferation that may impair the hair follicle matrix cells.[97]

Short anangen syndrome is an uncommon condition characterized by the inability to grow long hair and an increase in the number of hairs in telogen because of an idiopathic shortening of the duration of anagen.[98,99] It may be one mechanism behind the condition chronic TE and may also be associated with loose anagen syndrome.[100] Immediate telogen release is characterized by a shortening of normal telogen with shedding of club hairs as the follicles are stimulated to reenter anagen. Theoretically, it might be an extrinsic signal, such as a drug or other molecules, that precipitate a telogen-release event.[94] This is common in patients starting therapy with minoxidil because minoxidil can stimulate the telogen follicles resulting in rapid progression to anagen.[101] Delayed telogen release results from a prolonged telogen followed by transition to anagen.

Physiologic (eg, surgery, systemic illness/postfebrile illness) or psychoemotional (acute and chronic) stress may cause TE and excessive hair shedding.[102–105] Hair follicle cycling can be modulated by classic bioregulators of systemic stress responses.[106] A central stress response may induce the hair follicle itself to generate stress mediators and to express cognate receptors, which may be directly involved in the modulation of stress responses.[105,107–109] Some studies suggest that central stress responses may lead to local substance P release from sensory nerve fibers in the skin; Substance P along with nerve growth factor can mediate stress-induced hair growth-inhibitory effects, such as keratinocyte apoptosis, inhibition of proliferation, and premature hair follicle regression.[110]

HORMONES
Hormones and Hair Loss

Hair follicles can be sensitive to changes in systemic levels of hormones. Thyroid hormones, glucocorticoids, insulin-like growth factor I, and prolactin can have clinically significant effects on specific aspects of hair growth and systemic imbalances can trigger TE (see **Fig. 6**). The most common endocrine triggers of TE include hypothyreosis, hyperthyreosis, hyperprolactinemia, and polycystic ovary syndrome.[111,112] Even within the normal cycling of hair follicles, hormonal activity can have an impact. Prolactin and melatonin

regulate winter and summer coat molting of mammals.[113,114] To some extent, humans may also be receptive with seasonal shedding observed in some populations or people who suffer from jet lag.[94,115]

Further, postpartum hair loss is a delayed anagen release form of TE. Hair follicles that are androgen sensitive can be modulated by administration of estrogen.[5] In guinea pigs, estrogens were shown to prolong anagen.[116] During pregnancy, the estrogen level increases until delivery[117]; hair remains in prolonged anagen rather than cycling into telogen. Immediately after delivery, the estrogen levels drop significantly and the testosterone levels rise, triggering the postpartum hair loss.[118,119] If a large number of follicles are involved, postpartum telogen conversion will be accompanied by increased shedding some months later.

In addition to systemic hormone influences, local hormone synthesis, receptor expression and receptor binding, and metabolic activity in and around hair follicles can also be key determinants of hair cycling. In turn these factors may be mediated by genes (see **Fig. 6**). Hair follicles produce complete hormone cascades, which act on the different hair follicle cell populations in paracrine and autocrine manners. That hair follicles produce, and are very receptive to, local stress hormone activity is a good example.[120,121] Arguably, however, androgens are the primary class of hormones with significant impact on hair growth and disorder development involving both systemic and hair follicle localized activity.

Androgens and Hair Growth

Androgens have diverse effects on hair follicles in different body regions. The impact of androgens on hair growth vary from essentially nonexistent as with eyelashes, weak as with temporal and suboccipital region hair, moderate with arm and leg hair, to strong as with facial, parietal region, pubic, and axillary hair. The differential expression of receptors and enzymes likely provides the basis for the variable responsiveness to androgens in the different hair follicle types. In human sexual maturity, androgens cause enlargement of fine, vellus hair follicles into coarse, heavily pigmented terminal hair follicles. This dramatic stimulation of "vellus-terminal hair switch" is propagated by an increased level of circulating androgens bound to either sex hormone–binding globulin or albumin.[122–124]

Men can develop AGA with a normal level of androgens starting as early as their teens.[125,126] Women can also be affected by a more diffuse patterned hair loss. This highly prevalent condition, affects up to 70% of men and 40% of women in mid adult life.[127] As illustrated by the Norwood-Hamilton classification, the male pattern generally begins with bitemporal recession, followed by vertex baldness and mid-frontal hair loss; allowing the terminal hair follicles to be retained in the occipital scalp region.[126,127] This effect of androgens on specific areas of scalp is caused by differences in factors such as the distribution of androgen receptors, localized production of high-potency androgens, and the degradation rate of androgens.[128,129]

AGA: A Hormone-Mediated Hair Loss Disorder

Clinically, AGA is a result of altered hair growth cycling and hair follicle miniaturization, with the transformation of terminal to vellus hair follicles and the production of shorter, finer hair shafts.[39] In men with AGA, the duration of anagen reduces dramatically from 2 to 6 years to a few months, whereas the telogen stage continues to last for the same time or a prolonged period.[130] This accelerated pace of driving hair follicles out of anagen prematurely and the relative lengthening of telogen combine to produce a reduction in the anagen-to-telogen ratio from a normal 12:1 ratio to an aberrant 5:1 ratio,[27] while the proportion of telogen hair increases from 5-10% to 15-20%.[131] The time delay for hair follicles to rotate out of telogen and back to anagen allows for increased exogen shedding and progressive increase in the numbers of empty kenogen hair follicles.

At the cellular level, follicular miniaturization is potentially caused by a diminution in dermal papilla volume, which in turn is caused by a reduction in cell number per papilla.[39] The dermal papilla plays an important role in regulating keratinocyte cells in hair follicle growth and the determination of hair bulb matrix and hair shaft size.[132,133] Dermal papillae also alter their production of hair growth regulatory factors in the presence of androgens.[123] These regulatory factors are capable of influencing the growth and activity of other hair follicular components.[134] For example, in presence of androgens, dermal papilla cells inhibit the growth of keratinocyte cells by secretion of by transforming growth factor-β1.[135] The combined effects of dermal papilla miniaturization and compromised growth of other hair follicular cells instigate the follicle to produce finer, unpigmented vellus-like hair instead of large, pigmented terminal hair.

Molecular Mechanism of AGA

More than 60 years ago, Hamilton was the first to illustrate the essence of androgens as a prerequisite for the development of baldness in genetically susceptible men.[125] Adult men castrated at the prepubertal stage were able to retain a juvenile hair line and not go bald. However, castrated men were equally susceptible to baldness as the uncastrated population with the administration of testosterone. The alopecia condition did not advance or reverse once the administration of testosterone ceased. Based on these observations, Hamilton established that testosterone, or its metabolites, had a crucial role in the development of AGA.[124]

Testosterone is the major circulating androgen in men and its conversion to dihydrotestosterone (DHT) by the enzyme steroid 5α-reductase has been studied extensively in relation to hair growth.[124,136] Compared with testosterone, DHT has approximately 5-fold more potency for the androgen receptor.[128] A higher level of 5α-reductase has been found in frontal follicles than in occipital follicles of the same individual.[129] The type 2 isozyme of 5α-reductase is prominently expressed within the outer root sheath and inner root sheath and predominantly in dermal papillae in frontal hair follicles.[116,137] DHT exerts its effects by binding to androgen receptors. In balding scalp, increased expression of both 5α-reductases and androgen receptors are present, resulting in increased formation and activity of DHT–androgen receptor complexes. Such changes suggest this complex modulates the expression of androgen-sensitive genes.[129,138]

Genetics and AGA

It is well accepted that genetics play an important role in AGA, because it is a heritable condition (see **Fig. 6**).[139,140] The difference in prevalence and the degree of progression in different ethnic groups further support the significance of genetics in the development of AGA.[126] However, the nature of this genetic predisposition remains unclear. The concept of a polygenic inheritance is more accurate than a single gene model. If the mode of inheritance is regulated by only a single gene, these conditions should rarely occur at a frequency greater than 1 in 1000.[141] In AGA, multiple genes are likely involved to determine the age of onset, progression, patterning, and severity of hair loss.[142] Researchers have analyzed some potential candidate genes that might play an important role in AGA, such as 5α-reductase genes and the androgen receptor gene.

DHT is an important determinant in AGA.[143] The enzyme responsible for the conversion of testosterone into DHT, 5α-reductase, has 2 isoforms: type 1 and type 2,[144,145] encoded by separate genes, *SRD5A1*[146] and *SRD5A2*.[147] Individuals lacking a functional type 2 5α-reductase gene develop pseudohermaphroditism and do not develop AGA.[110] Surprisingly, however, studies show there is no significant difference in the distribution of *SRD5A1* and *SRD5A2* markers between balding men and nonbalding individuals.[148] The results suggest that there are no major linkages of these 2 genes to the development of AGA.

In contrast, androgen receptor expression evaluation in balding scalp[129,149] suggests mutations in the *AR* gene may be involved to AGA. Researchers were able to conclude that a restriction fragment length polymorphism in exon 1 of *AR* was present in 98.1% in young bald men but in only 76.6% of older men without the balding condition.[150] These data suggest this particular nonfunctional single nucleotide polymorphism in *AR* is important for AGA susceptibility. The other factors contributing to AGA may include other functional single nucleotide polymorphisms that exist in the noncoding region upstream of *AR*[151,152] or epigenetic modification such as DNA methylation.[153] Overall, the research strongly suggests AGA is predominantly a genetic condition, but the number and nature of genes involved have yet to be fully elucidated.

HAIR DISORDER TREATMENT DEVELOPMENT

Approaches for treating hair diseases are many and varied depending on the nature of the disease. However, the objectives of treatment are similar in all cases: to directly or indirectly return an individual's hair follicle size, density, and growth cycles to within normal parameters. Treatments and their development fall into one or more of three main categories: modifiers of the hair growth cycle (duration of anagen, duration of telogen, timing of exogen), modifiers of hair follicle size (terminal, intermediate, vellus), and/or normalizing hair follicle density (number of hair follicles per unit area). Treatment to remove a disorder initiating event, while not directly acting on the affected hair follicles, may enable the damaged follicles to recover through their inherent regenerative capacity. For example, finasteride, a synthetic azosteroid that is widely used to treat AGA, is a potent and highly selective type 2 5α-reductase inhibitor.[154] It reduces the conversion of testosterone to DHT by binding to the type 2 isozyme irreversibly and consequently diminishes the downstream action of androgens on hair growth. In 80% of those undergoing finasteride treatment, significantly increased hair counts, increased hair fiber size, and prolonged anagen hair growth duration are observed.[91] It may not be possible to

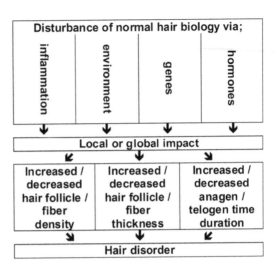

Fig. 7. Factors elicit hair disorders by modifying hair density, size, and hair growth cycle. One or more hair disorder-promoting/modulating factors, acting in a systemic or localized fashion, adversely alter normal hair follicle/fiber density, size/thickness, and/or growth cycling to elicit the disorder.

successfully target the underlying disease mechanism, yet treatment approaches that normalize hair growth parameters can still be used. For example, minoxidil is a direct hair growth stimulator, prolonging anagen and increasing hair fiber size.[155–158] Although officially used only for AGA, it is also sometimes used off label to treat TE and AA.[45,159] Even when hair follicles are irretrievably lost, new experimental treatments are being investigated for their ability to induce new follicle formation and increase hair density.[7,160]

- A hair disorder may be characterized as (1) a change in hair density, (2) a change in hair fiber thickness, and/or (3) a change in hair follicle growth cycles.
- Hair follicle embryogenesis can lead to a hair disorder when (1) hair follicle formation fails (congenital hypotrichoses), (2) hair follicles fail to maintain their biologic integrity (progressive hypotrichoses), or (3) inappropriately sized hair follicles grow in specific locations (congenital hypotrichoses/hypertrichoses).
- A hair disorder can be acquired when (1) hair follicles are destroyed reducing normal density (eg, scarring alopecia, AGA), (2) hair follicles change from vellus to terminal size (acquired hypertrichoses), and (3) hair follicles change from terminal to vellus size (eg, AGA).
- Hair follicle cycling can lead to a hair disorder when (1) anagen duration is significantly

increased (hypertrichoses), (2) anagen duration is significantly decreased (eg, AA), or (3) telogen duration is significantly increased associated with exogen shedding (most alopecias).

- The potential trigger factors for hair disorders can be attributed to one or more categories: inflammation, genetics, environment, and hormones.
- The basic objectives of hair disorder treatment development are to (1) modify anagen to normalize anagen duration, (2) modify telogen to normalize telogen duration, (3) modify the structure of damaged, miniaturized hair follicles to increase hair follicle size, (4) modify the structure of terminal hair follicles to reduce hair follicle size, and (5) replicate hair follicles and their characteristics to increase hair follicle density.

CONCLUSIONS

The basic mechanisms by which hair disorders occur can be categorized depending on whether the conditions affect hair follicle size, density, hair growth cycle, and, to a lesser extent, growth rate. These changes are mediated by one or more of the factors of inflammation, genetics, the environment, and hormones (**Fig. 7**). Hair follicles are complex skin appendages, the perturbations of which have an impact on physical and psychological human health disproportionate to their small dimensions. The causal mechanisms for the disordered hair follicle are many and varied but, with an understanding of the essential characteristics of these disorders, new treatment approaches may be revealed.

ACKNOWLEDGMENTS

This work was supported by grants from the Canadian Dermatology Foundation (CDF). EW and TB are recipients of a CIHR Skin Research Training Center (CIHR-SRTC) award. KJM is a recipient of Canadian Institutes of Health Research (MSH-95328) and Michael Smith Foundation for Health Research [CI-SCH-00480(06-1)] investigator awards.

REFERENCES

1. Dixson BJ, Vasey LV. Beards augment perceptions of men's age, social status, and aggressiveness, but not attractiveness. Behav Ecol 2012;23: 481–90.
2. Blume-Peytavi U, Hillmann K, Guarrera G. Hair growth assessment techniques. In: Blume-Peytavi U, Tosti A, Whiting DA, et al, editors. Hair growth and disorders. Berlin: Springer-Verlag; 2008. p. 125–58.
3. Vogt A, McElwee KJ, Blume-Peytavi U. Biology of the hair follicle. In: Blume-Peytavi U, Tosti A, Whiting DA, et al, editors. Hair growth and disorders. Berlin: Springer-Verlag; 2008. p. 1–22.
4. Millar SE. Molecular mechanisms regulating hair follicle development. J Invest Dermatol 2002;118: 216–25.
5. Stenn KS, Paus R. Controls of hair follicle cycling. Physiol Rev 2001;81:449–94.
6. Sinclair R, McElwee KJ. Hair physiology and its disorders. Drug Discov Today Dis Mech 2008;5: e163–71.
7. McElwee KJ, Kissling S, Wenzel E, et al. Cultured peribulbar dermal sheath cells can induce hair follicle development and contribute to the dermal sheath and dermal papilla. J Invest Dermatol 2003;121:1267–75.
8. Muller SA. Hair neogenesis. J Invest Dermatol 1971;56:1–9.
9. Billingham RE. A reconsideration of the phenomenon of hair neogenesis with particular reference to the healing of cutaneous wounds in adult mammals. In: Montagna W, Ellis RA, editors. Hair growth and disorders. New York: Academic Press; 1958. p. 451–68.
10. Yu M, Finner A, Shapiro J, et al. Hair follicles and their role in skin health. Expert Rev Dermatol 2006; 1:855–71.
11. Smith NP. Tufted folliculitis of the scalp. J R Soc Med 1978;71:606–8.
12. Rook A. Endocrine influences on hair growth. Br Med J 1965;1:609–14.
13. Rudolph KL, Chang S, Lee HW, et al. Longevity, stress response, and cancer in aging telomerase-deficient mice. Cell 1999;96:701–12.
14. Stenn KS, Paus R. What controls hair follicle cycling? Exp Dermatol 1999;8:229–33 [discussion: 33–6].
15. Geyfman M, Andersen B. Clock genes, hair growth and aging. Aging (Albany NY) 2010;2:122–8.
16. Hebert JM, Rosenquist T, Gotz J, et al. FGF5 as a regulator of the hair growth cycle: evidence from targeted and spontaneous mutations. Cell 1994;78:1017–25.
17. Pennycuik PR, Raphael KA. The angora locus (go) in the mouse: hair morphology, duration of growth cycle and site of action. Genet Res 1984;44:283–91.
18. Millar SE, Willert K, Salinas PC, et al. WNT signaling in the control of hair growth and structure. Dev Biol 1999;207:133–49.
19. Stenn K. Exogen is an active, separately controlled phase of the hair growth cycle. J Am Acad Dermatol 2005;52:374–5.
20. Hanakawa Y, Li H, Lin C, et al. Desmogleins 1 and 3 in the companion layer anchor mouse anagen hair to the follicle. J Invest Dermatol 2004;123:817–22.

21. Ma L, Liu J, Wu T, et al. 'Cyclic alopecia' in Msx2 mutants: defects in hair cycling and hair shaft differentiation. Development 2003;130:379–89.

22. Rebora A, Guarrera M. Kenogen. A new phase of the hair cycle? Dermatology 2002;205:108–10.

23. Guarrera M, Rebora A. Kenogen in female androgenetic alopecia. A longitudinal study. Dermatology 2005;210:18–20.

24. Trueb RM. Chemotherapy-induced alopecia. Semin Cutan Med Surg 2009;28:11–4.

25. Messenger AG, Slater DN, Bleehen SS. Alopecia areata: alterations in the hair growth cycle and correlation with the follicular pathology. Br J Dermatol 1986;114:337–47.

26. Hordinsky M. Cicatricial alopecia: discoid lupus erythematosus. Dermatol Ther 2008;21:245–8.

27. Whiting DA. Diagnostic and predictive value of horizontal sections of scalp biopsy specimens in male pattern androgenetic alopecia. J Am Acad Dermatol 1993;28:755–63.

28. Johnson E, Ebling FJ. The effect of plucking hairs during different phases of the follicular cycle. J Embryol Exp Morphol 1964;12:465–74.

29. Shafir R, Tsur H. Local hirsutism at the periphery of burned skin. Br J Plast Surg 1979;32:93.

30. Ravin N. New hair growth over fracture sites. N Engl J Med 1990;323:350.

31. Solomons B. Disorders of the hair and their treatment before the 18th century. Br J Dermatol 1966;78:113–20.

32. Schmitt A, Rochat A, Zeltner R, et al. The primary target cells of the high-risk cottontail rabbit papillomavirus colocalize with hair follicle stem cells. J Virol 1996;70:1912–22.

33. Boxman IL, Berkhout RJ, Mulder LH, et al. Detection of human papillomavirus DNA in plucked hairs from renal transplant recipients and healthy volunteers. J Invest Dermatol 1997;108:712–5.

34. Boxman IL, Hogewoning A, Mulder LH, et al. Detection of human papillomavirus types 6 and 11 in pubic and perianal hair from patients with genital warts. J Clin Microbiol 1999;37:2270–3.

35. Adachi A, Suzuki T, Tomita Y. Detection of human papillomavirus type 56 DNA, belonging to a mucous high-risk group, in hair follicles in the genital area of a woman no longer suffering from viral warts. Br J Dermatol 2004;151:212–5.

36. Walsh N, Boutilier R, Glasgow D, et al. Exclusive involvement of folliculosebaceous units by herpes: a reflection of early herpes zoster. Am J Dermatopathol 2005;27:189–94.

37. Akilov OE, Butov YS, Mumcuoglu KY. A clinico-pathological approach to the classification of human demodicosis. J Dtsch Dermatol Ges 2005;3:607–14.

38. Zichichi L, Asta G, Noto G. Pseudomonas aeruginosa folliculitis after shower/bath exposure. Int J Dermatol 2000;39:270–3.

39. Tobin DJ, Gunin A, Magerl M, et al. Plasticity and cytokinetic dynamics of the hair follicle mesenchyme during the hair growth cycle: implications for growth control and hair follicle transformations. J Investig Dermatol Symp Proc 2003;8:80–6.

40. Ito T, Meyer KC, Ito N, et al. Immune privilege and the skin. Curr Dir Autoimmun 2008;10:27–52.

41. Lu W, Shapiro J, Yu M, et al. Alopecia areata: pathogenesis and potential for therapy. Expert Rev Mol Med 2006;8:1–19.

42. Wang E, McElwee KJ. Etiopathogenesis of alopecia areata: why do our patients get it? Dermatol Ther 2011;24:337–47.

43. Ito T, Ito N, Bettermann A, et al. Collapse and restoration of MHC class-I-dependent immune privilege: exploiting the human hair follicle as a model. Am J Pathol 2004;164:623–34.

44. Petukhova L, Duvic M, Hordinsky M, et al. Genome-wide association study in alopecia areata implicates both innate and adaptive immunity. Nature 2010;466:113–7.

45. Alkhalifah A, Alsantali A, Wang E, et al. Alopecia areata update: part I. Clinical picture, histopathology, and pathogenesis. J Am Acad Dermatol 2010;62:177–88 [quiz: 89–90].

46. McElwee KJ, Hoffmann R, Freyschmidt-Paul P, et al. Resistance to alopecia areata in C3H/HeJ mice is associated with increased expression of regulatory cytokines and a failure to recruit CD4+ and CD8+ cells. J Invest Dermatol 2002;119:1426–33.

47. Perret C, Wiesner-Menzel L, Happle R. Immunohistochemical analysis of T-cell subsets in the peribulbar and intrabulbar infiltrates of alopecia areata. Acta Derm Venereol 1984;64:26–30.

48. Kang H, Wu WY, Lo BK, et al. Hair follicles from alopecia areata patients exhibit alterations in immune privilege-associated gene expression in advance of hair loss. J Invest Dermatol 2010;130:2677–80.

49. Botchkareva NV, Ahluwalia G, Shander D. Apoptosis in the hair follicle. J Invest Dermatol 2006;126:258–64.

50. Weedon D, Strutton G. Apoptosis as the mechanism of the involution of hair follicles in catagen transformation. Acta Derm Venereol 1981;61:335–9.

51. Eichmuller S, van der Veen C, Moll I, et al. Clusters of perifollicular macrophages in normal murine skin: physiological degeneration of selected hair follicles by programmed organ deletion. J Histochem Cytochem 1998;46:361–70.

52. McElwee KJ, Spiers EM, Oliver RF. In vivo depletion of CD8+ T cells restores hair growth in the DEBR model for alopecia areata. Br J Dermatol 1996;135:211–7.

53. McElwee KJ, Spiers EM, Oliver RF. Partial restoration of hair growth in the DEBR model for Alopecia

areata after in vivo depletion of CD4+ T cells. Br J Dermatol 1999;140:432–7.

54. McElwee KJ, Freyschmidt-Paul P, Hoffmann R, et al. Transfer of CD8(+) cells induces localized hair loss whereas CD4(+)/CD25(-) cells promote systemic alopecia areata and CD4(+)/CD25(+) cells blockade disease onset in the C3H/HeJ mouse model. J Invest Dermatol 2005;124:947–57.

55. Alsaleh QA, Nanda A, al-Hasawi F, et al. Concurrent appearance of alopecia areata in siblings. Pediatr Dermatol 1995;12:285–6.

56. Stankler L. Synchronous alopecia areata in two siblings: a possible viral aetiology. Lancet 1979;1: 1303–4.

57. McDonagh AJ, Tazi-Ahnini R. Epidemiology and genetics of alopecia areata. Clin Exp Dermatol 2002;27:405–9.

58. McElwee KJ, Tobin DJ, Bystryn JC, et al. Alopecia areata: an autoimmune disease? Exp Dermatol 1999;8:371–9.

59. Sundberg JP, Silva KA, Li R, et al. Adult-onset Alopecia areata is a complex polygenic trait in the C3H/HeJ mouse model. J Invest Dermatol 2004; 123:294–7.

60. Skinner RB Jr, Light WH, Bale GF, et al. Alopecia areata and presence of cytomegalovirus DNA. JAMA 1995;273:1419–20.

61. McElwee KJ, Boggess D, Burgett B, et al. Murine cytomegalovirus is not associated with alopecia areata in C3H/HeJ mice. J Invest Dermatol 1998; 110:986–7.

62. Wise RP, Kiminyo KP, Salive ME. Hair loss after routine immunizations. JAMA 1997;278:1176–8.

63. Sundberg JP, Silva KA, Zhang W, et al. Recombinant human hepatitis B vaccine initiating alopecia areata: testing the hypothesis using the C3H/HeJ mouse model. Vet Dermatol 2009;20:99–104.

64. McElwee KJ, Niiyama S, Freyschmidt-Paul P, et al. Dietary soy oil content and soy-derived phytoestrogen genistein increase resistance to alopecia areata onset in C3H/HeJ mice. Exp Dermatol 2003;12:30–6.

65. McElwee KJ, Silva K, Beamer WG, et al. Melanocyte and gonad activity as potential severity modifying factors in C3H/HeJ mouse alopecia areata. Exp Dermatol 2001;10:420–9.

66. Zhang X, Yu M, Yu W, et al. Development of alopecia areata is associated with higher central and peripheral hypothalamic-pituitary-adrenal tone in the skin graft induced C3H/HeJ mouse model. J Invest Dermatol 2009;129:1527–38.

67. Ito N, Sugawara K, Bodo E, et al. Corticotropin-releasing hormone stimulates the in situ generation of mast cells from precursors in the human hair follicle mesenchyme. J Invest Dermatol 2010;130: 995–1004.

68. Ito T. Hair follicle is a target of stress hormone and auto-immune reactions. J Dermatol Sci 2010;60:67–73.

69. McElwee KJ. Etiology of cicatricial alopecias: a basic science point of view. Dermatol Ther 2008;21:212–20.

70. Harries MJ, Paus R. The pathogenesis of primary cicatricial alopecias. Am J Pathol 2010;177:2152–62.

71. Hutchens KA, Balfour EM, Smoller BR. Comparison between Langerhans cell concentration in lichen planopilaris and traction alopecia with possible immunologic implications. Am J Dermatopathol 2011;33:277–80.

72. Chiarini C, Torchia D, Bianchi B, et al. Immunopathogenesis of folliculitis decalvans: clues in early lesions. Am J Clin Pathol 2008;130:526–34.

73. Meyer KC, Klatte JE, Dinh HV, et al. Evidence that the bulge region is a site of relative immune privilege in human hair follicles. Br J Dermatol 2008; 159:1077–85.

74. Harries MJ, Meyer KC, Chaudhry IH, et al. Does collapse of immune privilege in the hair-follicle bulge play a role in the pathogenesis of primary cicatricial alopecia? Clin Exp Dermatol 2010;35: 637–44.

75. Shapiro J. Cicatricial alopecias. Dermatol Ther 2008;21:211.

76. Karnik P, Tekeste Z, McCormick TS, et al. Hair follicle stem cell-specific PPARgamma deletion causes scarring alopecia. J Invest Dermatol 2009;129: 1243–57.

77. Ross EK, Tan E, Shapiro J. Update on primary cicatricial alopecias. J Am Acad Dermatol 2005;53:1–37 [quiz: 38–40].

78. Lipsker D, Boeckler P, Cribier B. Tick-borne lymphadenopathy/dermacentor-borne necrosis erythema lymphadenopathy: an infectious cause of cicatricial alopecia. Clin Exp Dermatol 2008;33:518–9.

79. Tosti A, Piraccini BM, Iorizzo M, et al. Frontal fibrosing alopecia in postmenopausal women. J Am Acad Dermatol 2005;52:55–60.

80. Kruk-Jeromin J, Janik J, Rykala J. Aplasia cutis congenita of the scalp. Report of 16 cases. Dermatol Surg 1998;24:549–53.

81. Trakimas C, Sperling LC, Skelton HG 3rd, et al. Clinical and histologic findings in temporal triangular alopecia. J Am Acad Dermatol 1994;31: 205–9.

82. Chassaing N, Bourthoumieu S, Cossee M, et al. Mutations in EDAR account for one-quarter of non-ED1-related hypohidrotic ectodermal dysplasia. Hum Mutat 2006;27:255–9.

83. Kere J, Srivastava AK, Montonen O, et al. X-linked anhidrotic (hypohidrotic) ectodermal dysplasia is caused by mutation in a novel transmembrane protein. Nat Genet 1996;13:409–16.

84. MacDermot KD, Winter RM, Malcolm S. Gene localisation of X-linked hypohidrotic ectodermal dysplasia (C-S-T syndrome). Hum Genet 1986;74: 172–3.

85. Zlotogorski A, Panteleyev AA, Aita VM, et al. Clinical and molecular diagnostic criteria of congenital atrichia with papular lesions. J Invest Dermatol 2002;118:887–90.

86. Roberts JL, Whiting DA, Henry D, et al. Marie Unna congenital hypotrichosis: clinical description, histopathology, scanning electron microscopy of a previously unreported large pedigree. J Investig Dermatol Symp Proc 1999;4:261–7.

87. Bondeson J, Miles AE. The hairy family of Burma: a four generation pedigree of congenital hypertrichosis lanuginosa. J R Soc Med 1996;89:403–8.

88. Lavker RM, Sun TT, Oshima H, et al. Hair follicle stem cells. J Investig Dermatol Symp Proc 2003; 8:28–38.

89. Lindner G, Botchkarev VA, Botchkareva NV, et al. Analysis of apoptosis during hair follicle regression (catagen). Am J Pathol 1997;151:1601–17.

90. Cece R, Cazzaniga S, Morelli D, et al. Apoptosis of hair follicle cells during doxorubicin-induced alopecia in rats. Lab Invest 1996;75:601–9.

91. Roberts JL, Fiedler V, Imperato-McGinley J, et al. Clinical dose ranging studies with finasteride, a type 2 5alpha-reductase inhibitor, in men with male pattern hair loss. J Am Acad Dermatol 1999;41:555–63.

92. Kaimal S, Thappa DM. Diet in dermatology: revisited. Indian J Dermatol Venereol Leprol 2010;76: 103–15.

93. Goldberg LJ, Lenzy Y. Nutrition and hair. Clin Dermatol 2010;28:412–9.

94. Headington JT. Telogen effluvium. New concepts and review. Arch Dermatol 1993;129:356–63.

95. Ruckert R, Lindner G, Bulfone-Paus S, et al. High-dose proinflammatory cytokines induce apoptosis of hair bulb keratinocytes in vivo. Br J Dermatol 2000;143:1036–9.

96. Trueb RM. Systematic approach to hair loss in women. J Dtsch Dermatol Ges 2010;8:284–97, 98.

97. Stout AJ, Gresser I, Thompson WD. Inhibition of wound healing in mice by local interferon alpha/beta injection. Int J Exp Pathol 1993;74:79–85.

98. Giacomini F, Starace M, Tosti A. Short anagen syndrome. Pediatr Dermatol 2011;28:133–4.

99. Barraud-Klenovsek MM, Trueb RM. Congenital hypotrichosis due to short anagen. Br J Dermatol 2000;143:612–7.

100. Shrivastava SB. Diffuse hair loss in an adult female: approach to diagnosis and management. Indian J Dermatol Venereol Leprol 2009;75:20–7 [quiz: 27–8].

101. Mori O, Uno H. The effect of topical minoxidil on hair follicular cycles of rats. J Dermatol 1990;17: 276–81.

102. Whiting DA. Chronic telogen effluvium: increased scalp hair shedding in middle-aged women. J Am Acad Dermatol 1996;35:899–906.

103. Gilmore S, Sinclair R. Chronic telogen effluvium is due to a reduction in the variance of anagen duration. Australas J Dermatol 2010;51:163–7.

104. Whiting DA. Chronic telogen effluvium. Dermatol Clin 1996;14:723–31.

105. Aoki E, Shibasaki T, Kawana S. Intermittent foot shock stress prolongs the telogen stage in the hair cycle of mice. Exp Dermatol 2003;12:371–7.

106. Hadshiew IM, Foitzik K, Arck PC, et al. Burden of hair loss: stress and the underestimated psychosocial impact of telogen effluvium and androgenetic alopecia. J Invest Dermatol 2004;123:455–7.

107. Slominski A, Wortsman J, Luger T, et al. Corticotropin releasing hormone and proopiomelanocortin involvement in the cutaneous response to stress. Physiol Rev 2000;80:979–1020.

108. Arck PC, Handjiski B, Hagen E, et al. Indications for a 'brain-hair follicle axis (BHA)': inhibition of keratinocyte proliferation and up-regulation of keratinocyte apoptosis in telogen hair follicles by stress and substance P. FASEB J 2001;15:2536–8.

109. Arck PC, Handjiski B, Peters EM, et al. Stress inhibits hair growth in mice by induction of premature catagen development and deleterious perifollicular inflammatory events via neuropeptide substance P-dependent pathways. Am J Pathol 2003;162:803–14.

110. Imperato-McGinley J, Guerrero L, Gautier T, et al. Steroid 5alpha-reductase deficiency in man: an inherited form of male pseudohermaphroditism. Science 1974;186:1213–5.

111. Baldari M, Guarrera M, Rebora A. Thyroid peroxidase antibodies in patients with telogen effluvium. J Eur Acad Dermatol Venereol 2010;24:980–2.

112. Kligman AM. Pathologic dynamics of human hair loss. I. Telogen effuvium. Arch Dermatol 1961;83: 175–98.

113. Foitzik K, Langan EA, Paus R. Prolactin and the skin: a dermatological perspective on an ancient pleiotropic peptide hormone. J Invest Dermatol 2009;129:1071–87.

114. Fischer TW, Slominski A, Tobin DJ, et al. Melatonin and the hair follicle. J Pineal Res 2008;44:1–15.

115. Randall VA, Ebling FJ. Seasonal changes in human hair growth. Br J Dermatol 1991;124:146–51.

116. Hoffmann R, Happle R. Finasteride is the main inhibitor of 5alpha-reductase activity in microdissected dermal papillae of human hair follicles. Arch Dermatol Res 1999;291:100–3.

117. Kornman KS, Loesche WJ. The subgingival microbial flora during pregnancy. J Periodontal Res 1980;15:111–22.

118. Riecher-Rossler A, Hafner H, Stumbaum M, et al. Can estradiol modulate schizophrenic symptomatology? Schizophr Bull 1994;20:203–14.

119. Baum MJ, Brand T, Ooms M, et al. Immediate postnatal rise in whole body androgen content in male

rats: correlation with increased testicular content and reduced body clearance of testosterone. Biol Reprod 1988;38:980–6.

120. Ito N, Ito T, Kromminga A, et al. Human hair follicles display a functional equivalent of the hypothalamic-pituitary-adrenal axis and synthesize cortisol. FASEB J 2005;19:1332–4.

121. Arck PC, Slominski A, Theoharides TC, et al. Neuroimmunology of stress: skin takes center stage. J Invest Dermatol 2006;126:1697–704.

122. Ebling FJ. The biology of hair. Dermatol Clin 1987; 5:467–81.

123. Randall VA. Androgens and human hair growth. Clin Endocrinol (Oxf) 1994;40:439–57.

124. Kaufman KD. Androgen metabolism as it affects hair growth in androgenetic alopecia. Dermatol Clin 1996;14:697–711.

125. Hamilton JB. Male hormone stimulation is prerequisite and an incitant in common baldness. Am J Anat 1942;71:451.

126. Hamilton JB. Patterned loss of hair in man; types and incidence. Ann N Y Acad Sci 1951;53:708–28.

127. Norwood OT. Male pattern baldness: classification and incidence. South Med J 1975;68:1359–65.

128. Kaufman KD. Androgens and alopecia. Mol Cell Endocrinol 2002;198:89–95.

129. Sawaya ME, Price VH. Different levels of 5alpha-reductase type I and II, aromatase, and androgen receptor in hair follicles of women and men with androgenetic alopecia. J Invest Dermatol 1997; 109:296–300.

130. Jackson EA. Hair disorders. Prim Care 2000;27: 319–32.

131. Courtois M, Loussouarn G, Hourseau C, et al. Hair cycle and alopecia. Skin Pharmacol 1994;7:84–9.

132. Van Scott EJ, Ekel TM. Geometric relationships between the matrix of the hair bulb and its dermal papilla in normal and alopecic scalp. J Invest Dermatol 1958;31:281–7.

133. Ibrahim L, Wright EA. A quantitative study of hair growth using mouse and rat vibrissal follicles. I. Dermal papilla volume determines hair volume. J Embryol Exp Morphol 1982;72:209–24.

134. Bahta AW, Farjo N, Farjo B, et al. Premature senescence of balding dermal papilla cells in vitro is associated with p16(INK4a) expression. J Invest Dermatol 2008;128:1088–94.

135. Itami S, Inui S. Role of androgen in mesenchymal epithelial interactions in human hair follicle. J Investig Dermatol Symp Proc 2005;10:209–11.

136. Wilson JD, Gloyna RE. The intranuclear metabolism of testosterone in the accessory organs of reproduction. Recent Prog Horm Res 1970;26:309–36.

137. Bayne EK, Flanagan J, Einstein M, et al. Immunohistochemical localization of types 1 and 2 5alpha-reductase in human scalp. Br J Dermatol 1999;141:481–91.

138. Janne OA, Palvimo JJ, Kallio P, et al. Androgen receptor and mechanism of androgen action. Ann Med 1993;25:83–9.

139. Nyholt DR, Gillespie NA, Heath AC, et al. Genetic basis of male pattern baldness. J Invest Dermatol 2003;121:1561–4.

140. Chumlea WC, Rhodes T, Girman CJ, et al. Family history and risk of hair loss. Dermatology 2004; 209:33–9.

141. Kuster W, Happle R. The inheritance of common baldness: two B or not two B? J Am Acad Dermatol 1984;11:921–6.

142. Ellis JA, Harrap SB. The genetics of androgenetic alopecia. Clin Dermatol 2001;19:149–54.

143. Schweikert HU, Wilson JD. Regulation of human hair growth by steroid hormones. II. Androstenedione metabolism in isolated hairs. J Clin Endocrinol Metab 1974;39:1012–9.

144. Harris G, Azzolina B, Baginsky W, et al. Identification and selective inhibition of an isozyme of steroid 5 alpha-reductase in human scalp. Proc Natl Acad Sci U S A 1992;89:10787–91.

145. Jenkins EP, Andersson S, Imperato-McGinley J, et al. Genetic and pharmacological evidence for more than one human steroid 5 alpha-reductase. J Clin Invest 1992;89:293–300.

146. Jenkins EP, Hsieh CL, Milatovich A, et al. Characterization and chromosomal mapping of a human steroid 5 alpha-reductase gene and pseudogene and mapping of the mouse homologue. Genomics 1991;11:1102–12.

147. Thigpen AE, Silver RI, Guileyardo JM, et al. Tissue distribution and ontogeny of steroid 5 alpha-reductase isozyme expression. J Clin Invest 1993;92:903–10.

148. Ellis JA, Stebbing M, Harrap SB. Genetic analysis of male pattern baldness and the 5alpha-reductase genes. J Invest Dermatol 1998;110:849–53.

149. Hibberts NA, Howell AE, Randall VA. Balding hair follicle dermal papilla cells contain higher levels of androgen receptors than those from non-balding scalp. J Endocrinol 1998;156:59–65.

150. Ellis JA, Stebbing M, Harrap SB. Polymorphism of the androgen receptor gene is associated with male pattern baldness. J Invest Dermatol 2001; 116:452–5.

151. Cobb JE, Zaloumis SG, Scurrah KJ, et al. Evidence for two independent functional variants for androgenetic alopecia around the androgen receptor gene. Exp Dermatol 2010;19:1026–8.

152. Brockschmidt FF, Hillmer AM, Eigelshoven S, et al. Fine mapping of the human AR/EDA2R locus in androgenetic alopecia. Br J Dermatol 2010;162: 899–903.

153. Cobb JE, Wong NC, Yip LW, et al. Evidence of increased DNA methylation of the androgen receptor gene in occipital hair follicles from men

with androgenetic alopecia. Br J Dermatol 2011;
165:210–3.

154. Drake L, Hordinsky M, Fiedler V, et al. The effects of
finasteride on scalp skin and serum androgen
levels in men with androgenetic alopecia. J Am
Acad Dermatol 1999;41:550–4.

155. Buhl AE, Waldon DJ, Miller BF, et al. Differences in
activity of minoxidil and cyclosporin A on hair
growth in nude and normal mice. Comparisons of
in vivo and in vitro studies. Lab Invest 1990;62:
104–7.

156. Iwabuchi T, Maruyama T, Sei Y, et al. Effects of
immunosuppressive peptidyl-prolyl cis-trans isom-
erase (PPIase) inhibitors, cyclosporin A, FK506,

ascomycin and rapamycin, on hair growth initiation
in mouse: immunosuppression is not required for
new hair growth. J Dermatol Sci 1995;9:64–9.

157. Sinclair R. Male pattern androgenetic alopecia.
BMJ 1998;317:865–9.

158. Otberg N, Finner AM, Shapiro J. Androgenetic
alopecia. Endocrinol Metab Clin North Am 2007;
36:379–98.

159. Duvic M, Lemak NA, Valero V, et al. A randomized
trial of minoxidil in chemotherapy-induced alopecia.
J Am Acad Dermatol 1996;35:74–8.

160. Ito M, Yang Z, Andl T, et al. Wnt-dependent de
novo hair follicle regeneration in adult mouse skin
after wounding. Nature 2007;447:316–20.

How to Diagnose Hair Loss

Adrianna J. Jackson, MD[a,b], Vera H. Price, MD, FRCPC[b,*]

KEYWORDS

- Cicatricial • Noncicatricial • Scarring • Pull test • Tug test • Hair Card • Hair mount

KEY POINTS

- At the start of the interview, evaluate for the presence or absence of follicular orifices, because history taking will be guided by whether the problem at hand is a noncicatricial or cicatricial alopecia.
- Determine whether the main issue is hair coming out "by the roots" or whether hair breakage is the main problem, because this will also guide the direction of history taking.
- For the clinical examination, position the patient with a hair problem in a chair, not on the examination table, to see the hair and scalp from above, and use magnified lighting from a close light source such as a portable magnifying lamp or a dermatoscope; daylight from a window or a lamp on the ceiling is not sufficient for the hair and scalp examination.
- The Hair Card, a 3 × 5-inch card, white on one side and black on the other, with a centimeter ruler along one edge, demonstrates new hair growth and miniaturized hair, and differentiates new hair from broken hair; the ruler portion is used for measuring length of new growth, temporal recession, and dimensions of hair loss.
- A scalp biopsy is the essential first step if a cicatricial alopecia is suspected, taken at or just beyond an active area of inflammation where hairs are still present, not a bare area.

INTRODUCTION

The hair follicle cycle is key to understanding hair loss because all causes of hair loss affect the hair cycle in some manner. The anatomic site of hair determines its size, and the diameter is determined by the size of the matrix. The 3 main phases of the hair follicle cycle include: (1) anagen or growth phase, which lasts 2 to 6 years; (2) catagen or involution phase, which lasts 2 to 3 weeks; and (3) telogen or resting phase, which lasts 2 to 3 months. The duration of anagen determines the hair length.[1]

Hair follicles grow in a nonsynchronized fashion. Approximately 85% to 90% of scalp hair follicles are in anagen, 10% to 15% in telogen, and fewer than 1% in catagen. Scalp hair grows approximately 0.35 mm/d or 1 cm/mo.[1] With 100,000 to 150,000 hairs on the scalp, the daily output of hair keratin protein is an impressive 35 m (0.35 mm/d × 100,000 hairs). Average normal daily scalp hair loss in an adult is 40 to 100 hairs on a nonshampoo day and 200 to 300 hairs on a shampoo day. Each hair that is shed is replaced by a new hair.

EVALUATING THE PATIENT
History

At the start of the interview, evaluate for the presence or absence of follicular orifices. Whether the problem at hand is a cicatricial (scarring) or noncicatricial alopecia guides history taking. The majority of this discussion focuses on noncicatricial alopecia, which accounts for most problems concerning hair loss.

Box 1 outlines the key features of history taking. Early in the interview, attempt to differentiate whether the hair is coming out "by the roots" or whether hair breakage is the issue.[2] If the hair is coming out by the roots, ask whether the main concern is increased shedding or increased

a Advanced Dermatology, 430 S. Mason Rd #101, Katy, TX 77450; b Department of Dermatology, University of California, San Francisco, 1701 Divisadero Street, 3rd Floor, San Francisco, CA 94115, USA
* Corresponding author.
E-mail address: PriceV@derm.ucsf.edu

Dermatol Clin 31 (2013) 21–28
http://dx.doi.org/10.1016/j.det.2012.08.007

derm.theclinics.com

<table>
<tr><td>

Box 1
Medical history

Age of onset

Duration

Is hair coming out by the roots or is it breaking?

Increased shedding or increased thinning?

Medications

Past health

Family history

Diet: is there adequate protein or iron intake?

Menses, pregnancies, menopause

Hair care/hair cosmetics

Occupation and hobbies

</td><td>

Box 2
Differential diagnosis of hair coming out by the roots

Telogen effluvium

Alopecia areata

Androgenetic alopecia

Hair loss due to oral contraceptives

　　While taking oral contraceptives

　　After stopping oral contraceptives

Syphilitic alopecia

</td></tr>
</table>

thinning. The patient's medical history, particularly 6 to 12 months before the onset, may be relevant for increased shedding; for example, febrile illnesses, hospitalizations, surgeries, and traumatic events. Inquire about a family history of the same type of condition (androgenetic alopecia or alopecia areata) or associated conditions (family history of autoimmune diseases in alopecia areata). In a patient with androgenetic alopecia, ask about thinning hair in each family member. Ask patients whether they eat a balanced diet and, if they are vegetarian, ask the source of their dietary protein. Hair is composed of approximately 98% keratin protein, and the average adult produces approximately 35 m of hair keratin protein per day (0.35 mm/d × 100,000 hairs), which emphasizes the importance of daily protein intake.

In female patients, assess menses, pregnancies, and menopause. Does she have a menstrual period every month, for how many days, and how heavy is her menstrual flow? Does she have a history of infertility or miscarriages? Postpartum effluvium occurs 1 to 3 months after delivery, but does not necessarily occur after every pregnancy in a given patient. With menopause, hormone replacement with progestins that have androgenic metabolites, or testosterone, may aggravate or cause hair loss, as does removal of both ovaries.

Hair coming out by the roots
Common causes of hair coming out by the roots are shown in **Box 2**. Distinguish whether there is increased shedding or increased thinning. Interest is focused on increased shedding that involves excessive hair drop-out on nonshampoo days. The sudden onset of markedly increased hair shedding is typical of telogen effluvium, and may last up to 6 months. In contrast, increased thinning

implies less and less coverage and a more visible scalp, and may not be associated with increased shedding. Keep in mind that hair density has to decrease by more than half before there is noticeable hair thinning (**Fig. 1**). Increased thinning is typical of androgenetic alopecia and age-related thinning.

Oral contraceptive pills (OCP) may cause hair loss either while taking the OCP or after stopping the OCP. Taking progestins with androgenic metabolites, or testosterone, may cause increased thinning, particularly in women predisposed to androgenetic alopecia. Hair loss after stopping OCP can simulate postpartum effluvium and can occur after stopping any OCP.[2]

Sometimes it is difficult to assess a patient's concern about shedding, and in this situation hair collections are used. Ask patients to collect all hairs shed on a nonshampoo day, from the time they wake up until bedtime, and to place the hairs in a plastic bag that is dated. Collections are repeated once every 2 weeks over an 8-week period, and the 4 collections mailed to the clinician. The patient's hair length must be documented ahead of time so that the volume of hair

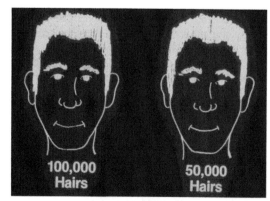

Fig. 1. Hair density has to decrease by more than half before there is noticeable hair thinning.

collected can be properly assessed. On a non-shampoo day, average daily hair loss is 40 to 100 hairs and on a shampoo day, 200 to 300 hairs. Do not count the hairs but rather make a visual estimate of each day's collection.

Hair breakage

Increased hair breakage implies increased hair fragility. The Hair Card, discussed later in this article, demonstrates whether the distal ends are tapered, as with new growth (**Fig. 2**), or whether they are blunt or straight, which indicates hair has been cut or broken (**Fig. 3**). Common diagnoses associated with hair breakage are noted in **Box 3**. The hallmark of tinea capitis is scalp scaling in an area of hair breakage. When tinea capitis is suspected, ask if schoolmates or other family members (such as grandmothers!) are affected. Trichotillomania, on the other hand, is not the result of innate fragility but rather of an extrinsic cause of hair breakage, such as a patient pulling or breaking hair. Hair-care practices and use of hair cosmetics do not cause significant hair breakage when carried out properly and according to directions. However, when done improperly they can cause damage and breakage. Examples of improper hair care practices include excessive heat used too frequently; bleaching, chemical relaxers, and permanent waves that are left on too long, or used too frequently; or chemical relaxers and permanent waves applied on the same day as hair coloring. Some individuals undoubtedly have a greater susceptibility to breakage than others.

Chemotherapeutic drugs including antimetabolites, alkylating agents, and mitotic inhibitors temporarily arrest mitotic activity in rapidly dividing cells. Because the cells of the hair matrix of anagen hairs contain rapidly dividing cells, mitotic arrest

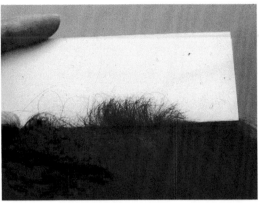

Fig. 3. A white background demonstrating blunt ends, which indicates hair has been cut or broken.

results in narrowing of the hair shaft. When the narrowed segment of hair shaft reaches the scalp surface, the hair breaks off. Because 85% to 90% of scalp hairs are in anagen phase, approximately 85% to 90% of hairs will break off. This impressive breakage occurs 1 to 3 weeks after chemotherapy is administered[2]; this is referred to as anagen arrest rather than anagen effluvium (**Fig. 4**).

Box 4 includes a list of structural hair-shaft anomalies, divided into those with increased fragility and those without increased fragility. This discussion does not permit a detailed review of these anomalies.[3,4]

Clinical Examination

Global examination

First, assess the global appearance of the patient (**Box 5**). These findings may be visible across the room.

Close examination

Position all patients with hair problems in a chair, not on the examination table, to see the hair and scalp from above (unless you are 7 ft tall!). Use good lighting or a magnifying light for close inspection. Alternatively, a dermatoscope also provides magnification.[5] The hair pull, hair tug,

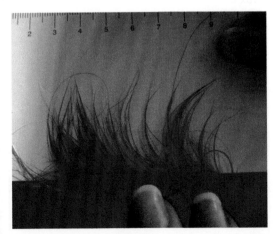

Fig. 2. The Hair Card demonstrating tapered ends, which indicates new hair growth.

Box 3
Differential diagnosis of hair breakage
Tinea capitis
Trichotillomania
Improper hair care and/or hair cosmetics
Anagen arrest
Structural hair-shaft anomalies

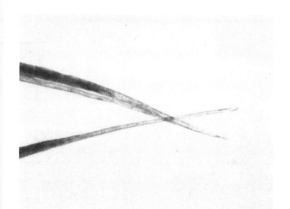

Fig. 4. Anagen arrest with chemotherapy. Mitotic arrest narrows the shafts and hairs break when they reach the scalp surface.

Hair Card, and hair mount are 4 simple tools that aid the assessment of a hair problem in the office (**Box 6**). The authors find the Hair Card (**Box 7,** see **Fig. 2**) essential when examining hair.

To assess hair density, serially part the hair starting at the frontal hairline, note the spacing between hairs, and repeat the parts at 1-inch (2.5-cm) intervals. Compare the hair density over the frontal scalp with the density over the occipital scalp. Make note of general erythema, perifollicular erythema,

---

Box 5
Global examination
Scalp visible?
Full coverage?
Distal ends skimpy?
Intact frontal hairline?
Hair loss diffuse or patchy?
Pattern and distribution of hair loss?
Hair curly or straight, color, length?
Cystic acne, virilization?

perifollicular scale, papules, pustules, crusting, telangiectasia, and tufting. If pustules are present, take a bacterial culture. Determine if follicular markings are present or absent. With patchy hair loss, note the color of the scalp: is it skin-colored, white, peach-colored, or erythematous? If scaling is present in a bare patch, include tinea capitis in your differential diagnosis.

With patchy hair loss, it is useful to document the extent of hair loss for comparison at subsequent visits. Divide the scalp into 4 quadrants and estimate the area that all the alopecic patches placed together would occupy.[6] The hair loss can be estimated as 0% to 25%, 26% to 50%, 51% to 75%, 76% to 99%, or 100%, and is a helpful reference for follow-up visits. Photographs are also useful to document the extent and distribution of hair loss. A diagram of the anatomic areas of the scalp is shown in **Fig. 5**.

Pull test A pull test is helpful in determining excessive hair shedding (**Fig. 6**). At the scalp level,

---

Box 4
Structural anomalies of the hair shaft
Hair-Shaft Disorders with Increased Fragility
Acquired
Bubble hair
Acquired trichorrhexis nodosa
Congenital
Congenital trichorrhexis nodosa (arginosuccinic aciduria)
Monilethrix
Pili torti (Björnstad, Menkes)
Trichorrhexis invaginata (Netherton syndrome)
Trichothiodystrophy
Hair-Shaft Disorders Without Increased Fragility
Congenital
Pili annulati
Pseudopili annulati
Woolly hair
Uncombable hair syndrome

Box 6
Close examination
Pull test
Tug test
Hair Card
Hair mount
Scalp:
Follicular markings present, diminished, or absent
Skin-colored, white, peach-colored, or erythematous
Perifollicular erythema, perifollicular scale, papules, pustules, crusting, telangiectasia, and tufting
Hair elsewhere: too much or too little

Box 7
The Hair Card

The Hair Card assists in the examination and visualization of hair on the scalp, brows, eyelashes, or else-where. The Hair Card is a 3 × 5-inch card, white on one side and black on the other, with a centimeter ruler along one edge. Any white background is a simple "make do" substitute, but will not help in the examination of white or blond hair.

What the Hair Card Does:

Demonstrates miniaturized hair

Demonstrates new hair growth

Differentiates new hair from broken hair

The ruler portion is used for:

    Measuring length of new growth

    Measuring temporal recession

    Measuring dimensions of area of hair loss

How to Use the Hair Card:

A good light source directed at the hair is essential when using the Hair Card

The black or white side is used to contrast with the color of the hair:

    If dark hair is examined, use white side

    If blond or white hair is examined, use black side

To visualize the hair, place the blank (without any writing) portion of the card under or behind the hair to be examined (the larger the blank portion of the card, the more useful it is)

Always place the Hair Card on the skin or as close to the skin surface as possible

To Demonstrate Miniaturized Hairs in Androgenetic Alopecia:

Select a thinning site on the scalp

Part the hair with your fingers

Place the Hair Card on the part you have created, directly on the scalp surface

A good light must be directed at the selected site

New short growth will be apparent against the contrasting color of the Hair Card, and miniaturized (thin) hair is easily identified and contrasted with the new short growth of normal size (girth)

To Differentiate New Hair Growth from Broken (or Cut) Hair:

Place the Hair Card under the distal ends of the hair in question

New growth is easily identified because the distal ends are tapered or pointed

Broken hair is easily identified because the distal ends are blunt or straight

To Measure Temporal Recession:

Using the ruler side of the Hair Card, measure the distance from the lateral end of the brow to the apex of the temporal recession. In a male without temporal recession, this distance is approximately 7 to 7.5 cm

---

grasp 30 to 40 closely grouped hairs between the thumb and index finger. Pull the grouped hairs firmly but gently away from the scalp. Repeat at 3 different locations on the scalp. With alopecia areata, pull at the margin of a patch, over new hair growth, and randomly over unaffected scalp. If a pull test yields anagen hair (positive anagen pull test), suspect a primary cicatricial alopecia.

Tug test A tug test is useful in demonstrating hair fragility (**Fig. 7**). In a tug test, grasp a cluster of hairs with one hand while the distal ends are pulled away with the other hand (like plucking feathers). Fragile hair breaks into small bits, which can be examined in a hair mount.

Hair mount Light microscopic examination of hair is an easy office procedure, much like a potassium

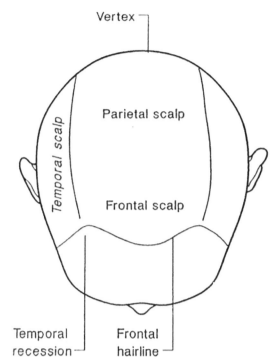

Fig. 5. The anatomic areas of the scalp.

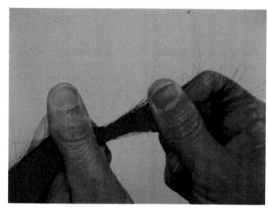

Fig. 7. How to do a tug test to demonstrate hair fragility.

fracture and longitudinal splitting.[4] In hair shaft anomalies associated with fragility, mount hair shaft segments to display the anomaly (see **Box 4**). In primary cicatricial alopecia, a pull test may extract anagen hairs, which then are mounted for confirmation. **Figs. 4**, **9**, and **10** illustrate the 3 situations whereby anagen hairs may be easily extracted or affected.

How to prepare a hair mount Use a black or white velvet background for selecting the bulbs

hydroxide (KOH) preparation, and often helps in diagnosis. Decide in advance if you want to look at hair bulbs or hair shafts. Telogen hair has no inner root sheath and the bulb has a distinctive club shape with reduced or absent melanin (**Fig. 8**). Anagen hairs, in contrast, are larger and have a dark pigmented bulb, and an inner root sheath (**Fig. 9**). With hair breakage, the small broken hairs from a tug test are useful to show trichorrhexis nodosa (TN). This most common cause of acquired hair breakage shows the typical

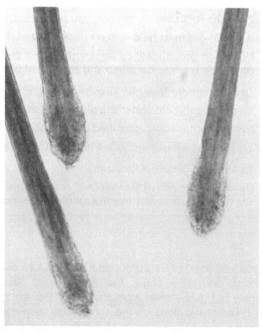

Fig. 8. Telogen hair when extracted has no inner root sheath, and the bulb has a distinctive club shape with reduced or absent melanin (Original magnification ×400).

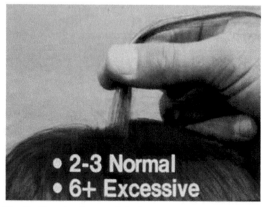

Fig. 6. How to do a pull test.

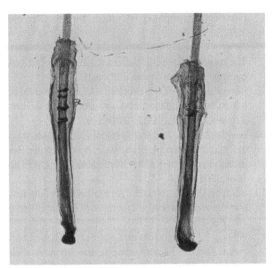

Fig. 9. Anagen hair has an inner root sheath and darkly pigmented bulb (Original magnification ×100).

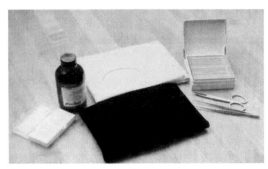

Fig. 11. Hair mount supplies.

or hair shaft segments you wish to mount (**Fig. 11**). A black background helps to identify white bulbs, and a white background helps to visualize dark hair. Velvet is used to keep the hairs from flying away. Good lighting is essential. Clip 1 cm segments of the hair and place them parallel on a glass slide. Place 1 to 2 drops of a mounting medium on the hairs and cover with a coverslip; try to avoid bubbles. (The mounting medium can be Permount from Fisher Scientific, Pittsburgh, PA or any mounting medium found in pathology laboratories). In a mounting medium, hair is seen sharply, light scatter is eliminated, and the mounted hair can be kept indefinitely. KOH, water, and oil are not satisfactory for a hair mount.[4]

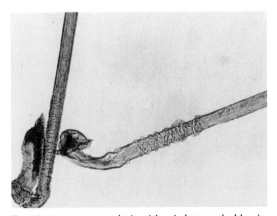

Fig. 10. Loose anagen hair with misshapen darkly pigmented bulb, short twisted segment immediately distal to the bulb, absent inner root sheath, and "ruffled" cuticle (Original magnification ×100).

One word of caution: if you suspect pili torti (as in Menkes kinky hair syndrome), examine the hair dry (unmounted) under a coverslip, otherwise the shadows of the twists will not be visualized.

LABORATORY TESTS

In patients with hair loss, order a complete blood count, ferritin, thyroid stimulating hormone, and vitamin D 25OH. Vitamin D 25OH and ferritin are important for a normal hair cycle.[7,8] In women, if the history and examination reveal severe cystic acne, hirsutism, galactorrhea, menstrual irregularities, infertility, or virilization, check the free or total testosterone, dehydroepiandrosterone sulfate, and prolactin levels. If any one of these tests are positive, refer the patient to an interested endocrinologist or gynecologist.

SCALP BIOPSY

Scalp biopsies offer additional information, and in a suspected cicatricial alopecia, a scalp biopsy is the essential first step. In cicatricial alopecia, perform the biopsy at or just beyond an early active area with inflammation and where hairs are still present; the site of a positive anagen pull test is ideal, but not always available. In alopecia areata and cicatricial alopecia, do not biopsy bare areas! Anesthetize with 1% lidocaine with epinephrine, and wait 10 minutes to allow time for adequate vasoconstriction. Take 1 or 2 4-mm punch biopsies down to subcutaneous fat. Depending on the preference of the dermatopathologist, request horizontal and/or vertical sections stained with hematoxylin and eosin. Horizontal sections have the advantage of assessing large numbers of follicles for hair density, terminal-to-vellus hair ratios, anagen-to-telogen hair ratios, and the extent of any inflammatory infiltrate.[9–11]

REFERENCES

1. Montagna W, Parakkal PF. The structure and function of skin. 3rd edition. New York: Academic Press; 1974. p. 186–219.
2. Price VH. Management of hair problems. Int J Dermatol 1979;19:95–103.
3. Mirmirani P, Huang KP, Price VH. A practical, algorithmic approach to diagnosing hair shaft disorders. Int J Dermatol 2011;50:1–12.
4. Price VH. Structural anomalies of the hair shaft. In: Orfanos CE, Rudolf H, editors. Hair and hair diseases. Berlin, Heidelberg (Germany), New York: Springer-Verlag; 1990. p. 363–422.
5. Tosti A. Dermoscopy of hair and scalp disorders with clinical and pathological correlations. London: Informa Healthcare Ltd; 2007.
6. Khoury EL, Price VH, Abdel-Salam MM, et al. Topical minoxidil in alopecia areata: no effect on the perifollicular lymphoid infiltration. J Invest Dermatol 1992;99:40–7.
7. Amor KT, Rashid RM, Mirmirani P. Does D matter? The role of vitamin D in hair disorders and hair follicle cycling. Dermatol Online J 2010;16:3.
8. Kantor J, Kessler LJ, Brooks DG, et al. Decreased serum ferritin is associated with alopecia in women. J Invest Dermatol 2003;121:985–8.
9. Headington JT. Transverse microscopic anatomy of the human scalp. A basis for a morphometric approach to disorders of the hair follicle. Arch Dermatol 1984;120:449–56.
10. Sperling LC, Winton GB. The transverse anatomy of androgenic alopecia. J Dermatol Surg Oncol 1990; 16:1127–33.
11. Whiting DA. Diagnostic and predictive value of horizontal sections of scalp biopsy specimens in male pattern androgenetic alopecia. J Am Acad Dermatol 1993;28:755–63.

Trichoscopy
How It May Help the Clinician

Lidia Rudnicka, MD, PhD[a,b,c,*], Adriana Rakowska, MD, PhD[a],
Malgorzata Olszewska, MD, PhD[d]

KEYWORDS

- Trichoscopy • Dermoscopy • Alopecia areata • Androgenetic alopecia • Telogen effluvium
- Trichotillomania • Cicatricial alopecia • Tinea capitis

KEY POINTS

- Trichoscopy (hair and scalp dermoscopy) may be performed with any handheld or digital dermoscope.
- This method may be used as a diagnostic aid in differential diagnosis of hair loss and scalp diseases and in monitoring therapy.
- Trichoscopy diagnosis is based on evaluation of hair shafts, follicular openings, and perifollicular epidermis.
- Characteristic trichoscopy features of several hair and scalp diseases are known. These diseases include alopecia areata, androgenetic alopecia, discoid lupus erythematosus, folliculitis decalvans, genetic hair shaft abnormalities, lichen planopilaris, scalp psoriasis, tinea capitis, and trichotillomania.

Trichoscopy (or dermoscopy of hair and scalp) is an easy in-office technique that may be performed with a handheld dermoscope or a digital videodermoscopy system. This method is gaining increasing popularity, because it may be widely applied in differential diagnosis of hair and scalp diseases.

Trichoscopy is based on analysis of structures that may be visualized with a dermoscope. These basic structures may be divided into 4 groups: (1) hair shafts, (2) hair follicle openings (dots), (3) perifollicular epidermis, and (4) blood vessels.

BASIC STRUCTURES
Evaluation of Hair Shafts

The authors have recently suggested a classification of hair shaft abnormalities that may be visualized by trichoscopy.[1,2] This classification distinguishes the following groups of hair shaft abnormalities: (1) hair shafts with fractures, (2) hair narrowings, (3) hairs with node-like structures, (4) curls and twists, (5) bands, and (4) short hairs. Only selected types of abnormalities are discussed in this article.

Many types of short hairs appear crucial for differential diagnosis of the most frequent types of hair loss in clinical practice. These are hairs that are less than 5 mm long. They include, among others, bent and hypopigmented vellus hairs, which are most characteristic of androgenetic alopecia.[3,4] Vellus hairs may be also present in long-lasting, severe alopecia areata.[5,6] Another type of short hairs is comma[7] and corckscrew hairs,[8,9] which are characteristic for tinea capitis. Short flame-like hairs are observed in trichotillomania.[1,2]

Micro–exclamation mark hairs are hairs with narrowings at the proximal end. This type of

Authors have no conflict of interest.
[a] Department of Dermatology, CSK MSWiA, Woloska 137, Warsaw 02-507, Poland; [b] Mossakowski Medical Research Centre, Polish Academy of Sciences, Pawińskiego 5, Warsaw 02-106, Poland; [c] Department of Clinical Nursing, Faculty of Health Sciences, Medical University of Warsaw, Ciolka 27 Room 106, Warsaw 01-445, Poland; [d] Department of Dermatology, Medical University of Warsaw, Koszykowa 82A, Warsaw 02-008, Poland
* Corresponding author. Department of Dermatology, CSK MSWiA, 02-507 Warsaw, Poland, Woloska 137.
E-mail address: lidia.rudnicka@euderm.eu

abnormality is observed in alopecia areata and in trichotillomania.[2]

Evaluation of Hair Follicle Openings (Dots)

With trichoscopy, whether hair follicle openings are normal, empty, fibrotic, or contain biologic material, such as hyperkeratotic plugs or hair residues, may be distinguished. *Dots* is a common term for hair follicle openings seen by trichoscopy.[10]

Black dots (formerly called cadaverized hairs) represent pigmented hairs broken or destroyed at scalp level.[10] They are observed in alopecia areata, dissecting cellulitis, tinea capitis, and trichotillomania.[2,11–13]

Yellow dots are hair follicle openings that contain keratosebaceous material.[2,10,14] They may be observed in alopecia areata,[11] discoid lupus erythematosus,[2] and female androgenic alopecia.[15] Rarely, yellow dots may be observed in telogen effluvium and trichotillomania.[1] Yellow dots, appearing as large 3-D soap bubbles imposed over dark dystrophic hairs, are specific for dissecting cellulitis.[16]

There are 2 types of white dots: classic, big, irregular white dots and pinpoint white dots.

Box 1
Classification of perifollicular and interfollicular skin surface abnormalities in trichoscopy (most common or characteristic occurrences shown in parentheses)

- Scaling
  - Diffuse
    - White (psoriasis, discoid lupus erythematosus, allergic dermatitis, dry skin)
    - Yellowish (seborrheic dermatitis, discoid lupus erythematosus, ichthyosis)
  - Perifollicular
    - Color of scales
      - White (lichen planopilaris)
      - Yellowish (folliculitis decalvans)
    - Shape of scale arrangement
      - Tubular (lichen planopilaris)
      - Tubular with collar formation (folliculitis decalvans)
- Color
  - Brown areas
    - Honeycomb hyperpigmentation (common)
    - Perifollicular; peripilar sign (female and male androgenetic alopecia, telogen effluvium, healthy individuals)
    - Scattered (discoid lupus erythematosus, actinic keratosis)
  - White areas (cicatricial alopecia, detached epidermis, edema)
  - Pink, strawberry ice cream–color areas (early fibrosis in cicatricial alopecia)
  - Yellow areas (dissecting cellulitis, follicular pustules, bacterial infection)
  - Red (inflammation, extravasation, erosion, vascular abnormalities)
  - Violaceous blue (lichen planopilaris, discoid lupus erythematosus)
- Discharge
  - Yellow and yellow-red (folliculitis decalvans, bacterial infections, dissecting cellulitis, tinea capitis)
  - White follicular spicules (monoclonal gammopathy)
- Surface structure
  - Starburst pattern hyperplasia (folliculitis decalvans)

Data from Rudnicka L, Olszewska M, Rakowska A, editors. Trichoscopy: dermoscopy of hair and scalp. Springer-Verlag; 2012.

Classic white dots represent areas of perifollicular fibrosis and are observed most commonly in lichen planopilaris.[2,10] Pinpoint white dots correspond to hair follicle openings and eccrine gland openings, observed within pigmented background. They are present in patients with dark skin phototypes, regardless of hair loss.[17,18]

Red dots are described in discoid lupus erythematosus and are considered a good prognostic finding, indicating possible hair regrowth.[19]

Regularly distributed gray or brown-gray dots are a characteristic finding in the eyebrow area of patients with frontal fibrosing alopecia.[1]

Evaluation of Perifollicular Epidermis

Abnormalities of scalp skin color or structure that may be visualized by trichoscopy include scaling, changes in color, abnormalities in skin surface structure, and presence of discharge. A new classification of these abnormalities is presented in **Box 1**, which indicates the clinical significance of individual abnormalities.

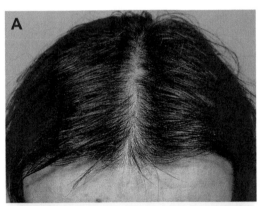

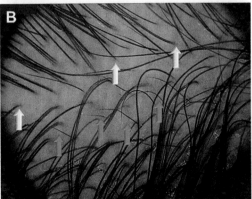

Fig. 1. Telogen effluvium. Clinical appearance (A) and trichoscopy (B). Trichoscopy shows multiple upright regrowing hairs (*blue arrows*) and predominance of follicular units with only 1 hair (*white arrows*). There is no hair shaft thickness heterogeneity, which allows excluding androgenetic alopecia.

Evaluation of Blood Vessels

Appearance of cutaneous microvessels in trichoscopy may vary in type, arrangement, and number, depending on disease. Analysis of blood vessel arrangement is of special importance in differential diagnosis of inflammatory scalp diseases, such as scalp psoriasis, seborrheic dermatitis, or discoid lupus erythematosus.[1]

DIFFERENTIAL DIAGNOSIS OF NONSCARRING ALOPECIA
Telogen Effluvium

The term, *telogen effluvium*, refers to a wide range of clinical situations with the common feature of abrupt, generalized shedding of telogen hairs. It is considered the most common type of hair loss, but only limited evidence-based knowledge is available.

Trichoscopy findings in telogen effluvium include presence of empty hair follicles, predominance of follicular units with only 1 hair, perifollicular discoloration (peripilar sign), and upright regrowing hairs (**Fig. 1, Table 1**). Trichoscopy results do not differ depending on the factor that induced telogen hair loss.

Androgenetic Alopecia

Male androgenetic alopecia and female androgenetic alopecia share similar trichoscopy features.

Table 1
Trichoscopy features of telogen effluvium and androgenetic alopecia

	Telogen Effluvium	Androgenetic Alopecia
Follicular units with only 1 hair	+	++
Upright regrowing hairs	++	±
Perifollicular discoloration (peripilar sign)	+	++
Vellus hairs	–	+
Hair shaft thickness heterogeneity	–	+
Predominance of abnormalities in the frontal region	–	+

+, Increased; ++, significantly increased.

Adapted from Rudnicka L, Olszewska M, Rakowska A, editors. Trichoscopy: dermoscopy of hair and scalp. Springer-Verlag; 2012.

Hair shaft thickness heterogeneity, with simultaneous presence of thin, intermediate, and thick hairs, is the most characteristic feature of androgenetic alopecia. It has been shown that hair diameter diversity reflects follicle miniaturization in androgenetic alopecia.[5,20] Hair thickness may be estimated when performing trichoscopy with a handheld dermoscope. With this method, hair shafts may classified as thin, intermediate, or thick. Some digital videodermoscopes possess software that allows detailed evaluation of hair shaft thickness in micrometers. Detailed evaluation of hair shaft thickness is not necessary for diagnosis and differential diagnosis in clinical practice but may be useful for monitoring treatment efficacy[21] and is indispensable for clinical trials.

Another trichoscopy feature of androgenetic alopecia is increased proportion of vellus hairs. The proportion of vellus hairs in the frontal scalp area of patients with female androgenetic alopecia is 20.9% ± 12%.[15] This is significantly more than the 6.15% ± 4.6% in healthy volunteers.[3,4,15] Multiple vellus hairs may be also present in severe alopecia areata.[11,13] Thus, sole presence of vellus hairs should not be mistaken for androgenetic alopecia.

The number of hairs in 1 follicular unit is decreased in androgenetic alopecia. Follicular units with only 1 hair predominate in these patients, especially in a late phase of disease. In the frontal area of patients with female androgenetic alopecia, average percentage of follicular units with only 1 hair is 65.2% ± 19.9%. The corresponding number in healthy individuals is 27.3% ± 13%.[22] The percentage of follicular units with only 1 hair is also increased in telogen effluvium (39.0% ± 13.4%) and in various forms of anagen hair loss.[4,15,22]

The authors' experience and study results of show presence of yellow dots a constant finding in androgenetic alopecia, but literature data are inconsistent.

In different studies, yellow dots were observed in 66%,[15] 30.5%,[23] 10% to 26%,[5] and 7%[10] of patients with androgenetic alopecia. The authors find an explanation for this discrepancy in that in androgenetic alopecia some yellow dots have only sebaceous content and not keratosebaceous material, as in other diseases. These sebaceous yellow dots may be washed away by a vigorous hair wash. Accordingly, when patients come for a trichoscopy examination directly after washing their hair, these yellow dots may not be detectable. In the authors' practice, in patients with noncicatricial alopecia, trichoscopy is always performed together with a trichogram. For this reason,

patients are asked to not wash their hair for 3 days before examination. The small, sebaceous yellow dots may develop during these 3 days. This hypothesis is partly confirmed by the authors' unpublished observations, showing that the number of sebaceous yellow dots in androgenetic alopecia is higher before than after hair washing. No other trichoscopy features depend on hair washing.

Brown perifollicular discoloration (peripilar sign)[24] is observed in 20% to 66% of patients with androgenetic alopecia.[5,15] A proportion of 32.4% ± 4.7% hair follicle openings are affected.[5,15] This feature may be also observed in some patients with telogen effluvium and in healthy individuals with the difference that in androgenetic alopecia the proportion of affected hair follicle openings is higher in the frontal compared with the occipital area. In healthy individuals and in patients with telogen effluvium, the proportion of affected hair follicle openings is

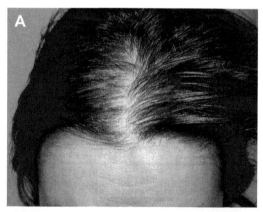

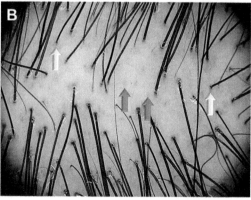

Fig. 2. Female androgenetic alopecia. Clinical appearance (A) and trichoscopy (B). Trichoscopy shows significant hair shaft thickness heterogeneity, yellow dots (*blue arrows*), and predominance of follicular units with only 1 hair (*white arrows*).

significantly lower and the distribution is proportional in all scalp areas.[4,22] **Table 1** summarizes the major differences between androgenetic alopecia and telogen effluvium. **Fig. 2** presents major trichoscopy features of androgenetic alopecia.

Trichoscopy of senescent (senile, involutionary) alopecia shares with androgenetic alopecia predominance of follicular units with only 1 hair, decreased hair shaft density with honeycomb pattern pigmentation, and slight tendency to form brown perifollicular discoloration (peripilar sign).[1]

Alopecia Areata

In most cases, alopecia areata is diagnosed based on clinical appearance.[25,26] Trichoscopy may be useful, however, for differential diagnosis of difficult cases, in particular in diffuse alopecia areata or in patients with total hair loss.

The hallmark trichoscopy features of alopecia areata are regularly distributed yellow dots, micro–exclamation mark hairs, tapered hairs, black dots, broken hairs, and regrowing hairs. Trichoscopy of alopecia areata may differ depending on diseases activity, severity, and duration. These differences were evaluated in multiple studies in recent years.

Lacarrubba and colleagues[14] investigated 200 patients with alopecia areata, subdivided into acute and chronic disease. This study identified 3 features of acute alopecia areata: micro–exclamation marks, black dots, and vellus hairs. Inui and colleagues[11] identified similar markers of disease activity (black dots, tapering hairs, and broken hairs) based on trichoscopy performed in 300 patients with alopecia areata. In this study, vellus hairs were found to be a marker of long-lasting, inactive disease. Ross and colleagues[10] divided 58 patients with alopecia areata into the following subgroups: patchy, ophiasis, diffuse, and alopecia totalis/universalis. Trichoscopy features were similarly expressed in all investigated subgroups. The authors' experience[2,27] shows that black dots are a most constant marker of disease activity in alopecia areata. A recent study from Turkey[23] performed with a handheld dermoscope confirmed earlier data obtained by digital videodermoscopy.

Some patients with active alopecia areata of long duration show monilethrix-like hairs with characteristic Pohl-Pinkus constrictions. In a study by Mane and colleagues[28] this type of abnormality was observed in 2 of 66 (3%) investigated patients with alopecia areata. Presence of hairs with Pohl-Pinkus constrictions may lead to misdiagnosis of monilethrix.

Features of hair regrowth include pigmented short upright regrowing hairs[11] and regularly

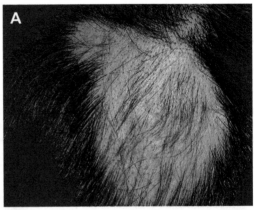
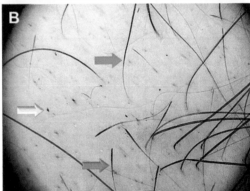
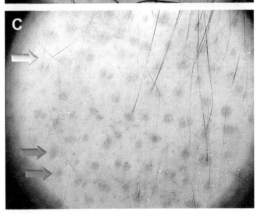

Fig. 3. Female androgenetic alopecia. Clinical appearance (*A*) and trichoscopy (*B, C*). Trichoscopy of active alopecia areata (*B*) shows micro–exclamation mark hairs (*blue arrow*), black dots (*white arrow*), and tapered hairs (*green arrow*), which differ from micro–exclamation mark hairs in that their distal end is not visible within 1 field on view of a dermoscope. In long-lasting inactive alopecia areata (*C*), regularly distributed yellow dots (*blue arrows*) and vellus hairs (*white arrows*) predominate in trichoscopy.

coiled pigtail hairs.[2] The authors used the term, *pigtail hairs*, in a publication[2] to describe hairs that form regular circular or oval structures as they grow. They have to be distinguished from irregularly coiled hairs of trichotillomania.

Trichotillomania is a common and the most difficult differential diagnosis of alopecia areata.[29] Trichoscopy features of alopecia areata are presented in **Fig. 3**.

Trichotillomania

Trichoscopy of trichotillomania shows decreased hair density, hairs broken at different lengths, short hairs with trichoptilosis (split ends), irregular coiled hairs, upright regrowing hairs, and black dots.[1,29–31] Yellow dots are generally not observed in trichotillomania.[29] Inui and colleagues[11] observed yellow dots in 1 patient with trichotillomania. These dots differed from yellow dots in other diseases by containing a black dot in their central part.[11] The authors' retrospective analysis of trichoscopy images confirms the presence of characteristic yellow dots with fine black peppering inside as a rare but highly characteristic trichoscopy feature of trichotillomania.[1,27] This finding has to be differentiated from yellow dots in dissecting folliculitis, which are bigger, bulging, and contain a single black hair shaft residue.

In a recent study,[27] the authors identified further characteristic trichoscopy features of trichotillomania. These are hair shaft residues, which appear in trichoscopy as flame hairs, tulip hairs, V-sign, and structureless hair residues (**Table 2**).

Micro–exclamation mark hairs are rare in trichotillomania,[2,32] but they may be a diagnostic pitfall and cause misdiagnosis of alopecia areata. The authors' experience shows that micro–exclamation mark hairs in trichotillomania tend to have a pigmented proximal end and a flat distal end, whereas most micro–exclamation mark hairs in

Table 2 Trichoscopy differential diagnosis of trichotillomania		
	Trichotillomania	Alopecia Areata
Broken hairs	++	+
Irregular coiled hairs/hook hairs	+	−
Short hairs with trichoptilosis (split ends)	+	−
Micro–exclamation mark hairs	+	++
Tapered hairs	+	++
Flame hairs	+	−
Tulip hairs	++	+
V-sign	++	±
Structureless hair residues	+	±
Black dots	+	++
Yellow dots	±	++
Yellow dots with black peppering	+	−
Regrowing pigtail hairs (circular or oval)	−	+
Hypopigmented vellus hairs	−	+

Adapted from Rudnicka L, Olszewska M, Rakowska A, editors. Trichoscopy: dermoscopy of hair and scalp. Springer-Verlag; 2012.

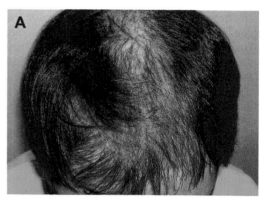
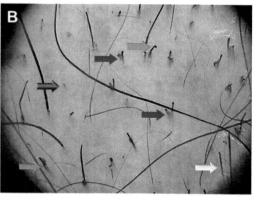

Fig. 4. Trichotillomania. Clinical appearance (*A*) and trichoscopy (*B*). Trichoscopy shows multiple faces of hair residues. These include broken hairs (*blue arrow*), micro–exclamation mark hairs (*white arrow*), black dots (*black arrow*), and hook hairs (*green arrow*), which reflect incomplete coiling of mechanically stretched hairs.

alopecia areata have a hypopigmented proximal end and a pointed distal end.[1,27]

Alopecia areata may be the initial trigger for trichotillomania and the 2 conditions may coexist,[33] which makes trichoscopic differential diagnosis even more challenging. **Table 2** summarizes main differences in trichoscopy between trichotillomania and alopecia areata. Trichoscopy features of trichotillomania are presented in **Fig. 4**.

DIFFERENTIAL DIAGNOSIS OF CICATRICIAL ALOPECIA

Cicatricial alopecia is less frequent in clinical practice compared with noncicatricial alopecia and differential diagnosis is rarely difficult.[34–36]

Trichoscopy may be helpful, however, in establishing correct diagnosis in doubtful cases. The most characteristic trichoscopy features of cicatricial alopecia are presented in **Table 3**. The table includes the most common types of primary cicatricial alopecia: discoid lupus erythematosus, classic lichen planopilaris, frontal fibrosing alopecia, dissecting cellulitis, and folliculitis decalvans.

Discoid Lupus Erythematosus

The most characteristic trichoscopy features of discoid lupus erythematosus of the scalp are thick arborizing vessels and large yellow dots.[2,16] Scattered brown discoloration of the skin may be

Table 3
Trichoscopy features of cicatricial alopecia

		Discoid Lupus Erythematosus	Classic Lichen Planopilaris	Frontal Fibrosing Alopecia	Dissecting Cellulitis	Folliculitis Decalvans
Vessels	Thick arborizing vessels	++	+	—	—	—
	Elongated vessels	+	++	—	—	
	Pinpoint-like vessels with whitish halo	—	—	—	++	+
Color	White and milky-red homogenous areas	+	++	++	—	++
	Dark-brown scattered discoloration	+	—	—	—	—
	Violaceous blue discoloration	+	++	—	—	—
	Structure-less yellow areas	—	—	—	+	—
Dots	3-D yellow dots (soap bubbles) with hairs residues	—	—	—	+	—
	Large yellow dots	+	—	—	—	—
	White dots	+	++	+	—	+
	Red dots	+	—	++	—	—
	Gray dots (eyebrows)	—	—	+	—	—
Scaling	Perifollicular scaling	—	++	+	—	+
Hyperplasia	Perifollicular hyperplasia with starburst pattern	—	—	—	—	+

++, Very common; +, common.

Adapted from Rakowska A, Slowinska M, Kowalska-Oledzka E, et al. Trichoscopy in cicatricial alopecia. J Drugs Dermatol 2012;11(6):753–8.

observed in some patients.[2,16] Yellow dots with radial, thin arborizing vessels emerging from the dot are considered characteristic for discoid lupus erythematosus. This feature is sometimes referred to as "red spider in yellow dot."[16] Red dots, described by Tosti and colleagues,[19] are considered a good prognostic factor for of hair regrowth. Long-lasting, inactive lesions differ from active lesions by presence of structureless milky-red areas, and lack of follicular openings (**Fig. 5**).

Classic Lichen Planopilaris

The most characteristic trichoscopy feature of classic lichen planopilaris is white perifollicular scaling with scales entangling hair shafts up to 2 mm to 3 mm above scalp surface. The authors call this phenomenon, *tubular scaling*.[2,16]

Other findings include perifollicular inflammation, elongated blood vessels, and violaceous blue interfollicular areas.[16,37,38]

In the fibrotic stage of lichen planopilaris, the predominating features are big, irregular (classic) white dots, which merge into white and/or milky-red areas.[16,37,39] The color and appearance of the milky-red areas, which correspond to fibrosis of recent onset, are described by some investigators as strawberry ice cream color (**Fig. 6**).

Frontal Fibrosing Alopecia

Trichoscopy findings in active frontal fibrosing alopecia include minor perifollicular scaling and predominance of follicular openings with only 1 hair (**Fig. 7**). Arborizing vessels were described in 1 study[37] but not confirmed by other investigators.[16,40,41]

Dissecting Cellulitis

In dissecting cellulitis (dissecting folliculitis, perifolliculitis capitis abscedens et suffodiens)

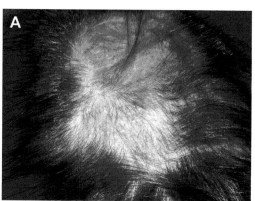

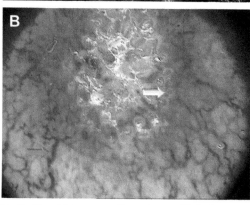

Fig. 5. Discoid lupus erythematosus. Clinical appearance (*A*) and trichoscopy (*B*). Trichoscopy shows multiple thick arborizing vessels (*blue arrow*), large yellow dots (*white arrow*), and fine scaling in the central part of the image.

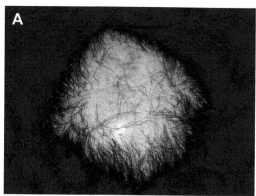

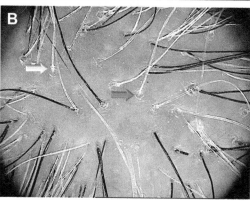

Fig. 6. Classic lichen planopilaris. Clinical appearance (*A*) and trichoscopy (*B*). Trichoscopy shows milky-red (strawberry ice cream color) area with a decreased number of follicular openings. Perifollicular scaling is visible (*blue arrow*). Scales may form tubular structures, which entangle the emerging hair shaft (*white arrow*). This feature is called tubular scaling.

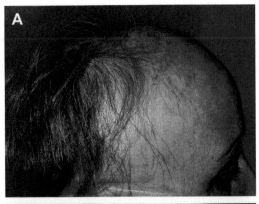

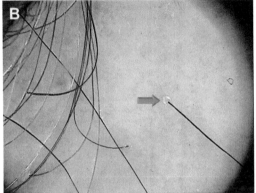

Fig. 7. Frontal fibrosing alopecia. Clinical appearance (*A*) and trichoscopy (*B*). Trichoscopy shows an ivory-white area with a significantly decreased number of follicular openings. Mild perifollicular scaling (*blue arrow*) and a solitary (lonely) hair is visible.

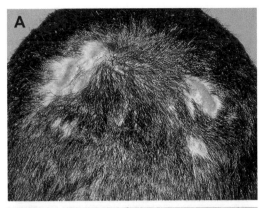

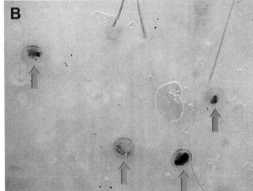

Fig. 8. Frontal fibrosing alopecia. Clinical appearance (*A*) and trichoscopy (*B*). Trichoscopy shows yellow structure-less areas and multiple 3-D yellow dots superimposed over black hair residues (soap bubbles) (*arrows*).

trichoscopy shows yellow, structureless areas. A characteristic finding is yellow dots with 3-D structure imposed over a thick, black, hair shaft residue. The authors consider the term, *soap bubbles*, used by Dr Sami Abdennader during a conference lecture, adequate to describe this feature (**Fig. 8**). Pinpoint-like vessels with a whitish halo were described in patients with dissecting folliculitis,[16] but they are not uncommon in other scalp diseases.[2] End-stage disease with scarring lesions is characterized by confluent ivory-white areas lacking follicular openings.

Folliculitis Decalvans

Folliculitis decalvans is characterized by presence of multiple hairs in 1 follicular unit.[42] These follicular tufts usually consist of 5 to 20 hairs.[42] This feature may be observed both clinically and by trichoscopy (**Fig. 9**). Additional trichoscopy findings include perifollicular hyperplasia arranged in a starburst pattern and follicular pustules.[43] Tubular scaling is observed in 66% of patients with folliculitis decalvans.[16] It differs from tubular scaling in patients with lichen planopilaris by a yellowish color and by a tendency to fold away from the hair shafts and form collar-like structures.[2]

In long-lasting lesions, white or milky-red (strawberry ice cream color) areas lacking follicular openings predominate.[16] White dots are rare.[44] There seems to be no characteristic vascular pattern, although Baroni and Romano[44] observed increased numbers of twisted red loops.

Pseudopelade Brocq

Trichoscopy features of classic pseudopelade of Brocq are nonspecific. These are white areas with no follicular openings. Solitary dystrophic hairs at the periphery of the lesion may be found. Thus, Brocq pseudopelade is a diagnosis of exclusion both clinically and by trichoscopy.[1,45]

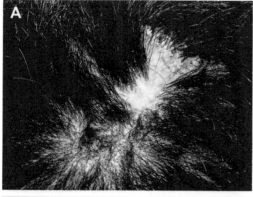

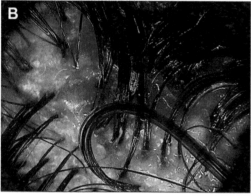

Fig. 9. Folliculitis decalvans. Clinical appearance (A) and trichoscopy (B). Trichoscopy shows tufts of hairs emerging from follicular units.

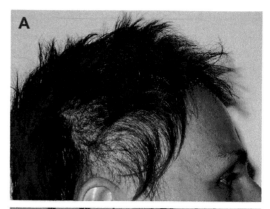

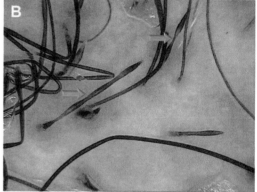

Fig. 10. Monilethrix. Clinical appearance (A) and trichoscopy (B). Trichoscopy shows monilethrix hairs (arrows) with constrictions at regular intervals. Hairs bend and fracture in constricted areas.

DIFFERENTIAL DIAGNOSIS OF HAIR SHAFT ABNORMALITIES

Trichoscopy is a perfect tool for noninvasive evaluation of most genetic hair shaft abnormalities.[12,46,47] It has been documented that trichoscopy allows detecting characteristic structure abnormalities of monilethrix (Fig. 10),[48–52] trichorrhexis invaginata,[51,53,54] trichorrhexis nodosa,[51] pili torti,[51] and pili annulati.[51] The first studies were performed with a digital video-dermoscopy system, but Silverberg and colleagues[55] showed that trichoscopy with a handheld dermoscope also may be applied as an in-office technique to diagnose genetic diseases of the hair.

OTHER APPLICATIONS OF TRICHOSCOPY

Kim and colleagues[56] performed a large study that documented that trichoscopy may be used for differential diagnosis of inflammatory scalp diseases, such as scalp psoriasis and seborrheic dermatitis, based predominantly on structure and arrangement of blood vessels.

Slowinska and colleagues[7] described comma hairs as a characteristic feature of tinea capitis (Fig. 11). Later, Hughes and colleagues[9] identified corckscrew hairs as another characteristic finding in patches of tinea capitis. Recent findings show also zigzag hairs and interrupted (Morse code–like) hairs are observed in these patients.[2]

Accumulating casuistic data indicate that trichoscopy may develop into a method of diagnosis beyond dermatology. Possible application of trichoscopy in identifying follicular spicules in multiple myeloma,[57] follicular mucinosis in lymphoproliferative disorders,[58] or scalp lesions in Langerhans cell histiocytosis[1] is feasible, but requires adequate, evidence-based confirmation.

UV-ENHANCED TRICHOSCOPY

UV-enhanced trichoscopy is a method of hair and scalp evaluation, first described by the authors' group in 2011.[2] This method differs from classic trichoscopy by replacing regular or polarized light

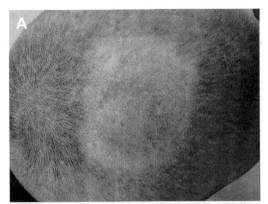

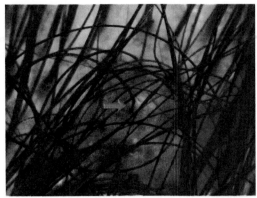

Fig. 12. UV-enhanced trichoscopy (UVET) differs from classic trichoscopy by application of UV light, at a wavelength covering the spectrum of a Wood lamp. The method may enhance the diagnostic potential of trichoscopy in tinea capitis and *Malassezia furfur (Pityrosporum ovale)* infections and may serve as aid in monitoring treatment efficacy in these infections. This image shows orange fluorescence in patients with pityrosporum folliculitis.

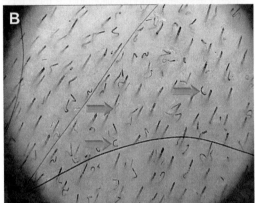

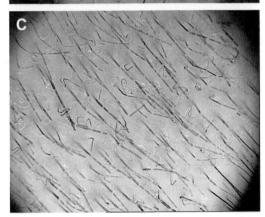

Fig. 11. Tinea capitis caused by *Microsporum canis.* Clinical appearance (*A*) and trichoscopy (*B, C*). Trichoscopy shows multiple comma hairs (*arrows*). Initial formation of corkscrew hairs, which represent comma hairs with multiple twists, is visible (*B*). Hairs with transverse bands (Morse code hairs) are presented (*B*). (*Courtesy of* Dr Monika Slowinska.)

with UV light, at a wavelength covering the spectrum of a Wood lamp. This method may enhance the diagnostic potential of trichoscopy in tinea capitis and *Malassezia furfur (Pityrosporum ovale)* infections (**Fig. 12**).

REFERENCES

1. Rudnicka L, Olszewska M, Rakowska A, editors. Trichoscopy: dermoscopy of hair and scalp. Springer-Verlag: London; 2012.
2. Rudnicka L, Olszewska M, Rakowska A, et al. Trichoscopy update 2011. J Dermatol Case Rep 2011;5:82–8.
3. Vogt A, McElwee KJ, Blume-Peytavi U. Biology of the hair follicle. In: Blume-Peytavi U, Tosti A, Whiting D, et al, editors. Hair; from basic science to clinical application. Berlin: Springer-Verlag; 2008. p. 1–22 ISBN: 3540469087.
4. Rakowska A. Trichoscopy (hair and scalp videodermoscopy) in the healthy female. Method standardization and norms for measurable parameters. J Dermatol Case Rep 2009;3:14–9.
5. Inui S, Nakajima T, Itami S. Scalp dermoscopy of androgenetic alopecia in Asian people. J Dermatol 2009;36:82–5.
6. Van Neste D. Natural scalp hair regression in preclinical stages of male androgenetic alopecia and its reversal by finasteride. Skin Pharmacol Physiol 2006;19:168–76.
7. Slowinska M, Rudnicka L, Schwartz RA, et al. Comma hairs: a dermatoscopic marker for tinea capitis: a rapid diagnostic method. J Am Acad Dermatol 2008;59:S77–9.
8. Sandoval AB, Ortiz JA, Rodriguez JM, et al. Dermoscopic pattern in tinea capitis. Rev Iberoam Micol 2010;27:151–2 [in Spanish].
9. Hughes R, Chiaverini C, Bahadoran P, et al. Corkscrew hair: a new dermoscopic sign for diagnosis

of tinea capitis in black children. Arch Dermatol 2011;147:355–6.

10. Ross EK, Vincenzi C, Tosti A. Videodermoscopy in the evaluation of hair and scalp disorders. J Am Acad Dermatol 2006;55:799–806.

11. Inui S, Nakajima T, Nakagawa K, et al. Clinical significance of dermoscopy in alopecia areata: analysis of 300 cases. Int J Dermatol 2008;47:688–93.

12. Rudnicka L, Olszewska M, Rakowska A, et al. Trichoscopy: a new method for diagnosing hair loss. J Drugs Dermatol 2008;7:651–4.

13. Inui S. Trichoscopy for common hair loss diseases: algorithmic method for diagnosis. J Dermatol 2011; 38:71–5.

14. Lacarrubba F, Dall'Oglio F, Rita Nasca M, et al. Videodermatoscopy enhances diagnostic capability in some forms of hair loss. Am J Clin Dermatol 2004; 5:205–8.

15. Rakowska A, Slowinska M, Kowalska-Oledzka E, et al. Dermoscopy in female androgenic alopecia: method standardization and diagnostic criteria. Int J Trichology 2009;1:123–30.

16. Rakowska A, Slowinska M, Kowalska-Oledzka E, et al. Trichoscopy of cicatricial alopecia. J Drugs Dermatol 2012;11(6):753–8.

17. de Moura LH, Duque-Estrada B, Abraham LS, et al. Dermoscopy findings of alopecia areata in an African-American patient. J Dermatol Case Rep 2008;2:52–4.

18. Abraham LS, Pineiro-Maceira J, Duque-Estrada B, et al. Pinpoint white dots in the scalp: dermoscopic and histopathologic correlation. J Am Acad Dermatol 2010;63:721–2.

19. Tosti A, Torres F, Misciali C, et al. Follicular red dots: a novel dermoscopic pattern observed in scalp discoid lupus erythematosus. Arch Dermatol 2009; 145:1406–9.

20. de Lacharriere O, Deloche C, Misciali C, et al. Hair diameter diversity: a clinical sign reflecting the follicle miniaturization. Arch Dermatol 2001;137:641–6.

21. Olszewska M, Rudnicka L. Effective treatment of female androgenic alopecia with dutasteride. J Drugs Dermatol 2005;4:637–40.

22. Slowinska M. [The value of videodermoscopy in differential diagnosis of androgenetic alopecia. Doctoral thesis]. Medical University of Warsaw; 2010.

23. Karadag Kose O, Gulec AT. Clinical evaluation of alopecias using a handheld dermatoscope. J Am Acad Dermatol 2012;67(2):206–14.

24. Deloche C, de Lacharriere O, Misciali C, et al. Histological features of peripilar signs associated with androgenetic alopecia. Arch Dermatol Res 2004; 295:422–8.

25. Shapiro J. Dermatologic therapy: alopecia areata update. Dermatol Ther 2011;24:301.

26. Alkhalifah A, Alsantali A, Wang E, et al. Alopecia areata update: part I. Clinical picture, histopathology,

and pathogenesis. J Am Acad Dermatol 2010;62: 177–88 [quiz: 89–90].

27. Rakowska A, Olszewska M, Rudnicka L. Differential diagnosis of alopecia areata versus trichotilomania by trichoscopy. J Dermatol Case Rep, in press.

28. Mane M, Nath AK, Thappa DM. Utility of dermoscopy in alopecia areata. Indian J Dermatol 2011; 56:407–11.

29. Abraham LS, Torres FN, Azulay-Abulafia L. Dermoscopic clues to distinguish trichotillomania from patchy alopecia areata. An Bras Dermatol 2010;85: 723–6.

30. Gallouj S, Rabhi S, Baybay H, et al. Trichotemnomania associated to trichotillomania: a case report with emphasis on the diagnostic value of dermoscopy. Ann Dermatol Venereol 2011;138:140–1 [in French].

31. Lee DY, Lee JH, Yang JM, et al. The use of dermoscopy for the diagnosis of trichotillomania. J Eur Acad Dermatol Venereol 2009;23:731–2.

32. Ihm CW, Han JH. Diagnostic value of exclamation mark hairs. Dermatology 1993;186:99–102.

33. Sah DE, Koo J, Price VH. Trichotillomania. Dermatol Ther 2008;21:13–21.

34. Otberg N, Wu WY, McElwee KJ, et al. Diagnosis and management of primary cicatricial alopecia: part I. Skinmed 2008;7:19–26.

35. Wu WY, Otberg N, McElwee KJ, et al. Diagnosis and management of primary cicatricial alopecia: part II. Skinmed 2008;7:78–83.

36. Olsen E, Stenn K, Bergfeld W, et al. Update on cicatricial alopecia. J Investig Dermatol Symp Proc 2003;8:18–9.

37. Duque-Estrada B, Tamler C, Sodre CT, et al. Dermoscopy patterns of cicatricial alopecia resulting from discoid lupus erythematosus and lichen planopilaris. An Bras Dermatol 2010;85:179–83.

38. Assouly P, Reygagne P. Lichen planopilaris: update on diagnosis and treatment. Semin Cutan Med Surg 2009;28:3–10.

39. Kossard S, Zagarella S. Spotted cicatricial alopecia in dark skin. A dermoscopic clue to fibrous tracts. Australas J Dermatol 1993;34:49–51.

40. Inui S, Nakajima T, Shono F, et al. Dermoscopic findings in frontal fibrosing alopecia: report of four cases. Int J Dermatol 2008;47:796–9.

41. Rubegni P, Mandato F, Fimiani M. Frontal fibrosing alopecia: role of dermoscopy in differential diagnosis. Case Rep Dermatol 2010;2:40–5.

42. Otberg N, Kang H, Alzolibani AA, et al. Folliculitis decalvans. Dermatol Ther 2008;21:238–44.

43. Trueb RM. Systematic approach to hair loss in women. J Dtsch Dermatol Ges 2010;8:284–97, 98.

44. Baroni A, Romano F. Tufted hair folliculitis in a patient affected by pachydermoperiostosis: case report and videodermoscopic features. Skinmed 2011;9: 186–8.

45. Alzolibani AA, Kang H, Otberg N, et al. Pseudopelade of Brocq. Dermatol Ther 2008;21:257–63.

46. Olszewska M, Rudnicka L, Rakowska A, et al. Trichoscopy. Arch Dermatol 2008;144:1007.

47. Mirmirani P, Huang KP, Price VH. A practical, algorithmic approach to diagnosing hair shaft disorders. Int J Dermatol 2011;50:1–12.

48. Rakowska A, Slowinska M, Czuwara J, et al. Dermoscopy as a tool for rapid diagnosis of monilethrix. J Drugs Dermatol 2007;6:222–4.

49. Liu CI, Hsu CH. Rapid diagnosis of monilethrix using dermoscopy. Br J Dermatol 2008;159:741–3.

50. Jain N, Khopkar U. Monilethrix in pattern distribution in siblings: diagnosis by trichoscopy. Int J Trichology 2010;2:56–9.

51. Rakowska A, Slowinska M, Kowalska-Oledzka E, et al. Trichoscopy in genetic hair shaft abnormalities. J Dermatol Case Rep 2008;2:14–20.

52. Wallace MP, de Berker DA. Hair diagnoses and signs: the use of dermatoscopy. Clin Exp Dermatol 2010;35:41–6.

53. Rakowska A, Kowalska-Oledzka E, Slowinska M, et al. Hair shaft videodermoscopy in netherton syndrome. Pediatr Dermatol 2009;26:320–2.

54. Burk C, Hu S, Lee C, et al. Netherton syndrome and trichorrhexis invaginata—a novel diagnostic approach. Pediatr Dermatol 2008;25:287–8.

55. Silverberg NB, Silverberg JI, Wong ML. Trichoscopy using a handheld dermoscope: an in-office technique to diagnose genetic disease of the hair. Arch Dermatol 2009;145:600–1.

56. Kim GW, Jung HJ, Ko HC, et al. Dermoscopy can be useful in differentiating scalp psoriasis from seborrhoeic dermatitis. Br J Dermatol 2011;164:652–6.

57. Tay LK, Lim FL, Ng HJ, et al. Cutaneous follicular hyperkeratotic spicules–the first clinical sign of multiple myeloma progression or relapse. Int J Dermatol 2010;49:934–6.

58. LeBoit PE. Alopecia mucinosa, inflammatory disease or mycosis fungoides: must we choose? And are there other choices? Am J Dermatopathol 2004;26:167–70.

Histopathology of Scarring and Nonscarring Hair Loss

John M. Childs, MD[a],*, Leonard C. Sperling, MD[b]

KEYWORDS

- Biopsy technique • Hair anatomy • Cicatricial alopecia • Non-cicatricial alopecia

KEY POINTS

Biopsy Technique

- Proper biopsy technique is essential for maximizing diagnostic yield and accuracy.
- 4 mm punch biopsies should be sectioned transversely to allow for the examination of all hairs in the specimen at various levels.

Hair anatomy

- Understanding normal hair anatomy and physiology is essential to discussing to the histopathology of alopecia.

Cicatricial alopecia

- Cicatricial alopecia can be defined as processes in which the follicular epithelium is replaced by connective tissue.
- Primary cicatricial alopecias share follicular destruction and scarring as a primary event in their pathogenesis.

Non-cicatricial alopecia

- Non-cicatricial alopecia does not include follicular destruction and scarring as a primary event.
- After many years of disease, however, permanent drop-out of follicles may occur.

INTRODUCTION

This review of the histologic findings of alopecia is preceded by a brief discussion of biopsy and processing techniques, the normal follicular anatomy and cycle, and expected findings in transverse sections. Subtle histologic abnormalities will be missed unless the normal follicular anatomy and follicular cycle, when viewed in transverse sections, are understood.

Disclosure: The views expressed in this article are those of the authors and do not necessarily reflect the official policy or position of the Department of the Navy, Army, Department of Defense, nor the US Government. We certify that all individuals who qualify as authors have been listed; each has participated in the conception and design of this work, the analysis of data, the writing of the document, and the approval of the submission of this version; that the document represents valid work; that if we used information derived from another source, we obtained all necessary approvals to use it and made appropriate acknowledgments in the document; and that each takes public responsibility for it. Nothing in the presentation implies any Federal/DOD/DON endorsement.

[a] Department of Pathology, Walter Reed National Military Medical Center, 8901 Wisconsin Avenue, Bethesda, MD 20889, USA; [b] Department of Dermatology, Uniformed Services University of the Health Sciences, 4301 Jones Bridge Road, Bethesda, MD 20814, USA
* Corresponding author.
E-mail address: john.childs2@med.navy.mil

Dermatol Clin 31 (2013) 43–56
http://dx.doi.org/10.1016/j.det.2012.08.001
0733-8635/13/$ – see front matter Published by Elsevier Inc.

BIOPSY AND PROCESSING TECHNIQUE

Proper biopsy technique is essential in maximizing diagnostic yield and accuracy. The ideal specimen should include a 4-mm punch biopsy of scalp, including subcutaneous fat and the deep-rooted terminal hair bulbs, from an involved area of alopecia. While a biopsy from the center of a lesion of alopecia areata or trichotillomania would be appropriate, biopsies from the center of a lesion of scarring alopecia are rarely helpful. In cicatricial alopecia, a biopsy of an involved margin is preferred. Biopsies from heavily inflamed or pustular lesions are likely to be nondiagnostic. When possible, a normal control biopsy should also be obtained for comparison; the occiput is the typical site for this. Despite excellent biopsy technique, sampling error occasionally results in nondiagnostic biopsies, and additional biopsies may be required to arrive at a specific diagnosis.

Once the plugs are removed, the specimens should be fixed in 10% neutral buffered formalin for at least 24 hours to ensure ideal fixation. Tissue for direct immunofluorescence microscopy should be submitted in appropriate transport media, such as Michel fixative. The specimens should then be sectioned transversely. This method allows for the examination of all hairs in a biopsy specimen at various levels, providing both qualitative and quantitative information. Transverse sections are currently the recommended technique of a working group of alopecia experts.[1] The authors' preferred sectioning technique involves dividing the specimen into 1-mm slices, inking the deep surfaces, and embedding the inked surfaces down. Once the ink is removed by the microtome, a single section including all slices is prepared. In this way, one section allows for viewing of multiple levels, and the remainder of the tissue is available for addition sections or special studies.[2] Other suitable techniques have also been described but are not discussed further here.[3,4]

Because some of the following disorders exhibit overlapping histologic features, careful clinical correlation is essential. Accordingly a thorough clinical history, including clinical photographs, should be submitted to the pathologist for a more complete and accurate diagnosis.

THE NORMAL SCALP

Pathologic processes are defined by a divergence from the normal state. Therefore, any discussion of the histology of alopecia must first include a description of the expected normal physiologic cycle and microanatomy of the follicle. The different sizes of hairs are terminal, indeterminate,

and vellus. Terminal hairs are large hairs with a diameter of greater than 0.06 mm and the hair bulb rooted deeply in the subcutaneous fat. Vellus hairs are smaller with a diameter of less than 0.03 mm, tend to be hypopigmented, and are rooted more superficially in the dermis. Vellus hairs can be readily identified because the diameter of the hair shaft will be less than the thickness of the inner root sheath. Indeterminate hairs are between 0.03 and 0.06 mm in diameter.

The phases of the hair cycle are anagen, catagen, and telogen. Anagen phase is the active growing phase of the hair and lasts between 2 and 7 years. Catagen phase is a brief transitional phase between anagen and telogen lasting only a few weeks. Telogen phase lasts approximately 100 days and is the phase during which the hair is shed. Although there is individual variation, at any given time 85% to 100% of terminal scalp hair is in the anagen phase, 0% to 15% is in the telogen phase, and only about 1% is in the catagen phase (**Fig. 1**).[5]

Anagen, catagen, and telogen hairs differ in their appearance at the different levels of the follicle, namely the hair bulb, the suprabulbar zone, the isthmus, and the infundibulum. Familiarity of these morphologies is important, especially when interpreting transverse sections. Terminal hairs and

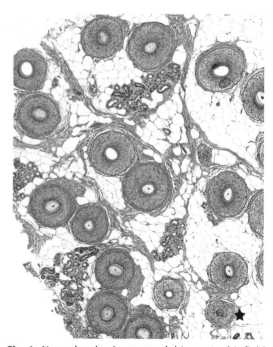

Fig. 1. Normal scalp, 4-mm punch biopsy. In this field, almost all follicles are uniformly-sized terminal anagen hairs. A single catagen/telogen follicle (*star*) puts the telogen count at 5% of the follicles shown (Original magnification ×40).

vellus hairs progress through all phases, although vellus hairs spend significantly less time in the anagen phase.

Anagen Hair Anatomy

The terminal hair bulb is usually located in the fat, and is composed of the germinative layer (hair matrix) and the hair papilla (mesenchymal structure derived from the dermis). The stalk of the papilla merges with the fibrous root sheath, which surrounds the entire follicle.

Superficial to the hair bulb is the suprabulbar zone. In this zone, the various layers begin to differentiate. Starting from the center of the follicle, the layers are: (1) the hair shaft medulla, (2) the hair shaft cortex, (3) the cuticular layer, (4) Huxley's layer of the inner root sheath, (5) Henley's layer of the inner root sheath, (6) the outer root sheath, (7) the glassy layer (vitreous layer), and (8) the fibrous root sheath. The cuticular layer comprises interlocking flattened cells of the hair-shaft cuticle and the inner root-sheath cuticle, and appears as a single anatomic layer.

Superior to the suprabulbar zone is the isthmus. The isthmus of the follicle is defined inferiorly by the insertion of the arrector pili muscle and superiorly by the insertion of the sebaceous duct. The bulge zone is located at the insertion of the arrector pili, and is the zone in which follicular stem cells reside. The "bulge" is anatomically inapparent in humans, and requires an immunohistochemical stain for cytokeratin-15 to clearly identify. The isthmus is an important zone for follicular keratinization: in the mid portion the inner root sheath desquamates, resulting in a separation between the hair shaft and the follicular wall. The cells of the outer root sheath then begin to cornify without formation of a granular cell layer (trichilemmal keratinization).

The most superficial portion of the follicle, the infundibulum, is defined inferiorly by the opening of the sebaceous duct and is superficially contiguous with the epidermal surface. Keratinization within the infundibulum forms with the presence of a granular cell layer.

Racial groups differ in the size and shapes of the hair shafts. Caucasian and Asian hairs tend to be round or slightly oval and centered within the follicle. African American hairs tend to be elliptical or reniform and are often eccentrically located within the follicle.

Catagen Hair Anatomy

Within a week of entering the catagen phase, the hair matrix disappears and is replaced by a thin rim of epithelial cells demonstrating nuclear pyknosis. The epithelium of the lower follicle also degenerates via apoptosis, and the vitreous layer becomes thickened and more prominent. The fibrous root sheath also thickens. As time passes, the hair papilla migrates upward following the disintegrating epithelial column, and comes to rest just below the bulge zone. As the disintegrating column of epithelial cells moves superficially, a collapsed fibrous root sheath is left behind (known as a stela or streamer). Immediately above the epithelial column, an expanded mass of epithelium forms the hair club as the cells begin to cornify from the center outward.

Telogen Hair Anatomy

At the beginning of telogen, the hair papilla is a condensed ball of spindle-shaped nuclei with a scant stroma. The papilla lies just deep to a nipple of epithelium called the secondary hair germ, which has an asterisk-like appearance in cross section. The secondary hair germ lies below the bulge zone, in close proximity to the follicular stem cells. Just superficial to this, the telogen club continues to cornify and expands to the full width of the follicle. After approximately 3 months, the clubbed hair is shed. Around the time of shedding, the transition back to the anagen phase begins. The new hair extends downward from the bulge zone and enters the anagen phase as previously described.

EXPECTED FINDINGS IN TRANSVERSE SECTIONS

In Caucasians (in a standard 4-mm punch biopsy), there should be approximately 25 to 30 terminal hairs when viewed at the level of the deep dermis (see **Fig. 1**). If counts are performed more superficially, the count will increase (on average by 5) owing to the presence of vellus hairs. Of the terminal hairs, an average of 6% will be in catagen/telogen phase. Individual variability results in a range of 0% to 15% telogen hairs. African Americans have fewer but larger follicles (21 total; 18 terminal and 3 vellus), with a telogen count of 6%. In Koreans, the average number of follicles is 16 (15 terminal and 1 vellus follicle) with a telogen count of 7%.[6,7]

Within the deep dermis and subcutaneous tissue, where the bulbar and suprabulbar portion of the follicles reside, the follicles are arranged individually (see **Fig. 1**). Within the mid dermis and superficial dermis, the hairs are arranged as follicular units with 2 to 5 hairs per unit. A 4-mm punch biopsy contains approximately 12 follicular units.

The terminal/vellus (T/V) ratio in the normal scalp should be at least 2:1, with most normal subjects having a ratio of greater than 4:1.[6] This number is variable among investigators, and likely differs because of the methodology used in classifying indeterminate (medium-sized) hairs.

CICATRICIAL ALOPECIA
Central Centrifugal Cicatricial Alopecia

The dominant and most important histologic finding in central centrifugal cicatricial alopecia (CCCA) is premature desquamation of the inner root sheath (PDIRS). While all affected follicles demonstrate this feature, PDIRS is not specific for CCCA when follicles are badly inflamed. The following histologic features are common in CCCA, but are nonspecific and can be seen in other cicatricial alopecias (**Fig. 2**): eccentric

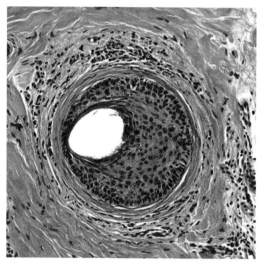

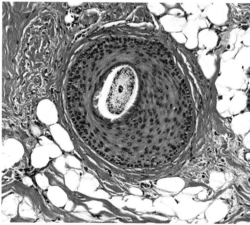

Fig. 2. Central, centrifugal cicatricial alopecia. These images depict a typical, "early" involved follicle. A section through the suprabulbar zone (*lower panel*) shows premature desquamation of the inner root sheath. A section through the isthmus (*upper panel*) shows eccentric epithelial thinning, concentric lamellar fibroplasias, and perifollicular chronic inflammation (Original magnification ×400).

epithelial atrophy with hair shafts in close proximity to the dermis; loss of sebaceous glands; concentric lamellar fibroplasia; and variably dense perifollicular inflammation, particularly at the level of the upper isthmus and infundibulum. Late changes include: follicular destruction with "naked" hair shafts in the dermis and an associated granulomatous inflammatory infiltrate; follicular scarring; and polytrichia (tufting).[8,9]

Essential to the pathogenesis and diagnosis of CCCA is PDIRS. It is thought that the inner root sheath serves as a physiologic barrier to external agents (bacteria, chemicals, and so forth), and when lost as in CCCA, the follicle is more prone to injury. PDIRS can be seen in noninflamed follicles, and may only be evident in a minority of follicles, justifying the need for the transverse sectioning method. The other findings commonly seen in CCCA are nonspecific, and are listed above.[9,10] It is worth noting that the inflammatory component in CCCA is variable. Highly inflammatory cases with pustule formation are synonymous with folliculitis decalvans. Similarly, most cases of "tufted alopecia" probably represent "burnt-out" CCCA.

The differential diagnosis includes acne keloidalis and lichen planopilaris (LPP). Because acne keloidalis can have similar histologic findings, the distinction is primarily clinical. LPP shares the peri-infundibular inflammation, perifollicular fibrosis, and follicular destruction with naked hair shafts. Interface alteration is not seen in CCCA, and when present favors a diagnosis of LPP. Other clues include the clefting between the follicular epithelium and the stroma in lichen planopilaris, and eccentric follicular atrophy in CCCA. LPP can have PDIRS, but this tends to be seen only in badly inflamed follicles.

Lichen Planopilaris

The dominant histologic finding in LPP is lichenoid interface dermatitis involving the infundibulum and superficial isthmus. One can also find (**Fig. 3**): concentric lamellar fibroplasia with clefting between the involved follicle and the dermis; an hourglass-shaped follicular silhouette when viewed with vertical sectioning; and PDIRS in involved follicles.[8]

These findings may involve a minority of follicles within the biopsy specimen, necessitating transverse sections to ensure evaluation of all follicular units.[11,12] The inflammation spares the lower third of the follicle; however, the interfollicular epithelium may be involved (25% of cases) and shows features typical of lichen planus. As in lichen planus, the interfollicular epithelium (when involved) exhibits acanthosis, hypergranulosis, hyperkeratosis, and sometimes clefting between the epithelium and

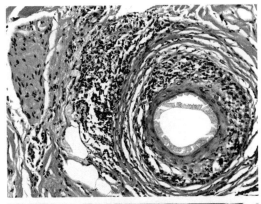

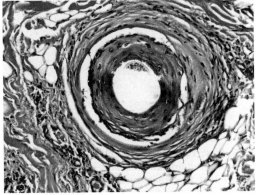

Fig. 3. Lichen planopilaris. Two different follicles are shown. In the lower panel, there is destruction of the basilar layer with artifactual epithelial/stromal clefting. In the upper panel, there is vacuolar interface alteration with perifollicular and intrafollicular lymphocytic inflammation (Original magnification ×400).

stroma.[13] The sebaceous lobules are lost, and eventually so is the entire folliculosebaceous unit. Naked hair shafts with associated granulomatous inflammation may be found within the dermis. The follicular scar is characteristically wedge shaped and devoid of elastin fibers (accentuated with elastin stains).[14]

The differential diagnosis includes CCCA, frontal fibrosing alopecia, fibrosing alopecia in a patterned distribution, and chronic cutaneous (discoid) lupus erythematosus. CCCA and LPP share PDIRS; however, noninflamed follicles exhibit PDIRS in CCCA, and some inflamed follicles in LPP have normal inner root sheaths. By contrast, CCCA can be excluded if inflamed follicles do not show PDIRS. In frontal fibrosing alopecia, the inflammation tends to be less dense with more apoptotic cells, and the interfollicular changes sometimes seen in LPP are absent. Fibrosing alopecia in a patterned distribution may have identical histologic findings, but tends to have a decreased T/V ratio, unlike LPP. Discoid lupus exhibits increased dermal mucin, perieccrine inflammation, and

interfollicular changes (vacuolar interface alteration, epidermal atrophy, and follicular plugging), none of which are seen in LPP. Direct immunofluorescence studies are also characteristic (linear junctional immunoglobulin (Ig)G, IgM, and C3 in lupus; colloid bodies highlighted with IgM in LPP).

Chronic Cutaneous (Discoid) Lupus Erythematosus

The dominant histologic finding in chronic cutaneous lupus erythematosus (CCLE) is vacuolar interface alteration of the follicular (infundibulum > isthmus) and interfollicular epithelium with epidermal atrophy. Also seen are (**Fig. 4**): thickening of the basement membrane; follicular plugging; a superficial and deep perivascular and perieccrine lymphoplasmacytic infiltrate; deep dermal mucin; and loss of sebaceous lobules.[8,13]

In CCLE, the follicular damage and destruction, like all causes of cicatricial alopecia, are due to

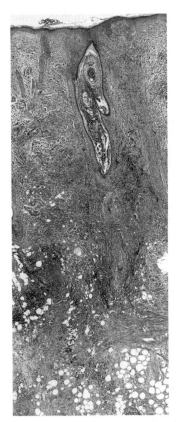

Fig. 4. Discoid lupus erythematosus (DLE). In this particularly well-developed lesion of DLE, there is epidermal thinning, infundibular distention, vacuolar interface alteration of the follicular epithelium, foci of dense and deep chronic inflammation, increased dermal mucin, and hyalinization of the superficial fat. The majority of DLE lesions will have some, but not all, of these features (Original magnification ×20).

inflammation at the level of the infundibulum and isthmus, resulting in permanent damage to the bulge zone follicular stem cells.[15] In biopsies from end-stage areas, the findings are similar to burnt-out scarring alopecia of any etiology. Direct immunofluorescence studies may be beneficial in this situation, as lesions of CCLE are more likely to be positive in long-standing lesions.[16]

Histologically, the major source of confusion is with LPP. Unlike lesions of CCLE that show epidermal atrophy, lesions of LPP shows epidermal acanthosis, hypergranulosis, and hyperkeratosis. CCLE also exhibits deep dermal mucin and a deep perivascular and perieccrine lymphoplasmacytic infiltrate. Direct immunofluorescence studies may also afford distinction (linear junctional IgG, IgM, and C3 in CCLE; colloid bodies highlighted with IgM in LPP).

Folliculitis Keloidalis (Acne Keloidalis)

The dominant histologic findings are perifollicular lymphoplasmacytic inflammation (peri-infundibular and peri-isthmic) and perifollicular lamellar fibroplasia (particularly peri-isthmic). One also sees disappearance of sebaceous glands in involved follicles; thinning of the follicular epithelium; PDIRS; follicular destruction with resulting naked hair shafts in the dermis; and follicular scarring.[8] Early biopsies, taken at the papular stage of the disease, show a lymphocytic folliculitis.[17,18] In addition, biopsies from clinically noninvolved areas may show follicular scarring, indicating subclinical disease.[17]

Because folliculitis keloidalis is a primary cicatricial alopecia, the findings listed in this summary are shared by other cicatricial alopecias. The follicular destruction and subsequent extrusion of naked hair shafts into the dermis leads to the hypertrophic scarring that may be found in later stages of the disease. Although these hair shafts may serve as a nidus for bacterial infection, few organisms are identified using special stains, indicating that bacterial overgrowth is not important in the pathogenesis.[17]

The differential diagnosis primarily includes CCCA and folliculitis decalvans. These conditions may be indistinguishable histologically and may represent different manifestations of related pathologic processes; hence, the distinction primarily depends on clinical correlation.

Dissecting Cellulitis

The dominant histologic findings in a well-developed lesion are (Fig. 5): deep perifollicular and lower dermal abscesses composed of lymphocytes, neutrophils, and plasma cells; increase in catagen/telogen hairs; intact sebaceous glands

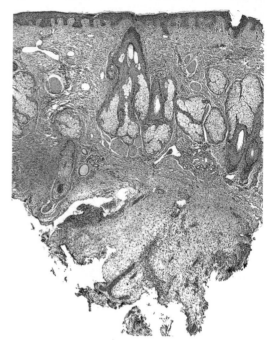

Fig. 5. Dissecting cellulitis of the scalp. An early lesion will show predominantly chronic inflammation below the level of the follicular bulbs, with an increased number of catagen/telogen hairs. Sebaceous glands and follicles are not destroyed until later in the course of the disease (Original magnification ×40).

(early disease); and eventually granulation tissue with squamous-lined true sinus tracts. Biopsies from early lesions show a deep perifollicular and subfollicular lymphocytic infiltrate.[8]

In early stages of the disease, the deep perifollicular and subfollicular inflammation does not primarily destroy follicles. Rather, the deep inflammation incites a conversion of terminal hairs from anagen to catagen/telogen, with subsequent shedding of hair. Thus, the hair loss in the early phase of the disease is temporary. The depth of the inflammation is also responsible for the preservation of sebaceous glands in early lesions. With time, the inflammation involves the entire dermis, and true follicular destruction ensues. At this stage, exuberant granulation tissue and squamous-lined sinus tracts may form.

The clinical and histologic findings are fairly characteristic; however, tinea capitis can occasionally mimic dissecting cellulitis. Histochemical stains for fungal organisms (Grocott methenamine-silver [GMS], periodic acid-Schiff [PAS]) combined with microbiological cultures allow for distinction. It is worth noting that histochemical stains are not 100% sensitive, and correlation with culture results is essential.[19]

Frontal Fibrosing Alopecia

The histologic findings are essentially identical to LPP and include: lichenoid inflammation involving the infundibulum and isthmus; apoptotic keratinocytes within the affected follicular epithelium; blurring of the epithelial-stromal junction; squamatization of the outer root sheath; and perifollicular concentric fibroplasia with clefting between the epithelium and the stroma.[8]

The histologic similarities between frontal fibrosing alopecia (FFA) and LPP are not surprising, because FFA may be a variant of LPP.[20,21] Although FFA and LPP cannot be reliably distinguished on histologic grounds, FFA tends to have less follicular inflammation, more necrotic keratinocytes, and characteristically spares the interfollicular epithelium.[22]

The differential diagnosis includes: LPP, fibrosing alopecia in a patterned distribution (FAPD), and discoid lupus erythematosus (DLE). The distinction between FFA and LPP is primarily clinical. FAPD shares the findings of FFA but also shows an increased T/V hair ratio. Unlike FFA, DLE shows superficial and deep perivascular and periadnexal inflammation (particularly perieccrine), increased dermal mucin, and (when present) characteristic epidermal changes including vacuolar interface alteration, epidermal atrophy, and follicular plugging.

Fibrosing Alopecia in a Patterned Distribution

The dominant histologic findings in FAPD are: increased numbers of vellus hairs; variably sized follicles; perifollicular lymphocytic inflammation of variable density; perifollicular fibroplasia; follicular destruction of both terminal and vellus hairs; and sparing of the interfollicular epitheium.[8] It is uncertain whether FAPD represents a unique clinicopathologic entity, or is just a variant of LPP superimposed on androgenetic alopecia.[23] Accordingly, the histologic findings show changes typical of androgenetic alopecia (variability in hair size with miniaturization) as well as changes indistinguishable from LPP. The inflammation tends to be limited to the upper half of the follicle, and seems to involve both terminal and vellus hairs; this differs slightly from LPP whereby terminal hairs are preferentially affected. The interfollicular epithelium is spared.

The differential diagnosis includes androgenetic alopecia, LPP, and DLE. Pure androgenetic alopecia does not exhibit scarring, follicular destruction, interface alteration, or significant inflammation. LPP has a similar inflammatory component, but differs in that few vellus hairs are affected. DLE shares the perifollicular inflammation but also shows deep inflammation often involving eccrine glands, occasional plasma cells, increased dermal mucin, and epidermal changes (vacuolar interface alteration and atrophy).

Tinea Capitis

The most important histologic finding in tinea capitis is the presence of fungal hyphae or spores surrounding or invading hair shafts. The amount of perifollicular inflammation is variable and may be composed of lymphocytes, neutrophils, and eosinophils.[8] Both endothrix (eg, *Trichophyton tonsurans*) and ectothrix (eg, *Microsporum canis*) infections result in mixed inflammation of variable intensity and distribution throughout the follicle. Lesions may appear relatively noninflammatory or may present as large crusted and purulent plaques (kerions). Regardless, diagnosis rests on the identification of the fungal organisms by special stains or culture.

When organisms are identified, the diagnosis is certain. However, in cases where organisms are not readily apparent, tinea capitis can mimic other cicatricial alopecias including dissecting cellulitis. Because a minority of follicles may be involved, transverse sections are recommended to increase diagnostic yield. Furthermore, cultures are essential because organisms may not be apparent histologically, particularly when inflammation is intense. The index of suspicion should be especially high when children or adolescents are involved, and microbiologic cultures should be performed in suspected cases.

NONCICATRICIAL, NONINFLAMMATORY FORMS OF ALOPECIA
Androgenetic Alopecia

The dominant histologic feature is marked variability in hair diameter with many miniaturized hairs (Fig. 6). There is a normal total number of hairs and an absence of significant inflammation, particularly deep or peribulbar inflammation.[8]

Androgenetic alopecia is characterized by a gradual reduction in the length of the anagen phase with subsequent miniaturization after successive cycles.[24,25] Biopsies from affected areas (vertex, crown, and frontal) show a normal number of follicles when counted at the superficial dermis with scattered vellus hairs. The T/V ratio is typically decreased to less than 2:1, although in some patients even 3:1 or 4:1 might be abnormal and correlation with a normal control biopsy (see Fig. 6) is required. Because each follicle cycles independently, the miniaturized hairs will be randomly scattered among normal follicles. Because of the increased proportion of vellus

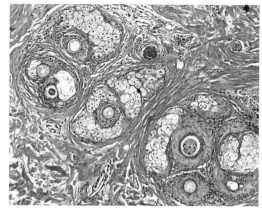

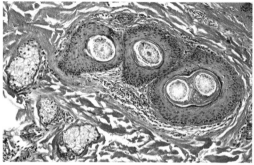

Fig. 6. Androgenetic alopecia (*top panel*) is characterized by the variably of shaft diameters, indicating hair miniaturization, which is clearly evident when compared with normal occipital scalp (*bottom panel*) from the same patient (Original magnification ×100).

follicles, deeper follicular counts at the dermal-fat junction are decreased and fibrous streamers (or stelae) are present.[26] These fibrous streamers are anatomically situated below the miniaturized hairs. Genetic and hormonal factors cause androgenetic alopecia, deep inflammation is absent, and sebaceous glands remain intact. It is noteworthy that mild chronic inflammation within the superficial dermis is nonspecific and is frequently encountered even in normal biopsies, particularly in African American women.[5,6] The telogen count may be slightly increased (15%–20%). The gradual but progressive course of the disease allows for increased sun exposure with solar elastosis seen in established cases.

Other entities in the differential diagnosis include alopecia areata and chronic telogen effluvium. In alopecia areata, the telogen count is typically much higher (>50%) with frequent "nanogen" hairs. A characteristic peribulbar lymphocytic inflammation is also usually present. Telogen effluvium also shows a normal number of total hairs and an increased telogen count (although typically a higher percentage), but can be distinguished by the lack of miniaturization. Evaluation of a clinically

normal occipital biopsy can aid in determining the presence of a concurrent telogen effluvium.

Telogen Effluvium

The dominant histologic finding is an increase in the percentage of terminal catagen/telogen hairs (typically fewer than 50%; **Fig. 7**). One also sees a normal total number of hairs; normal follicular size; a preserved T/V ratio; fibrous streamers below telogen hairs; and importantly, the absence of significant inflammation or miniaturization.[8]

In a pure telogen effluvium, the only abnormality is an increase in the percentage of terminal telogen hairs (typically 20%–50%); however, depending on any given patient's normal telogen percentage, a percentage of telogen hairs less than 20% may still be abnormal.[5] Although the total number of hairs is normal when viewed at the level of the mid dermis, when transverse sections are viewed at the level of the subcutis, the number of terminal hairs will appear to be reduced owing to the presence of fibrous streamers replacing the lower segments of the telogen hairs. Miniaturization does not occur in telogen effluvium, so the T/V ratio is preserved. No significant inflammation is identified.

The differential diagnosis includes other disorders with an increase in the percentage of catagen/telogen hairs, including: acute traction alopecia and trichotillomania, androgenetic alopecia, and alopecia areata incognita. Unlike acute traction alopecia and trichotillomania, telogen effluvium should not exhibit pigment casts or disrupted follicular anatomy. Miniaturization is typical

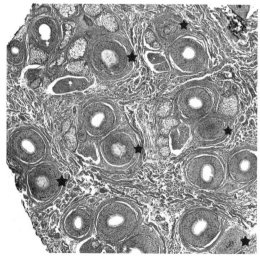

Fig. 7. Telogen effluvium. Almost all follicles are uniformly sized terminal hairs, but 33% of all follicles seen in this field are in the catagen/telogen phase (*stars*) (Original magnification ×40).

in androgenetic alopecia but is characteristically absent in telogen effluvium, unless the patient has both conditions. Alopecia areata usually has an even higher percentage of catagen/telogen hairs (>50%), and exhibits prominent miniaturization as well as focal peribulbar lymphocytic inflammation.

Trichotillomania

The dominant histologic finding is distorted follicular anatomy.[5] There is often a slight increase in catagen/telogen hairs; lack of peribulbar lymphocytic inflammation; pigment casts; trichomalacia; melanin pigment in collapsed fibrous root sheaths; fractured hair shafts; and intrafollicular and perifollicular hemorrhage[8] (**Fig. 8**).

The most distinctive finding, seen in up to 50% of transversely sectioned biopsies, is distorted follicular anatomy admixed with anatomically normal hairs.[5] The inner root sheath may be collapsed, indicating extraction before tissue processing. Pigment casts, consisting of partially extracted cortex material and fragments of pigmented hair matrix, may be seen in dilated follicular lumens. Distorted or extracted hair bulbs are diagnostic of trichotillomania, but are only seen in 20% of cases.[27,28] It is worth noting that absent hair shafts without distortion of the inner root sheath can be an artifact of processing and should not be confused with the aforementioned findings. The traumatic hair removal of trichotillomania also leads to an alteration of hair cycling with a variable increase in the catagen/telogen percentage.

The differential diagnosis includes acute traction alopecia, alopecia areata, and telogen effluvium. While the histologic changes may be similar in acute traction alopecia, the clinical presentation is usually distinctive. Alopecia areata shares the increased catagen/telogen counts, but the percentage is usually higher in alopecia areata (>50%). In alopecia areata the follicular distortion is absent and the characteristic peribulbar inflammation is present. Telogen effluvium lacks the distorted follicular anatomy of trichotillomania.

Traction Alopecia

The histologic findings in acute traction alopecia and long-standing traction alopecia differ significantly. In acute traction alopecia, the dominant findings are similar to mild trichotillomania and include: normal numbers and size of hairs; increased catagen/telogen hairs; absence of significant inflammation; and occasional pigment casts with rarely distorted follicular anatomy. In long-standing traction alopecia, the dominant finding is a reduction in the number of terminal hairs with retention of vellus hairs and intact sebaceous glands. One also sees an absence of significant inflammation, and occasional fibrous tracts at sites of former follicles.[8]

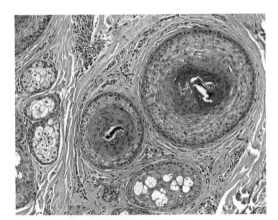

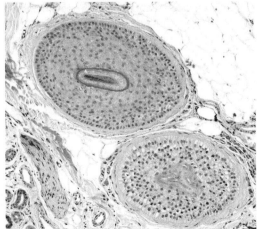

Fig. 8. Trichotillomania. Distorted, incomplete follicles lacking shafts (*bottom panel*, original magnification ×200) are diagnostic of mechanical alopecia from plucking. Pigment casts and trichomalacia (*upper panel*, original magnification ×400) are additional clues.

Given the histologic overlap with trichotillomania, acute traction alopecia is not discussed further here. End-stage, chronic or burnt-out traction alopecia is the most commonly biopsied form of disease. At this stage, there is a marked reduction in the number of terminal hairs. In many cases, distinct columns of connective tissue replace some follicles, leaving "blank spaces" devoid of follicles. In other cases, the hairs seem to simply disappear with retention of otherwise normal-appearing dermal collagen. The most striking feature is the retention of sebaceous lobules despite the marked loss of terminal follicles (**Fig. 9**).

The differential diagnosis of chronic traction alopecia includes temporal triangular alopecia

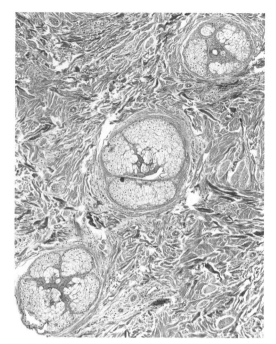

Fig. 9. Traction alopecia (end-stage). The three follicular units shown have intact sebaceous glands but no terminal hairs. A single vellus hair is present in one unit (*upper right*) (Original magnification ×100).

and androgenetic alopecia. Clinical information can usually differentiate chronic traction alopecia and temporal triangular alopecia. Androgenetic alopecia shows a normal number of follicles and hair miniaturization.

Temporal Triangular Alopecia

The dominant histologic findings in temporal triangular alopecia are a normal total number of hairs, with a predominance of vellus hairs and only rare terminal hairs. One also sees an absence of significant inflammation and an absence of fibrous streamers.[8]

Because of the striking number of vellus hairs without associated fibrous streamers, the vellus hairs in temporal triangular alopecia are thought to be primary vellus hairs, in accord with the congenital presentation of the disease. Even in the reported noncongenital cases, fibrous streamers are absent below the vellus hairs. To confirm that the total number of hairs is normal the transverse sectioning method is required, and most vellus hairs can be found at the level of the superficial dermis. All other adnexal structures and the surrounding stroma appear normal.

The differential diagnosis includes end-stage traction alopecia and androgenetic alopecia. In both end-stage traction alopecia and temporal triangular alopecia, there is a predominance of vellus hairs with intact sebaceous lobules. However, the presence of fibrous tracts below the vellus hairs favors traction alopecia. Androgenetic alopecia shows miniaturization with an admixture of small, medium, and large hairs as well as underlying stelae.

Postoperative, Pressure-Induced Alopecia

The dominant histologic findings, best appreciated within the first 2 to 3 weeks of onset, are: a normal number of follicles; nearly all hairs in the catagen/telogen phase; trichomalacia; melanin in collapsed outer root sheath; vascular thrombosis with necrosis; subcutaneous fat necrosis; and secondary infiltration with macrophages and lymphocytic inflammation. Biopsies of "late" cases show end-stage cicatricial alopecia.[8]

Secondary to the precipitating event (usually pressure from the surgical table), the primary pathologic process involves vascular thrombosis, subcutaneous necrosis, and reactive inflammation. With respect to the follicles, the most obvious abnormality is the striking synchronous shift to catagen/telogen phase of nearly all the follicles. Trichomalacia may be present, as well as pigment in collapsed root sheaths; however, incomplete or distorted follicular anatomy is not seen. The inflammation appears mild with respect to the degree of tissue necrosis, and includes macrophages and lymphocytes within the subcutaneous fat and dermis. The inflammation is not centered on the follicle, and is usually present in association with areas of tissue necrosis.

The differential diagnosis includes trichotillomania, which does have overlapping histologic features. Although trichomalacia is seen in postoperative, pressure-induced alopecia, distorted follicular anatomy is not observed. The striking synchronizing shift to catagen/telogen and deep dermal and subcutaneous inflammation and necrosis are not typical of trichotillomania. Biopsies from long-standing cases with alopecia show end-stage cicatricial alopecia. Of course, clinical correlation is essential.

NONCICATRICIAL, INFLAMMATORY FORMS OF ALOPECIA
Alopecia Areata

The dominant histologic findings in acute and subacute alopecia areata are (**Figs. 10** and **11**): a normal total number of hairs; increased number of miniaturized hairs; increased numbers of terminal catagen and telogen hairs (may exceed 50% in subacute cases); and peribulbar mononuclear cell infiltrate with occasional exocytosis into the bulbar epithelium. Focal trichomalacia may

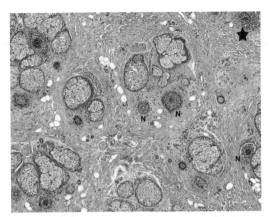

Fig. 10. Alopecia areata. In a well-established lesion, most or all follicles have miniaturized and a high percentage are in the catagen/telogen phase. In this field, several miniaturized hairs producing little or no shaft (nanogen hairs; N) are seen, as well as an inflamed nanogen hair (*star*) (Original magnification ×40).

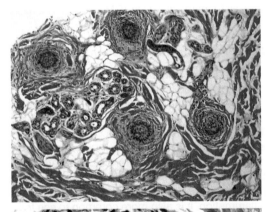

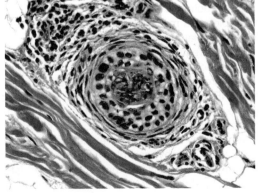

Fig. 11. Alopecia areata. (*Lower panel*, original magnification ×100) High-power view of a miniaturized (nanogen) and inflamed follicle, sectioned just above the bulb. This follicle is not producing any shaft. The central core consists of dystrophic inner root sheath. (*Upper panel*, original magnification ×400) All follicles have been converted to the catagen/telogen phase.

also be present. In chronic disease, the findings also include a marked increased in catagen and telogen hairs (approaching 100%); numerous nanogen hairs (miniaturized hairs with aberrant morphologies); and occasionally a lack of peribulbar inflammation if telogen hairs predominate.[8]

At the onset of disease, there is a peribulbar mononuclear inflammatory cell infiltrate that may invade the peribulbar epithelium and result in a disorganized appearance to the hair matrix, necrosis of matrical cells, and vacuole formation above the upper pole of the dermal papilla.[5,29] Amorphous pigment may be seen in the follicular epithelium. Within weeks, the involved follicles either enter the catagen or telogen phase, or miniaturize. By the second or third month, the number of catagen/telogen hairs is greatly increased (often more than 50% of follicles) and the T/V ratio begins to decrease, indicating miniaturization. Stelae or fibrous streamers are present below these miniaturized hairs. Inflammation tends to subside as hairs enter the catagen phase, and as a result inflammation is typically absent around catagen/telogen follicles. Some follicles remain in the anagen phase and continue to produce hairs, although the shafts of these hairs show trichomalacia and are fragile and constricted, resulting in the clinical shedding of "pencil-point hairs".[8]

With chronicity, anagen hairs are few in number and inflammation may be absent. While the total number of hairs remains normal, nearly all of the follicles are miniaturized with nanogen morphology (mixed anagen and telogen features, making them difficult to categorize; see **Fig. 11**).[30] When inflammation is present, it tends to involve the anagen or early catagen bulbs of miniaturized or nanogen hairs. A dominance of telogen hairs may result in an appearance of noninflammatory alopecia. As in other noncicatricial alopecias, the sebaceous glands are preserved.

The mimics of alopecia areata include syphilitic alopecia and lupus erythematosus. Exclusion of these entities requires careful clinical correlation including serologic studies, although some histologic clues may aid in differentiation. Syphilitic alopecia classically has plasma cells in the inflammatory infiltrate. The findings of increased dermal mucin, perieccrine inflammation with rare plasma cells, and vacuolar interface alteration of follicular epithelium suggest lupus erythematosus.

Psoriatic Alopecia

The dominant histologic findings are (**Fig. 12**): preserved follicular density; most hairs in the catagen/telogen phase; follicular miniaturization; conspicuous absence or atrophy of sebaceous

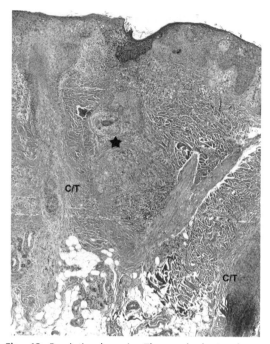

Fig. 12. Psoriatic alopecia. The marked atrophy or apparent absence of sebaceous glands helps differentiate this disorder from alopecia areata. The presence of psoriasiform epidermal hyperplasia also helps in this regard. An increase in catagen/telogen follicles (C/T) and hair miniaturization (*star*) are features shared with alopecia areata (Original magnification ×40).

glands; focal peribulbar, peri-isthmic, and peri-infundibular lymphocytic inflammation; and typical changes of psoriasis within the interfollicular epithelium (sometimes a seborrheic dermatitis-like inflammatory pattern).[8] Less commonly, there may be destruction of isolated follicles.

Given the clinical impression of a psoriatic plaque on the scalp with associated alopecia, it is not surprising that histologic changes typical of psoriasis are evident in psoriatic alopecia. These features include dilated papillary dermal blood vessels, psoriasiform epidermal hyperplasia, loss of the granular cell layer, broad zones of parakeratosis, and collections of neutrophils within the stratum corneum. However, the changes will not be appreciated if an alopecic, but nonerythematous zone is selected for biopsy.

The most obvious follicular abnormality is the shift of the majority follicles into the catagen/telogen phase.[31] In addition, there is often miniaturization with underlying fibrous streamers. Focal areas of peribulbar, peri-isthmic, and peri-infundibular inflammation can also be identified; however, follicular destruction is not often seen. A finding seemingly unique to psoriatic alopecia is atrophy of the sebaceous lobules, sometimes to the point

that recognition of any sebaceous structure can be difficult (see **Fig. 12**). This finding can even be seen in patients without clinical alopecia, and does not correlate with clinical outcome.[32] Although sebaceous gland destruction and atrophy are considered features of cicatricial alopecia, psoriatic alopecia is generally nonscarring and clinical hair regrowth after treatment is the norm. Premature desquamation of the inner root sheath may also occur.

The differential diagnosis includes: alopecia areata, tumor necrosis factor (TNF)-α inhibitor-associated psoriatic alopecia, and tinea capitis. Alopecia areata and psoriatic alopecia share a marked increase in the catagen/telogen percentage, miniaturization, and peribulbar inflammation; however, striking atrophy of the sebaceous lobules is not a feature of alopecia areata. Epidermal changes are not present in alopecia areata. The TNF-α inhibitor-associated cases share the features listed above but also exhibit superficial and deep inflammation with conspicuous plasma cells and eosinophils. Tinea capitis can be excluded with histochemical stains (GMS, PAS), microbiologic cultures, and good clinical correlation.

TNF-α Inhibitor–Induced Psoriatic Alopecia

The dominant histologic findings are similar to primary psoriatic alopecia (see earlier discussion); however, both the intensity and character of the inflammatory infiltrate are more prominent in TNF-α inhibitor–induced cases.[8] The inflammation is both superficial and deep with admixed plasma cells and eosinophils.[33] Peribulbar inflammation tends to be more conspicuous and contains plasma cells. Because of the intensity of the inflammation, it is also more common to see follicular destruction in TNF-α inhibitor–induced cases. The epidermis may be spongiotic and may have lichenoid inflammation.[34]

The differential diagnosis includes classic psoriatic alopecia, alopecia areata, and tinea capitis. The differences between classic psoriatic alopecia and TNF-α inhibitor–induced cases are presented above. Alopecia areata shares the marked shift to catagen/telogen, miniaturization, and peribulbar inflammation; however, the epidermal changes, sebaceous atrophy, and plasma cell infiltrate are absent. Tinea capitis can be excluded by histochemical stains (GMS, PAS), microbiologic cultures, and good clinical correlation.

Syphilitic Alopecia

Syphilitic alopecia may result as a consequence of the typical cutaneous papulosquamous lesions of syphilis (symptomatic syphilitic alopecia), diffuse alopecia secondary to a telogen effluvium, or as "essential" syphilitic alopecia with the classically described "moth-eaten" clinical appearance.[8] Because the histologic findings in cases that present as telogen effluvium are indistinguishable from other causes of telogen effluvium, it is not discussed further here.

The dominant histologic findings in symptomatic syphilitic alopecia are typical of other cutaneous lesions of secondary syphilis, and include epidermal hyperplasia with spongiosis and interface alteration, neutrophilic infiltrate within the epidermis, a superficial and sometimes deep perivascular lymphohistiocytic infiltrate with admixed plasma cells, and dilated and swollen endothelial cells.[35] In cases of essential syphilitic alopecia, the dominant findings are a marked increase in the catagen/telogen percentage, miniaturization, and peribulbar inflammation with admixed plasma cells. Immunohistochemical stains for treponemes may demonstrate organisms within the peribulbar region or follicular matrix.[36]

The differential diagnosis includes telogen effluvium and alopecia areata. Telogen effluvium should not show miniaturization or peribulbar inflammation. The closest mimic of essential syphilitic alopecia is alopecia areata. Both syphilitic alopecia and alopecia areata show a marked increase in the catagen/telogen percentage, miniaturization, and peribulbar inflammation; however, alopecia areata should not show peribulbar plasma cells. Close clinical correlation and correlation with serologic studies may be required to separate these 2 conditions.

Noncicatricial Alopecia Caused by Systemic Lupus Erythematosus

Although the most familiar form of alopecia in systemic lupus erythematosus is the classic cicatricial form, noncicatricial patterns can also be seen, and include a telogen effluvium (discussed earlier) and a patchy nonscarring alopecia in patients with active, systemic disease. The dominant histologic findings in the latter pattern are: miniaturization of follicles; an increase in the catagen/telogen percentage in involved areas; dense peribulbar mononuclear cell inflammation; and findings typical of systemic lupus erythematosus (superficial and deep perivascular and periadnexal inflammation, increased dermal mucin, and vacuolar interface alteration).[8]

The differential diagnosis includes syphilitic alopecia and alopecia areata; however, some findings can help distinguish lupus erythematosus from its mimics. Increased dermal mucin is often identifiable on routine hematoxylin-eosin–stained sections, but can be highlighted with histochemical stains for mucin (colloidal iron). In addition to peribulbar inflammation, which is denser than that seen in alopecia areata, there is also perivascular and perieccrine lymphocytic inflammation. Finally, focal basal vacuolar alteration can be seen. When these 3 entities cannot be distinguished on histologic grounds, close clinical correlation and the result of serologic studies can clarify the situation.

REFERENCES

1. Olsen EA, Bergfeld WF, Cotsarelis G, et al. Summary of North American Hair Research Society (NAHRS)-sponsored Workshop on Cicatricial Alopecia, Duke University Medical Center, February 10 and 11, 2001. J Am Acad Dermatol 2003;48(1):103–10.
2. Frishberg DP, Sperling LC, Guthrie VM. Transverse scalp sections: a proposed method for laboratory processing. J Am Acad Dermatol 1996;35(2 Pt 1): 220–2.
3. Elston D, McCollough M, Angeloni V. Vertical and transverse sections of alopecia biopsy specimens: combining the two techniques to maximize diagnostic yield. J Am Acad Dermatol 1995;32:454–7.
4. Nguyen JV, Hudacek K, Whitten JA, et al. The HoVert technique: a novel method for the sectioning of alopecia biopsies. J Cutan Pathol 2011;38(5):401–6.
5. Sperling LC, Lupton GP. Histopathology of nonscarring alopecia. J Cutan Pathol 1995;22(2):97–114.
6. Sperling L. Hair density in African-Americans. Arch Dermatol 1999;135:656–8.
7. Lee HJ, Ha SJ, Lee JH, et al. Hair counts from scalp biopsy specimens in Asians. J Am Acad Dermatol 2002;46(2):218–21.
8. Sperling LC, Cowper SE, Knopp EA. An atlas of hair pathology with clinical correlations. 2nd edition. London: Informa Healthcare; 2012.
9. Sperling L, Solomon A, Whiting D. A new look at scarring alopecia. Arch Dermatol 2000;136:235–42.
10. Templeton S, Solomon A. Scarring alopecia: a classification based on microscopic criteria. J Cutan Pathol 1994;21:97–109.
11. Mehregan DA, Van Hale HM, Muller SA. Lichen planopilaris: clinical and pathologic study of forty-five patients. J Am Acad Dermatol 1992;27(6 Pt 1): 935–42.
12. Mobini N, Tam S, Kamino H. Possible role of the bulge region in the pathogenesis of inflammatory scarring alopecia: lichen planopilaris as the prototype. J Cutan Pathol 2005;32(10):675–9.
13. Sperling LC, Cowper SE. The histopathology of primary cicatricial alopecia. Semin Cutan Med Surg 2006;25(1):41–50.
14. Elston DM, McCollough ML, Warschaw KE, et al. Elastic tissue in scars and alopecia. J Cutan Pathol 2000;27(3):147–52.

15. Headington JT. Cicatricial alopecia. Dermatol Clin 1996;14(4):773–82.

16. Jordon RE. Subtle clues to diagnosis by immunopathology. Scarring alopecia. Am J Dermatopathol 1980;2(2):157–9.

17. Sperling LC, Homoky C, Pratt L, et al. Acne keloidalis is a form of primary scarring alopecia. Arch Dermatol 2000;136(4):479–84.

18. Herzberg AJ, Dinehart SM, Kerns BJ, et al. Acne keloidalis. Transverse microscopy, immunohistochemistry, and electron microscopy. Am J Dermatopathol 1990;12(2):109–21.

19. Twersky JM, Sheth AP. Tinea capitis mimicking dissecting cellulitis: a distinct variant. Int J Dermatol 2005;44(5):412–4.

20. Kossard S, Lee MS, Wilkinson B. Postmenopausal frontal fibrosing alopecia: a frontal variant of lichen planopilaris. J Am Acad Dermatol 1997;36(1):59–66.

21. Faulkner CF, Wilson NJ, Jones SK. Frontal fibrosing alopecia associated with cutaneous lichen planus in a premenopausal woman. Australas J Dermatol 2002;43(1):65–7.

22. Poblet E, Jimenez F, Pascual A, et al. Frontal fibrosing alopecia versus lichen planopilaris: a clinicopathological study. Int J Dermatol 2006;45(4):375–80.

23. Zinkernagel MS, Trueb RM. Fibrosing alopecia in a pattern distribution: patterned lichen planopilaris or androgenetic alopecia with a lichenoid tissue reaction pattern? Arch Dermatol 2000;136(2):205–11.

24. Olsen EA, Messenger AG, Shapiro J, et al. Evaluation and treatment of male and female pattern hair loss. J Am Acad Dermatol 2005;52(2):301–11.

25. Sundberg JP, Beamer WG, Uno H, et al. Androgenetic alopecia: in vivo models. Exp Mol Pathol 1999;67(2):118–30.

26. Horenstein MG, Jacob JS. Follicular streamers (stelae) in scarring and non-scarring alopecia. J Cutan Pathol 2008;35(12):1115–20.

27. Muller SA. Trichotillomania: a histopathologic study in sixty-six patients. J Am Acad Dermatol 1990;23(1):56–62.

28. Lachapelle JM, Pierard GE. Traumatic alopecia in trichotillomania: a pathogenic interpretation of histologic lesions in the pilosebaceous unit. J Cutan Pathol 1977;4(2):51–67.

29. Whiting DA. Histopathologic features of alopecia areata: a new look. Arch Dermatol 2003;139(12):1555–9.

30. Headington J, Mitchell A, Swanson N. New histopathologic findings in alopecia areata studied in transverse section. 42nd Annual Meeting of the Society for Investigative Dermatology. San Francisco, 1981.

31. Runne U, Kroneisen-Wiersma P. Psoriatic alopecia: acute and chronic hair loss in 47 patients with scalp psoriasis. Dermatology 1992;185(2):82–7.

32. Headington JT, Gupta AK, Goldfarb MT, et al. A morphometric and histologic study of the scalp in psoriasis. Paradoxical sebaceous gland atrophy and decreased hair shaft diameters without alopecia. Arch Dermatol 1989;125(5):639–42.

33. Doyle LA, Sperling LC, Baksh S, et al. Psoriatic alopecia/alopecia areata-like reactions secondary to anti-tumor necrosis factor-alpha therapy: a novel cause of noncicatricial alopecia. Am J Dermatopathol 2011;33(2):161–6.

34. Seneschal J, Milpied B, Vergier B, et al. Cytokine imbalance with increased production of interferon-alpha in psoriasiform eruptions associated with antitumour necrosis factor-alpha treatments. Br J Dermatol 2009;161(5):1081–8.

35. Jeerapaet P, Ackerman A. Histologic patterns of secondary syphilis. Arch Dermatol 1973;107:373–7.

36. Nam-Cha SH, Guhl G, Fernandez-Pena P, et al. Alopecia syphilitica with detection of Treponema pallidum in the hair follicle. J Cutan Pathol 2007;34(Suppl 1):37–40.

How to Diagnose and Treat Medically Women with Excessive Hair

Ulrike Blume-Peytavi, MD

KEYWORDS

- Hypertrichosis • Hirsutism • Excessive hair • Pharmacologic treatment • Laser epilation

KEY POINTS

- Excessive hair growth in women can present as localized or diffuse hypertrichosis or as hirsutism with a male pattern hair growth distribution.
- Excessive hair growth in hirsute women can be due to adrenal, ovarian, or central endocrine abnormalities or also be drug induced or of idiopathic origin.
- Hirsutism can present an important psychological burden with loss of self-esteem and loss of femininity.
- Management of excessive hair should comprise a holistic approach, including pharmaceuticals, epilation methods, and aesthetic approaches, and emotional coping as well as lifestyle modifications.

INTRODUCTION

Excessive hair growth in women is not uncommon. Approximately 5% to 10% of women in reproductive age are hirsute with a Ferriman-Gallwey score higher than 8[1,2]; more than 40% of all women experience some degree of unwanted facial hair during their lifetime.[3] Excessive hair growth, especially in the face, can represent an important psychological burden with loss of self-esteem and loss of femininity to many women. Still, excessive female hair has not gained much attention in medical research.

Excessive hair growth in women can be the result of various causes, including adrenal, ovarian, or central endocrine abnormalities and also can be drug induced or of idiopathic origin. Considering the broad pathogenic spectrum, the diagnostic work-up is crucial for success in managing these patients, including the choice of the adequate treatment. Thus, the panel of treatments options is likewise broad and ranges from pharmaceuticals to physical, chemical, and laser epilation combined with psychological coping strategies. The central task for every treating doctor is to rectify any causal hormonal balance to slow down or stop excessive hair growth and improve the esthetic appearance of female patients, thereby positively affecting their quality of life.

DIAGNOSING EXCESSIVE HAIR GROWTH

Excessive hair growth in women presents clinically as hypertrichosis (localized or diffuse) or hirsutism (**Table 1**).[4] Hypertrichosis has a broad clinical presentation and depends on ethnic factors, frequently with no pathologic background.[3] It is androgen independent and presents with generalized or localized vellus hair growth distributed in a nonsexual pattern over the body. Hypertrichosis may be familial, drug related, or due to different metabolic or other nonendocrine disorders, such

The author declares no conflicts of interest.
Department of Dermatology and Allergy, Clinical Research Center for Hair and Skin Science, Charité–Universitätsmedizin Berlin, Charitéplatz 1, Berlin D-10117, Germany
E-mail address: ulrike.blume-peytavi@charite.de

Dermatol Clin 31 (2013) 57–65
http://dx.doi.org/10.1016/j.det.2012.08.009
0733-8635/13/$ – see front matter © 2013 Elsevier Inc. All rights reserved.

derm.theclinics.com

Table 1
Clinical characteristics of hypertrichosis and hirsutism

Hypertrichosis	Hirsutism
Male and female	Only female
Independent of age	Onset at puberty or later
Terminal or vellus hair	Terminal hair in male pattern distribution
Non–androgen-dependent body sites	Androgen-dependent body sites

Date from Blume-Peytavi U. An overview of unwanted female hair. Br J Dermatol 2011;165:19–23.

as anorexia nervosa.[5] In many cases, cosmetic treatments may be the most suitable.[3]

In cases of hirsutism, the clinical characteristics in female patients present as excess terminal (coarse) hairs with a male pattern distribution. The clinical history, including ethnic factors and complete physical examination, should be established to confirm the male pattern hair growth. Disorders that may potentially contribute to excessive hair growth, such as ovulatory dysfunction, adrenal hyperplasia, diabetes, or thyroid hormone abnormalities,[6] should be excluded. Hirsutism also can be caused by nonandrogenic factors or excessive androgen, although nonandrogenic causes are rare. Androgenic causes include polycystic ovary syndrome (PCOS), affecting 70% to 80% of hirsute women; rarely, hyperandrogenic insulin-resistant acanthosis nigricans syndrome[7] and 21-hydroxylase–deficient nonclassic adrenal hyperplasia; and, very rarely, ovarian or adrenal androgen-secreting neoplasms.[8–10]

When diagnosing female patients with excessive hair growth, the negative impact on patient quality of life[11] and possible psychological and psychosocial distress, especially in cases of facial hair, should also be taken into consideration. Complaints may include depression, social phobia, or body dysmorphic disorders.[12,13] Therefore, an interdisciplinary holistic treatment approach, which includes, in addition to pharmacologic management and possible cosmetic hair removal methods, emotional coping strategies and ongoing support and lifestyle modifications, may be advisable.[3]

The Skin Academy hirsutism subgroup developed a diagnostic evaluation form in 2009 for women with excessive hair growth, which is used in Europe, especially in the United Kingdom, Germany, and Switzerland. The diagnostic evaluation form has 3 parts (history, clinical examination, and investigations), each divided into subsections.[5]

History

In the history section, factors, such as patient age, ethnicity, family history, and medication, are taken into consideration. Non-neoplastic hirsutism is usually seen at puberty with increasing androgen secretion after weight gain or after discontinuing oral contraceptives.[14,15] In regards to patients' ethnic background, it should be determined what kind of hair growth is deemed normal and excessive. Furthermore, the speed of onset of the hair growth is assessed; in most women, a slow physiologic depilation is seen after menopause. Facial hair, on the contrary, tends to increase.

In some women, hirsutism rapidly develops or worsens in puberty, particularly if there are disturbances in androgen production. Rapid onset or worsening of hirsutism may be a sign of neoplasia-induced androgen excess. Some medications, for example, danazol; anticonvulsant drugs, such as valproic acid; and anabolic or androgenic steroids taken by athletes and patients with endometriosis or sexual dysfunctions, can cause hirsutism. The regularity of the menstrual cycle should be found out and the presence of PCOS ruled out. Most women with at least a 2-fold increase in androgen levels experience some degree of hirsutism or symptoms, such as acne vulgaris, seborrhea, and pattern alopecia. If no hyperandrogenemia is present, the condition is called idiopathic hirsutism.[16]

Clinical Examination

In the clinical examination section, the distribution of hair on the face and the body as well as the androgen dependency of the hairs is assessed. If excessive hair grows on the upper back, shoulders, and upper abdomen, an increase in androgen production should be suspected. If the hair growth is mild (8–15 in the Ferriman-Gallwey score, depending on a patient's ethnic background) and a patient's menstrual cycle is regular, the hirsutism is likely idiopathic.[17,18] This is the case in 5% to 15% of hirsute women,[19,20] and in some of them the skin and hair follicles' 5α-reductase activity is overactive, which results in hirsutism, although circulating androgen levels are normal.

Because increased androgen levels may also lead to pilosebaceous responses, such as acne, excessive sebum secretion, or diffuse or localized loss of hair, a dermatologic examination is mandatory. Obesity, a common feature often associated with PCOS, is assessed by calculating the body mass index, (weight/height^2).[5]

Thickening and darkening of the skin on the neck and inguinal region are assessed, because they may be a sign of acanthosis nigricans, related to high blood insulin levels or obesity. The genetic disorder, hyperandrogenic insulin-resistant acanthosis nigricans, includes many different genetic syndromes,[21] from which approximately 3% of hyperandrogenic women suffer. Insulin resistance is also common in PCOS, which is one of the most common causes of hirsutism, and can lead to hyperglycemia and dyslipidemia.[5]

The Ferriman-Gallwey score helps assess the extent of a patient's hirsutism; if the score is at least 8, a woman is considered hirsute.[1] Although well known, the Ferriman-Gallwey score has limitations: it is subjective and can be time-consuming. If, however, a clinician has experience with the method, it can be a good documentation technique in hirsute patients.

Patients should also be asked about quality-of-life changes and examined for symptoms of depression (such as sleeping difficulties, loss of energy, and drive). Feelings of disgust; changes in sexual activity, life behavior, and life-events; and signs of body dysmorphic disorder should also be evaluated. If necessary, additional counseling or psychotherapy should be considered.[5]

Investigations

Laboratory investigations should include a free androgen index to assess biochemical hyperandrogenemia; in cases of a normal total testosterone level, a diagnosis of idiopathic hirsutism is more likely but does not rule out other origin of androgen excess. In addition, prolactin, 17 hydroxyprogesterone, and a 24-hour urine cortisol to exclude Cushing syndrome, should be tested. In women with absent or irregular menstruation, pregnancy should be ruled out before initiating any treatment. Thyroid function should be assessed, although hypothyroidism is usually more the cause of coarsening of the hair rather than androgen excess–induced hirsutism.[5] PCOS is the most likely explanation for hirsutism but, nevertheless, other likely causes, such as hyperprolactinemia, should be ruled out.[22] Pelvic ultrasound, preferably transvaginal, including an examination of the ovaries, adrenal glands, or both, helps in examining possible presence of neoplasms.[23]

MEDICAL TREATMENT OF HIRSUTISM

Medical treatment of hirsutism aims at correcting any hormonal imbalances, thereby improving patient quality of life. The choice of therapy depends on the underlying cause, the location and extent of excessive hair growth, patient preferences, and access and affordability of the products. Monotherapy with oral contraceptices that have antiandrogenic activity is recommended as a first-line treatment of hirsutism for most premenopausal women. If a patient shows no clinical improvement, a combination therapy of oral contraceptives with antiandrogens is recommended. Any pharmacologic therapy for hirsutism, however, should be continued for 6 to 9 months before changing either dosage or drug category.

In women who also suffer from both hyperandrogenism and insulin resistance, insulin sensitizers also improve hirsutism. Topical eflornithine is used in conjunction with systemic medications or with laser epilation or photoepilation.[24] Classification of different treatment options are summarized in **Table 1** and guidelines on the medical treatment options for hirsutism in **Tables 2** and **3**.

Antiandrogens

Antiandrogens (cyproterone acetate [CPA], chlormadinone acetate [CMA], dienogest, drospirenone,

Table 2 Treatment of hirsutism	
Medical treatment of hirsutism: classification by the working mechanism of the different drugs	
Antiandrogens	• CPA • CMA • Dienogest • Drospirenone • Spironolactone • Flutamide and bicalutamide
Enzyme inhibitors	• Finasteride • Eflornithine
Insulin-sensitizing agents	• Metformin • [Rosiglitazone, pioglitazone][a]
Gonadotropin-releasing hormone analogs	• Leuprolide • Nafarelin
Adjuvants to medical treatment	
Epilation methods	• Physical and chemical epilation (tweezer, shaving, waxing, sugaring, or threading) • Electrolysis or electroepilation • Laser epilation/photoepilation

[a] Rosiglitazone was withdrawn from the European and Swiss markets in 2010 due to increased cardiovascular risks; Pioglitazone withdrawn in France 2011.

From Blume-Peytavi U, Hahn S. Medical treatment of hirsutism. Dermatol Ther 2008;21:329–39.

Table 3
Drugs used to treat hirsutism

Drug	Dosage	Schedule
CPA	2–100 mg	Cycle days 5–14 (combination with estrogens needed in women with uterus), also available as a combination oral contraceptive pill[b]: 2 mg CPA + 35 μg ethinyl estradiol
CMA	1–2 mg	Available only as a combination oral contraceptive pill[b] either as an OCP with 2 phases—first phase 1 mg CMA + 50 μg ethinyl estradiol and second phase 2 mg CMA + 50 μg ethinyl estradiol—or as a single-phase OCP 2 mg CMA + 30 μg ethinyl estradiol for 21 d
Dienogest	2 mg	Available only as a combination oral contraceptive pill[b]: 2 mg dienogest + 30 μg ethinyl estradiol
Drospirenone (DRSP)	3 mg	Available only as a combination oral contraceptive pill[b]: 3 mg DRSP + 30 μg ethinyl estradiol or 3 mg DRSP + 20 μg ethinyl estradiol
Spironolactone	50–200 mg/d	Continuously[a,c]
Flutamide	62.5–500 mg/d	Continuously[a]
Finasteride	1–5 mg/d	Continuously[a]
Metformin	1000–2000 mg/d	Continuously

[a] Should always be combined with effective contraception.
[b] Licensed for use in women in several countries.
[c] Over 21 days when combined with OCP, in menopause without interruption.
From Blume-Peytavi U, Hahn S. Medical treatment of hirsutism. Dermatol Ther 2008;21:329–39.

spironolactone, flutamide, and bicalutamide) prevent androgen cellular action by blocking intracellular androgen receptors.[24]

Cyproterone acetate, chlormadione acetate, anad dienogest

CPA, CMA, and dienogest have antiandrogenic activity. They block androgen receptors in target organs but also reduce 5α-reductase, which converts testosterone to 5α-dihydrotestosterone, a more potent androgen. CMA and CPA reduce ovarian and adrenal androgen production.[24]

CPA has steroidal side effects and can cause abnormalities in liver function and menstrual irregularity. Because of its progestin activity, it needs to be combined with estrogens in women who have a uterus. In CMA, the antiandrogenic potential is considered lower compared with CPA.[24]

A systematic review[25] of 9 randomized controlled trials using CPA for hirsutism in different doses (either 2 mg in an oral contraceptive pill or 25–100 mg). For all doses, a subjective improvement compared with placebo was seen. Clinical differences in the outcome were not observed between CPA and the other drugs included in the review (ketoconazole, spironolactone, flutamide, finasteride, and gonadotropin-releasing hormone analogs).

A randomized controlled trial[26] comparing the therapeutic efficacy of different medical treatments of hirsutism showed that a combination of CPA and estradiol (first week 0.01 mg/d, second week 0.02 mg/d, third week 0.01 mg/d, pause of 7 days, and 12.5 mg/d CPA during the first 10 days of every month) reduced hair growth more rapidly and showed the greatest decrease in hair growth after 12 months of treatment compared with flutamide (250 mg/d), fiansteride (5 mg/d), and ketoconazole (300 mg/d). A combination of oral contraceptives containing CMA (2 mg) or CPA (2 mg) and ethinyl estradiol (30–35 μg) resulted in an improvement in 36% of hirsutism patients.[27]

Spironolactone

Spironolactone is an aldosterone antagonist and androgen receptor antagonist and an effective treatment of hirsutism when given in doses of 50 mg/d to 200 mg/d. A cyclic dosage (2 × 50 mg or 3 × 75 mg 21 days on and 7 days off during menses when combined with oral contraceptives) is used.[28] Spironolactone is more effective when combined with oral contraceptives.[29]

Spironolactone is usually well tolerated with few side effects; these tend to increase at doses above 100 mg. When spironolactone is used alone, women may develop more frequent menses. Spironolactone can also elevate potassium levels by blocking aldosterone on the kidneys, and it should not be used in women with renal insufficiency or hyperkalemia. Blood pressure and potassium concentrations should be screened every 4 weeks, especially in the first months of treatment.[24]

A systematic review[30] of the use of spironolactone to treat hirsutism and/or acne concluded that spironolactone (100 mg/d for 6 months) resulted in a statistically significant subjective improvement with a decrease in the Ferriman-Gallwey score compared with placebo. Spironolactone (100 mg/d) was also found more effective in hyperandrogenism-related hirsutism than finasteride (5 mg/d) and CPA (12.5 mg/d, first 10 days of the cycle) up to 12 months after cessation of treatment.

Among hirsute women treated with low-dose spironolactone (75–100 mg/d), 72% showed improvement in an open-label trial.[28] Another trial[31] compared the efficacy of spironolactone (50 mg/d) and metformin (1000 mg/d) in women with PCOS and found both drugs equally effective in the management of PCOS; however, the number of menstrual cycles increased significantly. Although spironolactone was more successful in the treatment of hirsutism, serum luteinizing hormone/follicle-stimulating hormone and testosterone decreased in both groups. Spironolactone increased the menstrual cycles more and decreased testosterone more rapidly.

Drospirenone

The progestin, drospirenone, used in many oral contraceptives, is a weak antiandrogen. A dose of 3 mg (in oral contraceptives) is the equivalent of 25 mg of spironolactone or 1 mg of CPA. A nonrandomized study[32] investigating hirsute women treated with drospirenone (3 mg) oral contraceptive in combination with ethinyl estradiol (30 μg) showed that this combination improved hirsutism clinically through antiandrogenic and antimineralocorticoid action and biochemical manifestations. Total and free testosterone in serum decreased significantly, and sex hormone–binding globulin increased.

Flutamide and bicalutamide

The nonsteroidal compound, flutamide, acts as the androgen receptor site and is, therefore, considered a pure antiandrogen.[29] There are, however, also some data suggesting that flutamide might reduce androgen synthesis.

Flutamide is used in doses of 62. 5 mg/d to 500 mg/d. Because liver toxicity is a potential, albeit rare, side effect, serum transaminases should be measured frequently. Other side effects that have been reported include dry skin, diarrhea, nausea, and vomiting.

Bicalutamide (a dosage of 25 mg/d) is a new and potent, well-tolerated nonsteroidal pure antiandrogen. It was developed for treating prostate cancer (at a dosage of 50 mg/d). It has been shown effective in the treatment of patients with PCOS-induced and idiopathic hirsutism with no significant side effects.[33] Hepatotoxic effects have been reported starting at doses of 50 mg/d.

Flutamide has been found more effective than finasteride in treating hirsute patients with PCOS and with idiopathic hirsutism.[34] When comparing low-dose flutamide, finasteride, ketoconazole, and cyproterone acetate/estrogen regimens in hirsute women, flutamide and CPA in combination with estradiol were found the most effective and well tolerated.[26] Another trial[35] that compared the efficacy of flutamide (250 mg, for the first 10 days of the cycle) and spironolactone (100 mg/d) in combination with an oral contraceptive containing CPA (2 mg) and ethinyl estradiol (35 μg) in the treatment of moderate to severe idiopathic hirsutism showed a significant decrease in the Ferriman-Gallwey score, similar in both groups.

Enzyme Inhibitors

Finasteride

Because of its 5α-reductase blocking features, which inhibit the conversion of testosterone into 5α-dihydrotestosterone, finasteride is usually considered an antiandrogen. It reduces the amount of hormones available for interaction with the androgen receptor but does not cause changes in ovarian or adrenal androgen secretion.

Finasteride is used (in doses of 1 mg/d to 5 mg/d) in treating women with hirsutism and its efficacy has been evaluated in different clinical trials. Finasteride is able to decrease hirsutism scores by up to 60%, and, in addition, it reduces the average hair diameter. In trials including women with hirsutism due to different causes, finasteride was found as effective as antiandrogens while causing fewer side effects. A placebo-controlled trial[36] assessed the clinical and hormonal effects of finasteride in women with idiopathic or PCOS-related hirsutism; Ferriman-Gallwey scores were significantly lower after 6 months of finasteride (5 mg/d) compared with placebo. In another study,[26] comparing low-dose flutamide, finasteride, ketoconazole, and cyproterone acetate/estrogen regimens, finasteride showed a significant reduction in Ferriman-Gallwey score, hair diameter, and daily hair growth rate. Finasteride had the slowest onset of action; however, it reduced the hair diameter more than the other products included in the study and caused fewer side effects.

Using any antiandrogens for the treatment of hirsutism in women in reproductive age requires a safe and effective method of contraception due to the feminization risk of a male fetus. Considering the half-life of the drugs (listed previously), pregnancy seems safe 10 days after discontinuation of the therapy, but from a practical aspect the authors recommend having at least 1 normal cycle before becoming pregnant.[24]

Eflornithine

Eflornithine is an irreversible ornithine decarboxylase inhibitor. It catalyzes the rate-limiting step in follicular polyamine synthesis, necessary for hair growth. It does not remove the hair but reduces its growth speed. A topical eflornithine hydrochloride cream (13.9%) is approved in many countries for treating unwanted facial hair in women. Systemic absorption is low[37,38] and irritation of skin has been reported only with overuse in experimental conditions. Side effects in clinical use include itching and dry skin.[38,39]

In a placebo-controlled study[40] evaluating the efficacy of eflornithine cream twice daily in facial hirsutism over 24 weeks, the cream was generally well tolerated and significantly reduced unwanted facial hair growth, hair length, and hair mass compared with placebo. Eflornithine seems to reduce the growth rate and appearance of facial hair, and it helps improve patient quality of life. When treatment with the cream is discontinued, the hair returns to pretreatment levels in approximately 8 weeks. When comparing laser of the upper lip and chin in combination with either eflornithine cream or placebo,[41,42] a more significant decrease in hair count was observed when laser was combined with eflornithine.

Insulin-Sensitizing Agents

Insulin-sensitizing agents, metformin, are standard medications for treating type 2 diabetes mellitus. In diabetics, they decrease the elevated sugar levels; in nondiabetics, they decrease insulin levels, whereas blood sugar remains unaltered. They improve insulin action through raising insulin sensitivity. Metformin reduces the production of hepatic glucose and lowers insulin levels; thiazolidinediones improve insulin action in the liver, skeletal muscle, and adipose tissue. Both may also decrease adrenal and ovarian androgen biosynthesis, increase sex hormone–binding globulin levels, and improve secretion of gonadotropin.[43,44] Insulin-sensitizing agents may improve hirsutism by reducing insulin levels and, therefore, the circulating free and biologically active androgens.

Pioglitazone and rosiglitazone, however, have been reported associated with increased cardiovascular risks or elevated cancer risk,[45] leading to rosiglitazone withdrawn from the European and Swiss markets in 2010 and pioglitazone in 2011.

Monitoring liver enzyme levels is recommended when insulin-sensitizing agents are used.[43,44] Because there are insufficient epidemiologic data, metformin should not be used during pregnancy. Insulin-sensitizing agents have not been licensed for use in women with hirsutism or PCOS.[24]

In a comparison[46] of metformin (850 mg twice daily) with rosiglitazone (4 mg/d) in patients with hirsutism and PCOS, Ferriman-Gallwey scores decreased in both groups but significantly more so in the rosiglitazone group. But with today's knowledge only metformin can be recommended.

OTHER TREATMENT OPTIONS

When developing a treatment plan to improve a patient's quality of life and psychological well-being, epilation methods should be considered in combination with medical treatment, especially if a more rapid response is desired. These methods include for example shaving, waxing, sugaring or threading, using tweezers, depilatory creams, electrolysis (electroepilation), and laser epilation. In choosing a technique, patient preferences, skin region, and hair color should be taken into consideration. Particularly for laser epilation, the treatment costs should also be considered.[24]

Physical and Chemical Epilation

Although many women shave their legs and axillary region, they are reluctant to shave the face. Shaving is a quick and cheap method but needs to be repeated daily. In addition, folliculitis often develops when the hairs grow back on the inner thigh region. Electric epilating devices and cold or warm waxes also epilate the hair shaft and thus lead to a longer-lasting effect; the procedure needs to be repeated only every 2 to 6 weeks. The disadvantages of the techniques include pain, inefficient epilation of short hairs, skin irritation, and folliculitis. Sugaring is a variant of waxing from the Near East, where a mixture of lemon acid, sugar, glucose, and purified water is mixed, applied on the skin region, and then removed with a rapid movement.

In chemical epilation, the hair is dissolved by separating the disulfide bonds and peptides of the hair keratin. Most depilatory creams are based on thioglycolates (2%–4%). The cream is left on for 5 to 15 minutes and then removed together with the dissolved hair shafts. Ca++ salts of the thioglycolates have a low irritating effect, however; because not only the hair shaft but also the upper layers of the epidermis may be affected, irritation may occur. The method should be only used on the legs and not in the skin folds. Excess hair can be made less visible by bleaching, which is suitable for upper lip, chin, and arms. Hydrogen peroxide preparations (12%) are available for home use and are applied for 30 minutes; however, a test on a small skin region should be done first. Disadvantages include irritation and sensitization potential of peroxide/sulfates.[24]

Electrolysis (Electroepilation)

Electroepilation (electrolysis) includes different methods that put electric current delivered by a probe in contact with the hair; the epilation probe is introduced in the hair follicle opening and damages the follicle by direct current (galvanic electrolysis) or high-frequency alternating current (thermolysis), which destroys the follicle with heat. The regrowing rate is approximately 40%. Disadvantages of the technique include potential pain, follicular hyperpigmentation, and risk of scarring. In order to obtain satisfying results, the technique should be performed by an experienced and well-trained clinician.[47]

Laser Epilation/Photoepilation

The development of laser devices suitable for epilation has progressed greatly in recent years. Selective photothermolysis is based on selective damage of the pigmented part of the hair follicle; the surrounding skin is not damaged. Laser epilation and photoepilation are widely used, often in combination with a scanning mode to reduce the duration of treating large surfaces. Mostly used are the 755-nm alexandrite laser, 800-nm diode laser, and 1064-nm Nd:YAG laser and pulsed light sources.[48–51] All of these interrupt hair growth temporarily, but permanent results depend on the number of sessions, fluence, and hair color intensity; optimal target is dark hair on fair skin, whereas blond, red, and white hairs are not suitable for laser. The regrowing hairs are usually finer and lighter, and a reduction of 10% to 40% can be achieved per session.

HOLISTIC TREATMENT APPROACH

A holistic treatment approach for female patients with excessive hair should include, in addition to pharmaceutical and/or possible cosmetic treatments, emotional coping and support strategy and lifestyle modifications.[52–54]

Weight loss may have several benefits—apart from obvious health benefits—in terms of improving hirsutism. It decreases serum insulin, ovarian androgen production, and the conversion of androstenedione to testosterone and regulates increased sex hormone–binding globulin production and periods. Healthy nutrition and physical exercise also help reduce insulin levels.[52]

SUMMARY

Excessive hair growth in women is common and has several causes, including adrenal, ovarian, ventral endocrine abnormalities, or idiopathic backgrounds. When diagnosing excessive hair growth in women, the clinical characteristics need to be taken into consideration to determine whether a patient is suffering from the non–androgen-dependent hypertrichosis or androgen-dependent hirsutism.

Treatment options,[55] depending on the cause, range from pharmaceuticals, including antiandrogens, enzyme inhibitors, and insulin-sensitizing agents, to various physical and chemical epilation methods as well as laser hair removal. Monotherapy with oral contraceptives that have antiandrogenic activity is usually the first choice. Especially if a quick improvement is desired, pharmaceutical treatment can be combined with the epilation method of preference.

Because excessive hair growth in women may cause psychological and psychosocial problems, a holistic treatment approach, including support and emotional coping strategies, can be recommended.

REFERENCES

1. Hatch R, Rosenfeld RL, Kim MH, et al. Hirsutism: implications, etiology, and management. Am J Obstet Gynecol 1981;140:815–30.
2. Heithardt AB, Barnes RB. The diagnosis and management of hirsutism. Semin Reprod Med 2003;21:285–93.
3. Blume-Peytavi U. An overview of unwanted female hair. Br J Dermatol 2011;165:19–23.
4. Hillmann K, Blume-Peytavi U. Diagnosis of hair disorders. Semin Cutan Med Surg 2009;28:33–8.
5. Blume-Peytavi U, Atkin S, Shapiro J, et al. European consensus on the evaluation of women presenting with excessive hair growth. Eur J Dermatol 2009; 19:597–602.
6. Azziz R. The evaluation and management of hirsutism. Obstet Gynecol 2003;101:995–1007.
7. Sanchez LA, Knochenhauer ES, Gatlin R, et al. Differential diagnosis of clinically evident hyperandrogenism: experience with over 1000 consecutive patients. Fertil Steril 2001;76:S111.

8. O'Driscoll JB, Mamtora H, Higginson J, et al. A prospective study of the prevalence of clear-cut endocrine disorders and polycystic ovaries in 350 patients presenting with hirsutism or androgenic alopecia. Clin Endocrinol 1994;41:231–6.

9. Morán C, Tapia MC, Hernández E, et al. Etiologic review of hirsutism in 250 patients. Arch Med Res 1994;25:311–4.

10. Waggoner W, Boots LR, Azziz R. Total testosterone and DHEAS levels as predictors of androgen-secreting neoplasms: a populational study. Gynecol Endocrinol 1999;13:1–7.

11. Sonino N, Fava GA, Mani E, et al. Quality of life of hirsute women. Postgrad Med J 1993;69:186–9.

12. Barth JH, Catalan J, Cherry CA, et al. Psychological morbidity in women referred for treatment of hirsutism. J Psychosom Res 1993;37:615–9.

13. Hahn S, Janssen OE, Tan S, et al. Clinical and psychological correlates of quality-of-life in polycystic ovary syndrome. Eur J Endocrinol 2005;153:853–60.

14. Fruzzetti F, Perini D, Lazzarini V, et al. Adolescent girls with polycystic ovary syndrome showing different phenotypes have a different metabolic profile associated with increasing androgen levels. Fertil Steril 2009;92(2):626–34.

15. Codner E, Cassoria F. Puberty and ovarian function in girls with type 1 diabetes mellitus. Horm Res 2009;71:12–21.

16. Souter I, Sanchez LA, Perez M, et al. The prevalence of androgen excess among patients with minimal unwanted hair growth. Am J Obstet Gynecol 2004;191:1914–20.

17. Azziz R, Carmina E, Sawaya ME. Idiopathic hirsutism. Endocr Rev 2000;21:347–62.

18. Reingold SB, Rosenfield RL. The relationship of mild hirsutism or acne in women to androgens. Arch Dermatol 1987;123:209–12.

19. Azziz R, Waggoner WT, Ochoa T, et al. Idiopathic hirsutism: an uncommon cause of hirsutism in Alabama. Fertil Steril 1998;70:274–8.

20. Carmina E. Prevalence of idiopathic hirsutism. Eur J Endocrinol 1998;139:421–3.

21. Barbieri RL, Ryan KJ. Hyperandrogenism, insulin resistance, and acanthosis nigricans syndrome: a common endocrinopathy with distinct pathophysiologic features. Am J Obstet Gynecol 2012;147:90–101.

22. Martin KA, Chang RJ, Ehrmann DA, et al. Evaluation and treatment of hirsutism in premenopausal women: an Endocrine Society Clinical Practice Guideline. J Clin Endocrinol Metab 2008;93:1105–20.

23. Wajchenberg BL, Albergaria Pereira MA, Medonca BB, et al. Adrenocortical carcinoma: clinical and laboratory observations. Cancer 2000;88:711–36.

24. Blume-Peytavi U, Hahn S. Medical treatment of hirsutism. Dermatol Ther 2008;21:329–39.

25. Van der Spuy ZM, le Roux PA. Cyproterone acetate for hirsutism. Cochrane Database Syst Rev 2003:CD003053.

26. Venturoli S, Marescalchi O, Colombo FM, et al. A prospective randomized trial comparing low dose flutamide, finasteride, ketoconazole and cyproterone acetate-oestrogen regimens in the treatment of hirsutism. J Clin Endocrinol Metab 1999;84:1304–10.

27. Raudrant D, Rabe T. Progestogens with antiandrogenic properties. Drugs 2003;63:463–92.

28. Crosby PD, Rittmaster RS. Predictors of clinical response in hirsute women treated with spironolactone. Fertil Steril 1991;55:1076–81.

29. Swiglo BA, Cosma M, Flynn DN, et al. Antiandrogens for the treatment of hirsutism: a systematic review and meta-analyses of randomized controlled trials. J Clin Endocrinol Metab 2008;93:1153–60.

30. Farquhar C, Lee O, Toomath R, et al. Spironolactone versus placebo or in combination with steroids for hirsutism and/or acne. Cochrane Database Syst Rev 2003:CD000194.

31. Ganie MA, Khurana ML, Eunice M, et al. Comparison of efficacy of spironolactone with metformin in the management of polycystic ovary syndrome: an open-label study. J Clin Endocrinol Metab 2004;89:2756–62.

32. Gregoriou O, Papadias K, Konidaris S, et al. Treatment of hirsutism with combied pill containing drospirenone. Gynecol Endocrinol 2008;24:220–3.

33. Muderris II, Bayram F, Ozcelik B, et al. New alternative treatment in hirsutism: bicalutamide 25 mg/day. Gynecol Endocrinol 2002;16:63–6.

34. Falsetti L, Gambera A, Legrenzi L, et al. Comparison of finasteride versus flutamide in the treatment of hirsutism. Eur J Endocrinol 1999;141:361–7.

35. Inal MM, Yildirim Y, Taner CE. Comparison of the clinical efficacy of flutamide and spironolactone plus Diane 35 in the treatment of idiopathic hirsutism: a randomized controlled study. Fertil Steril 2005;84:1693–7.

36. Lakryc EM, Motta EL, Soares JM Jr, et al. The benefits of finasteride for hirsute women with polycystic ovary syndrome or idiopathic hirsutism. Gynecol Endocrinol 2003;17:57–63.

37. Malhotra B, Noveck R, Behr D, et al. Percutaneous absorption and pharmacokinetics of eflornithine HCL 13.9% cream in women with unwanted facial hair. J Clin Pharmacol 2001;41:972–8.

38. Hickman JG, Huber F, Palmisano M. Human dermal safety studies with eflornithine HCl 13.9% cream (Vaniqa), a novel treatment for excessive facial hair. Curr Med Res Opin 2001;16:235–44.

39. Balfour JA, McClellan K. Topical eflornithine. Am J Clin Dermatol 2001;2:197–201.

40. Wolf JE Jr, Shander D, Huber F, et al. Randomized, double-blind clinical evaluation of the efficacy and safety of topical eflornithine HCl 13.9% cream in the treatment of women with facial hair. Int J Dermatol 2007;46:94–8.

41. Smith SR, Piacquadio DJ, Beger B, et al. Eflornithine cream combined with laser therapy in the management of unwanted facial hair growth in women: a randomized trial. Dermatol Surg 2006;32:1237–43.

42. Hamzavi I, Tan E, Shapiro J, et al. A randomized bilateral vehicle-controlled study of eflornithine cream combined with laser treatment versus laser treatment alone for facial hirsutism in women. J Am Acad Dermatol 2007;57:54–9.

43. Lord JM, Flight IH, Norman RJ. Insulin-sensitizing drugs (metformin, troglitazone, rosiglitazone, pioglitazone, d-chiroinositol) for polycystic ovary syndrome. Cochrane Database Syst Rev 2003:CD003053.

44. Cosma M, Swiglo BA, Flynn DN, et al. Insulin sensitizers for the treatment of hirsutism: as systematic review and meta-analysis of randomized controlled trials. J Clin Endocrinol Metab 2008;93:1135–42.

45. Nissen SE, Wolski K. Effect of rosiglitazone on the risk of myocardial infarction and death from cardiovascular causes. N Engl J Med 2007;356(24):2457–71.

46. Dereli D, Dereli T, Bayraktar F, et al. Endocrine and metabolic effects of rosiglitazone in non-obese women with polycystic ovary disease. Endocr J 2005;52:299–308.

47. Yilmaz M, Karakoc A, Toruner FB, et al. The effects of rosiglitazone and metformin on menstrual cyclicity and hirsutism in polycystic ovary syndrome. Gynecol Endocrinol 2005;21:154–60.

48. Olsen EA. Methods of hair removal. J Am Acad Dermatol 1999;40:143–55.

49. Kopera D. Hair reduction: 48 months of experience with 800 nm diode laser. J Cosmet Laser Ther 2003;5:146–9.

50. Ash K, Lord J, Newman J, et al. Hair remocal using a long-pulsed alexandrite laser. Dermatol Clin 1999;17:387–99.

51. Nanni CA, Alster TS. Optimizing treatment parameters for hair removal using a topical carbon-based solution and 1064-nm Q-switched neodymium: YAG laser energy. Arch Dermatol 1997;133:1546–9.

52. Sanchez LA, Perez M, Azziz R. Laser hair reduction in the hirsute patient: a critical assessment. Hum Reprod Update 2002;8:169–81.

53. Guzzick DS. Polycystic ovary syndrome. Obstet Gynecol 2004;103:181–93.

54. Tang T, Lord JM, Norman RJ, et al. Insulin-sensitising drugs (metformin, rosiglitazone, pioglitazone, D-chiro-inositol) for women with polycystic ovary syndrome, oligo amenorrhoea and subfertility. Cochrane Database Syst Rev 2012;5:CD003053.

55. Franks S. The investigation and management. J Fam Plann Reprod Health Care 2012;38(3):182–6.

Drugs and Hair Loss

Mansi Patel, MBChB[a], Shannon Harrison, MBBS, MMed[b],
Rodney Sinclair, MBBS, MD, PhD[c],*

KEYWORDS

- Telogen effluvium • Anagen effluivum • Drug-induced alopecia • Hair loss
- Chemotherapy-induced alopecia

KEY POINTS

- Medications may cause hair loss by a variety of mechanisms including anagen arrest, telogen effluvium, or in the case of exogenous androgens, by accentuation of androgenetic alopecia.
- Drug-induced cicatricial or scarring alopecia is uncommon.
- Hair loss, and in particular telogen effluvium, may also occur in response to a number of triggers including fever, hemorrhage, severe illness, stress, and childbirth, and a thorough exclusion of these potential confounders is necessary before the hair loss can be attributed to the medication. In addition, androgenetic alopecia is commonly punctuated by an episode of increased hair shedding that lasts 2 to 4 months, and this shedding may further confuse the clinical picture.
- Many reports in the literature that attribute hair loss to particular medications have not adequately explored the nature of the hair loss and excluded other potential unrelated causes of hair loss; therefore, they are difficult to interpret.
- Anagen effluvium is a form of diffuse hair loss that follows administration of anticancer chemotherapeutic agents, radiation treatment, and various chemicals. The degree of hair loss is dependent on the route, dose and schedule of the chemotherapy agent.
- Drug-induced telogen effluvium mainly involves premature interruption of hair growth with an early entry of anagen follicles into the resting phase, leading to a noticeable increase in hair shedding 2 to 3 months later.
- In almost all cases, there is recovery of hair loss within 3 months following discontinuation of the medication. Many medications have been suspected of causing hair loss. A high index of suspicion should be maintained regarding medication-induced alopecia, especially if other causes have been excluded.

INTRODUCTION

Hair loss is a common complaint, both in men and women, and use of prescription medications is widespread. When there is a temporal association between the onset of hair loss and commencement of a medication, the medication is commonly thought to have caused the hair loss. However, hair loss, and in particular telogen effluvium, may occur in response to a number of triggers including fever, hemorrhage, severe illness, stress, and childbirth, and a thorough exclusion of these potential confounders is necessary before the hair loss can attributed to the medication. In addition, androgenetic alopecia is commonly punctuated by episodes of increased hair shedding that last 2 to 4 months, and this shedding may further confuse the clinical picture.

Many reports in the literature that attribute hair loss to particular medications have not adequately explored the nature of the hair loss and excluded

[a] Department of Medicine, St. Vincent's Hospital, University of Melbourne, Aikenhead Wing, 41 Victoria Parade, Fitzroy, Melbourne, Victoria 3065, Australia; [b] St. Vincent's Hospital, Aikenhead Wing, 41 Victoria Parade, Fitzroy, Melbourne, Victoria 3065, Australia; [c] St. Vincent's Hospital, University of Melbourne, Aikenhead Wing, 41 Victoria Parade, Fitzroy, Melbourne, Victoria 3065, Australia
* Corresponding author.
E-mail address: rod.sinclair@svhm.org.au

Dermatol Clin 31 (2013) 67–73
http://dx.doi.org/10.1016/j.det.2012.08.002

other potential unrelated causes of hair loss; therefore, they are difficult to interpret.

Nevertheless, certain medications are known to cause hair loss by various mechanisms, including anagen arrest, telogen effluvium, or accentuation of androgenetic alopecia by androgens.

Drug-induced cicatricial or scarring alopecia is uncommon.

NORMAL HAIR CYCLE AND HAIR SHEDDING

An understanding of the normal hair cycle is critical in interpreting whether hair loss might be related to medication use. When looking for a trigger of increased telogen hair shedding, it is important to consider events and medications introduced 2 to 3 months earlier that may have triggered a premature entry of the hair into catagen. In such cases, hair shedding is delayed until telogen release, which may precede or coincide with the onset of anagen.

The normal human hair cycle consists of 3 phases: anagen growth phase, catagen involutional phase, and telogen resting phase. As hair growth during anagen is relatively constant (1 cm/mo), anagen duration is the main determinant of the final length of the hair. The average duration of anagen is approximately 3 years in a normal human scalp. The hair follicle begins to involute as it enters catagen. Catagen lasts 2 weeks, during which time the lower two-thirds of the follicle undergoes complete involution. Telogen follows catagen, and a club-shaped structure is formed by keratinization of proximal hair shaft. The hair follicle remains in the telogen phase for approximately 3 months. During telogen, the hair fiber is shed from the scalp in a process called exogen. Telogen terminates with the commencement of the next anagen phase of the next hair cycle.[1]

Hair follicle activity within anatomic regions is not synchronous in adults, meaning the scalp hair follicles are not all in the same phase of the hair cycle. Trichograms of the scalp demonstrate that 86% of hairs are in anagen, 1% in catagen and 13% are in telogen.[2] In comparison, horizontal scalp biopsies show a higher ratio of anagen-to-telogen scalp hairs, indicating fewer hairs in telogen[3] than the trichogram data. About 50 to 150 hairs are shed daily, the number varying with age and season.[4] Many factors including genetics, hormone profiles, and immune system can interfere with the normal hair cycle and hair production and in some cases may also cause hair follicle destruction.

DRUGS AND ALOPECIA

In patients presenting with increased hair shedding, a careful clinical history is essential. History should include information on any potential triggers from the 3 months before the development of hair loss.[5] It is important to enquire about any drug intake, systemic illness, weight loss, family history of hair loss and also any gynecological problems in women. Clinical examination should determine if the scalp hair density is normal or decreased and whether there is evidence of diffuse or patchy alopecia.[6] Diagnostic techniques, such as the hair pull test may be used to assess the severity of hair shedding. The pull test is an examination technique to crudely assess active hair shedding. It involves grasping 50 to 60 strands of hairs in 3 separate areas of the scalp by thumb, index, and middle fingers and gently sliding the fingers along the hair shafts. With this gentle traction, if more than 10% (6 or more hairs from a single area) of grasped hairs are pulled out, then the test is positive. A positive test indicates increased telogen hairs, which may be the case in chronic telogen effluvium or androgenetic alopecia.[7]

Clinically, drug-induced hair loss presents with a diffuse, nonscarring, reversible alopecia that most commonly involves the scalp. Axillary, pubic, and total body hair are rarely affected. Generally it is not associated with other symptoms. Also, there is an absence of follicular or interfollicular inflammation. Women appear to be affected more frequently than men.[8] Medications may cause hair loss through interruption of normal hair growth cycle by 2 main mechanisms: anagen effluvium or telogen effluvium.[9]

ANAGEN EFFLUVIUM

Anagen effluvium is a form of diffuse hair loss that follows administration of anticancer chemotherapeutic agents, radiation treatment, and various chemicals.[10] Chemotherapy-induced alopecia (CIA) has an estimated incidence of 65% and is considered one of the most traumatic aspects of chemotherapy by female patients.[11] CIA results from the direct toxic insult to the rapidly dividing hair follicle cells in anagen, leading to abrupt cessation of mitotic activity. As a result, the growing hair shaft is only partially keratinized, causing hair fiber breakage. Chemotherapy-induced hair shedding begins 1 to 3 weeks after initiation of treatment and is usually complete at 1 to 2 months.[11] Anagen effluvium differs from telogen effluvium in that it is not dependent on the transition of hair follicles from anagen to telogen with subsequent release of telogen hairs. As most scalp hairs are in anagen at any given time, the resulting hair loss from anagen effluvium is copious and apparent. CIA affects mostly scalp hairs and to a variable degree terminal hairs at other sites such as eyebrows, eyelashes, axillary, and pubic hairs. CIA is usually reversible; hair regrowth takes place at the cessation of treatment.[12] A change in hair color and texture as it regrows is commonly reported among patients.[10] Permanent diffuse hair loss is known to occur following busulfan chemotherapy in patients undergoing bone marrow transplantation.[13]

Anagen effluvium is induced by antineoplastic medications, most commonly alkylating agents, antimetabolites, vinca alkaloids, and topoisomerase inhibitors.[14,15] The degree of hair loss is dependent on the route, dose, and schedule of the chemotherapy agent.[16] Doxorubicin-containing chemotherapy regimens result in total alopecia in most patients receiving this treatment.[17] Hair loss is seen more frequently and is more severe with combination chemotherapy than with a single chemotherapy agent.[18]

Minoxidil, used to treat androgenetic alopecia in both men and women, has been shown to reduce the duration of alopecia caused by chemotherapy. However, minoxidil is not effective in preventing initial alopecia due to chemotherapy agents.[17] Scalp cooling has been reported as an effective method of preventing chemotherapy-induced alopecia, especially when anthracyclines or taxanes are used.[19] It involves cooling of the scalp with cold air or liquid. It produces vasoconstriction of the scalp vessels, leading to reduced blood flow to hair follicles during chemotherapy, thus minimizing exposure to antineoplastic agents in plasma. It is also thought to decrease hair follicle biochemical activity, making it less susceptible to damage by cytotoxic agents. Guidelines on optimal method, temperature, and duration of scalp cooling do not exist at present. Minoxidil should not be used in patients with haematological malignancies undergoing chemotherapy with a curative intent.[19]

TELOGEN EFFLUVIUM

The term telogen effluvium refers to excessive loss of telogen hairs due to an abnormality of hair cycling.[1] Drug-induced telogen effluvium mainly involves premature interruption of hair growth with an early entry of anagen follicles into the resting phase, leading to a noticeable increase in hair shedding 2 to 3 months later. There is an increase in the proportion of telogen hairs on the scalp in telogen effluvium.[9] The choice of investigations to ascertain the cause of telogen hair loss is guided by history including history of known triggers and duration of hair loss at presentation. Some of the common causes of telogen effluvium include thyroid disease, childbirth, and medications.

Acute telogen effluvium is defined as hair loss present for less than 6 months, whereas in chronic telogen effluvium, excessive hair shedding lasts for longer than 6 months. Several conditions and physiologic states lead to acute telogen effluvium including systemic disease, drugs, fever, psychoemotional stress, weight loss, –childbirth, iron and vitamin D deficiencies, and inflammatory scalp disorders.[20] Interruption of oral contraceptives may also cause an acute telogen effluvium. Management of acute telogen effluvium is focused on identifying and treating the underlying cause.

Chronic telogen effluvium is an idiopathic disease entity characterized by chronic and fluctuating increases in telogen hair shedding without any loss of hair density.[21] Women may present with increased telogen hair shedding of more than 6 months duration, but with no visible reduction in hair density over the crown. The diagnosis of drug-induced telogen hair loss is made by demonstrating compatible chronology of drug exposure and the onset of hair loss and exclusion of other causes of alopecia. If a particular drug is suspected, testing involves cessation of the drug for at least 3 months. Regrowth following withdrawal of the drug and recurrence of hair loss on re-exposure to it supports the diagnosis of medication-induced alopecia.[22]

Several medications have been shown to induce telogen hair loss.

Psychotropics

Psychotropic medications including mood stabilisers (lithium and sodium valproate) and antidepressants can cause hair loss as an adverse effect of the medication. Several established mood stabilizers including lithium and sodium valproate are potential causes of hair loss. Lithium, commonly used to treat bipolar affective disorder, has a 12% incidence of alopecia[23] and a higher incidence of hair thinning.[24] Alopecia usually occurs 4 to 6 months after starting the medication. Lithium produces an increase in telogen shedding, although the exact mechanism of this remains unknown.[25] Patients also report a change in hair texture while taking lithium.[24] Thyroid function must be checked in these patients presenting with hair loss, as lithium can cause hyperthyroidism and hypothyroidism, the effects of which can manifest as hair changes.[22]

Sodium valproate has also been reported to cause alopecia,[26] which seems to be dose dependent, as reducing the dose reduces the frequency of valproate-induced alopecia[27] and also leads to hair regrowth in patients experiencing valproate-related hair loss.[28] Valproate-associated transient hair loss has also been described in the pediatric population.[28,29] Unlike with lithium and valproate, carbamazepine-induced hair loss is very rare.[18]

Antidepressants may also induce telogen hair loss. Fluoxetine, a selective serotonin reuptake inhibitor, is the most commonly reported antidepressant to cause a telogen hair loss.[30] Increased hair shedding occurs few months to sometimes even a year after starting the mediation.[18] Drug-induced hair loss has been reported in a male teenager treated for depression with low-dose sertraline. The hair loss stopped on cessation of sertraline. The presentation of hair loss is this case was unique in that the patient noticed hair loss several years after starting sertraline.[31] Tricyclic antidepressants may occasionally cause hair loss.[32] Monoamine oxidase inhibitors do not cause hair loss.[18]

Clinicians need to be aware of the potential for some psychotropics to induce hair loss, as this may contribute to noncompliance. Dose reduction or discontinuation of the medication almost always leads to complete hair regrowth.

Anticoagulants

Low molecular weight heparins such as enoxaparin have been known to induce hair loss. The telogen effluvium caused by enoxaparin results from premature transformation of growing hair follicles into the resting phase. Characteristically, there is a latent period of few weeks between drug exposure and increased hair shedding and hair loss.[33] Other low molecular weight heparins, dalteparin[34,35] and tinzaparin,[36] have also been reported to cause patchy alopecia. Less commonly, warfarin-induced alopecia has been described in literature.[37,38]

Cardiovascular Drugs

Beta-adrenoceptor antagonists, commonly used to treat hypertension, have been reported to be associated with alopecia. Metoprolol[39] and propranolol[40–42] have both been described to lead to reversible hair loss from a telogen effluvium. Another group of antihypertensives, the angiotensin-converting enzyme inhibitors, may also be associated with alopecia. Captopril is 1 of several drugs in this group and has been shown to induce a diffuse hair loss.[43] Often the hair loss is in association with other known cutaneous adverse effects. Amiodarone, a popular antiarrhythmic medication, has rarely been reported to be associated with alopecia.[44,45] Hair regrowth was reported on cessation of the medication.

Oral Contraceptives

Telogen effluvium is commonly observed following interruption of long-term oral contraceptive therapy. It has been postulated that the estrogen contained in the contraceptives prolongs anagen duration.[18,46] An alternate proposition is that certain oral contraceptives contain antiandrogens such as drosperidone or cyproterone acetate that arrest androgenetic alopecia, and that cessation of these agents leads to a resumption of a previously unrecognized tendency to androgentic alopecia. Some progesterone-based preparations, including those containing levonorgestrel, norgestrel, and norethisterone, as well as tibolone, may induce or worsen androgenetic alopecia.[47]

Retinoids

Retinoids routinely used in dermatology for a number of conditions, including acne vulgaris and psoriasis, may cause hair loss with visible alopecia in a high proportion of patients. The hair loss is dose-related, and body hair may also be affected. In a few cases, alopecia is severe. Vitamin supplements containing vitamin A commonly induce mild hair loss.[18] In addition, acitretin may also induce changes in hair color, including repigmentation and texture.[48]

Antimicrobials

Isoniazide is an important medication used in combination for the treatment of tuberculosis. Isoniazide-induced hair loss has been reported in a 30-year-old woman receiving combination treatment for pulmonary tuberculosis. Hair loss was reported a month after initiating treatment with isoniazide, and after stopping the treatment, hair regrowth was observed at 2 months. The exact mechanism of isoniazide-induced alopecia is not understood.[49] Other antituberculosis medications may also cause alopecia.[50]

Antiretroviral agents used in the treatment of human immunodeficiency virus (HIV) infection may also cause hair loss. Indinavir therapy has been reported to cause a generalized alopecia, which was reversible on withdrawal of the medication.[51] Combination therapy with more than one antiretroviral agent is associated with severe hair loss.[52]

Androgen Hormones

Androgenetic alopecia is accelerated by androgens. Medical use of testosterone, illicit use of anabolic steroids, and use of proandrogenic vitamin supplements such as DHEA (dihydroepiandosteroine) are relatively widespread in the community and may not be recognized. Oral contraceptives may contain progestogens with proandrogen effects. Also, the Mirena Intrauterine contraceptive device contains levonorgesterol. Alopecia is listed as an adverse event on the product information literature and may be due to exacerbation of androgenetic alopecia.[53]

CICATRICIAL (SCARRING) HAIR LOSS

Several cases of lichen planopilaris of the scalp associated with the use of biologics have been reported. Two cases of new-onset lichen plano-pilaris have been described with etanercept (tumor necrosis factor [TNF]-alpha antagonist) therapy.[54,55] Hair loss started at week 32 of eta-nercept treatment in an adult, and after ceasing the etanercept for 3 months, the scalp began to improve.[54] On reintroduction of the etanercept, the scalp lesions recurred.[54] Lichen planopilaris is rare in children,[56] but a case has been reported during etanercept treatment for psoriasis in an 8 year-old child.[55] Infliximab, another TNF-alpha inhibitor, has also been associated with a case of lichen planopilaris of the scalp and eyebrows in an adult with psoriasis.[57]

The human epidermal receptor (HER) and the epidermal growth factor receptor (EGFR) inhibitors are used with increasing frequency in the treat-ment of various malignancies.[58] The HER family of receptors is a group of tyrosine kinase receptors that affects cell growth and differentiation and includes the HER1 and HER2 receptors.[58] Erlotinib and gefitinib are HER1 tyrosine kinase inhibitors while cetuximab, and panitumab are monoclonal antibodies directed against EGFR (TKIs).[58] Lapati-nib is a HER1 and HER2 TKI.[58] Trastuzumab and pertuzumab are HER2 monoclonal antibody inhib-itors.[58] The HER1 TKIs have been reported to cause a variety of cutaneous adverse effects including nonscarring alopecia.[59,60] Now reports of possible drug-related scarring alopecia have been associated with gefitinib and erlotinib.[61,62] The scalp biopsies of these patients were similar, showing chronic folliculitis and perifolliculitis with lymphocytes, plasma cells, and a few eosinophils and neutrophils, as well as perifollicular fibrosis of the upper follicle consistent with scarring, suggestive of a drug-related scarring alopecia.[61,62] In the case of erlotinib, cessation of the drug for 3 weeks caused an improvement in the scalp and reintroduction a recurrence of the scalp lesions.[62] Folliculitis decalvans has also been reported during erlotinib treatment and responded to animicrobial and topical corticosteroid therapy, allowing the er-lotinib to be continued.[63] Tufted hair folliculitis has been reported during treatment with lapatinib and trastuzumab.[58,64] In the case of lapatinib, there was clinical improvement with dose reduction.[64]

SUMMARY

Drug-induced alopecia usually presents as a diffuse, nonscarring alopecia most commonly involving the scalp. In almost all cases there is recovery of hair loss after discontinuation of the medication. A high index of suspicion should be maintained regarding medication-induced alopecia, especially if other causes have been excluded.

REFERENCES

1. Harrison S, Sinclair R. Telogen effluvium. Clin Exp Dermatol 2002;27(5):389–95.
2. Kligman AM. The human hair cycle. J Invest Derma-tol 1959;33:307–16.
3. Whiting DA. Chronic telogen effluvium. Dermatol Clin 1996;14(4):723–31.
4. Paus R, Cotsarelis G. The biology of hair follicles. N Engl J Med 1999;341(7):491–7.
5. Harrison S, Bergfeld W. Diffuse hair loss: its triggers and management. Cleve Clin J Med 2009;76(6):361–7.
6. Gordon KA, Tosti A. Alopecia: evaluation and treat-ment. Clin Cosmet Investig Dermatol 2011;4:101–6.
7. Blume-Peytavi U, Blumeyer A, Tosti A, et al. S1 guideline for diagnostic evaluation in androgenetic alopecia in men, women and adolescents. Br J Der-matol 2011;164(1):5–15.
8. Pillans PI, Woods DJ. Drug-associated alopecia. Int J Dermatol 1995;34(3):149–58.
9. Mercke Y, Sheng H, Khan T, et al. Hair loss in psycho-pharmacology. Ann Clin Psychiatry 2000;12(1):35–42.
10. Yun SJ, Kim SJ. Hair loss pattern due to chemotherapy-induced anagen effluvium: a cross-sectional observa-tion. Dermatology 2007;215(1):36–40.
11. Trueb RM. Chemotherapy-induced alopecia. Semin Cutan Med Surg 2009;28(1):11–4.
12. Trueb RM. Chemotherapy-induced anagen effluvium: diffuse or patterned? Dermatology 2007;215(1):1–2.
13. Tosti A, Piraccini BM, Vincenzi C, et al. Permanent alopecia after busulfan chemotherapy. Br J Derma-tol 2005;152(5):1056–8.
14. Koppel RA, Boh EE. Cutaneous reactions to chemo-therapeutic agents. Am J Med Sci 2001;321(5):327–35.
15. Espinosa E, Zamora P, Feliu J, et al. Classification of anticancer drugs–a new system based on thera-peutic targets. Cancer Treat Rev 2003;29(6):515–23.
16. Selleri S, Arnaboldi F, Vizzotto L, et al. Epithelium–mesenchyme compartment interaction and oncosis on chemotherapy-induced hair damage. Lab Invest 2004;84(11):1404–17.
17. Duvic M, Lemak NA, Valero V, et al. A randomized trial of minoxidil in chemotherapy-induced alopecia. J Am Acad Dermatol 1996;35(1):74–8.

18. Tosti A, Pazzaglia M. Drug reactions affecting hair: diagnosis. Dermatol Clin 2007;25(2):223–31.

19. Grevelman EG, Breed WP. Prevention of chemotherapy-induced hair loss by scalp cooling. Ann Oncol 2005;16(3):352–8.

20. Tosti A, Piraccini BM, Sisti A, et al. Hair loss in women. Minerva Ginecol 2009;61(5):445–52.

21. Gilmore S, Sinclair R. Chronic telogen effluvium is due to a reduction in the variance of anagen duration. Australas J Dermatol 2010;51(3):163–7.

22. Mortimer PS, Dawber RP. Hair loss and lithium. Int J Dermatol 1984;23(9):603–4.

23. Orwin A. Hair loss following lithium therapy. Br J Dermatol 1983;108(4):503–4.

24. Mccreadie RG, Morrison DP. The impact of lithium in South-west Scotland. I. Demographic and clinical findings. Br J Psychiatry 1985;146:70–4.

25. Dawber R, Mortimer P. Hair loss during lithium treatment. Br J Dermatol 1982;107(1):124–5.

26. Jeavons PM, Clark JE. Sodium valproate in treatment of epilepsy. Br Med J 1974;2(5919):584–6.

27. Despland PA. Tolerance to and unwanted effects of valproate sodium. Praxis (Bern 1994) 1994;83(40): 1132–9 [in French].

28. Henriksen O, Johannessen SI. Clinical and pharmacokinetic observations on sodium valproate—a 5-year follow-up study in 100 children with epilepsy. Acta Neurol Scand 1982;65(5):504–23.

29. Egger J, Brett EM. Effects of sodium valproate in 100 children with special reference to weight. Br Med J (Clin Res Ed) 1981;283(6291):577–81.

30. Ogilvie AD. Hair loss during fluoxetine treatment. Lancet 1993;342(8884):1423.

31. Rais T, Singh T, Rais A. Hair loss associated with long-term sertraline treatment in teenager. Psychiatry (Edgmont) 2005;2(7):52.

32. Warnock JK. Psychotropic medication and drug-related alopecia. Psychosomatics 1991;32(2):149–52.

33. Wang YY, Po HL. Enoxaparin-induced alopecia in patients with cerebral venous thrombosis. J Clin Pharm Ther 2006;31(5):513–7.

34. Barnes C, Deidun D, Hynes K, et al. Alopecia and dalteparin: a previously unreported association. Blood 2000;96(4):1618–9.

35. Apsner R, Horl WH, Sunder-Plassmann G. Dalteparin-induced alopecia in hemodialysis patients: reversal by regional citrate anticoagulation. Blood 2001;97(9):2914–5.

36. Sarris E, Tsele E, Bagiatoudi G, et al. Diffuse alopecia in a hemodialysis patient caused by a low molecular- weight heparin, tinzaparin. Am J Kidney Dis 2003;41(5):E15.

37. Nagao T, Ibayashi S, Fujii K, et al. Treatment of warfarin-induced hair loss with ubidecarenone. Lancet 1995;346(8982):1104–5.

38. Umlas J, Harken DE. Warfarin-induced alopecia. Cutis 1988;42(1):63–4.

39. Graeber CW, Lapkin RA. Metoprolol and alopecia. Cutis 1981;28(6):633–4.

40. Hilder RJ. Propranolol and alopecia. Cutis 1979; 24(1):63–4.

41. Scribner MD. Propranolol therapy. Arch Dermatol 1977;113(9):1303.

42. Martin CM, Southwick EG, Maibach HI. Propranolol induced alopecia. Am Heart J 1973;86(2): 236–7.

43. Leaker B, Whitworth JA. Alopecia associated with captopril treatment. Aust N Z J Med 1984;14(6): 866.

44. Samuel LM, Davie M, Starkey IR. Amiodarone and hair loss. Postgrad Med J 1992;68(803):771.

45. Mcgovern B, Garan H, Kelly E, et al. Adverse reactions during treatment with amiodarone hydrochloride. Br Med J (Clin Res Ed) 1983;287(6386): 175–80.

46. Hair loss and contraceptives. Br Med J 1973; 2(5865):499–500.

47. Se W. Comprehensive dermatological drug therapy. Saunders Elsevier; 2007. p. 431.

48. Seckin D, Yildiz A. Repigmentation and curling of hair after acitretin therapy. Australas J Dermatol 2009;50(3):214–6.

49. Gupta KB, Kumar V, Vishvkarma S, et al. Isoniazid-induced alopecia. Lung India 2011;28(1):60–1.

50. Fitzgerald JM, Turner MT, Dean S, et al. Alopecia side effect of antituberculosis drugs. Lancet 1996; 347(8999):472.

51. Harry TC, Matthews M, Salvary I. Indinavir use: associated reversible hair loss and mood disturbance. Int J STD AIDS 2000;11(7):474–6.

52. Ginarte M, Losada E, Prieto A, et al. Generalized hair loss induced by indinavir plus ritonavir therapy. AIDS 2002;16(12):1695–6.

53. Mirena. Product information leaflet. Bayer HealthCare Pharmaceuticals; 2009.

54. Garcovich S, Manco S, Zampetti A, et al. Onset of lichen planopilaris during treatment with etanercept. Br J Dermatol 2008;158(5):1161–3.

55. Abbasi NR, Orlow SJ. Lichen planopilaris noted during etanercept therapy in a child with severe psoriasis. Pediatr Dermatol 2009;26(1):118.

56. Handa S, Sahoo B. Childhood lichen planopilaris: a study of 87 cases. Int J Dermatol 2001;40:461.

57. Fernandez-Torres R, Paradela S, Valbuna L, et al. Infliximab-induced lichen planopilaris. Ann Pharmacol 2010;44:1501–3.

58. Rosman HS, Anadkat MJ. Tufted hair folliculitis in a woman treated with trastuzumab. Target Oncol 2010;5:295–6.

59. Myskowski PL, Halpern AC. Skin reactions to the new biologic anticancer drugs. Curr Opin Support Palliat Care 2009;3:294–9.

60. Graves JE, Jones BF, Lind AC, et al. Nonscarring alopecia associated with the epidermal growth

factor receptor inhibitor gefitinib. J Am Acad Dermatol 2006;55:349–53.

61. Donovan JC, Ghazarian DM, Shaw JC. Scarring Alopecia Associated with use of the epidermal growth factor receptor inhibitor gefitinib. Arch Dermatol 2008;144(11):1524–5.

62. Hepper DM, Wu P, Anadkat MJ. Scarring alopecia associated with the epidermal growth factor receptor inhibitor erlotinib. J Acad Dermatol 2011; 64(5):996–8.

63. Hoekzema R, Drillenburg P. Folliculitis decalvans associated with erlotinib. Clin Exp Dermatol 2010; 35:916–8.

64. Ena P, Fadda GM, Ena L, et al. Tufted hair folliculitis in a woman treated with lapatinib for breast cancer. Clin Exp Dermatol 2008;33:776–94.

Autoimmune Disease and Hair Loss

Siamak Moghadam-Kia, MD[a], Andrew G. Franks Jr, MD*,[b]

KEYWORDS

- Autoimmune disease • Hair loss • Scalp discoid lupus erythematosus • Lichen planopilaris

KEY POINTS

- Once systemic disease is in remission, it is prudent to recognize the importance of alopecia in the patient's overall sense of well-being and quality-of-life clinical outcome.
- Scarring alopecia (scalp discoid lupus erythematosus) can be the presenting manifestation of systemic lupus erythematosus (SLE).
- Diffuse nonscarring alopecia in lupus is ultimately responsive to treatment of the active systemic disease.
- Severe, often intractable burning pruritus of the scalp is a frequent complaint in dermatomyositis.
- Lichen planopilaris may overlap with or mimic other autoimmune forms of scarring alopecia.
- Alopecia can also be caused or aggravated by medications used to treat systemic autoimmune disease and fibromyalgia.

ALOPECIA IN SYSTEMIC AUTOIMMUNE DISEASE

Patients with systemic autoimmune systemic disease who also have hair loss show lower quality of life (QOL) and mental health scores than patients without this cutaneous manifestation. Patients in remission from their global systemic disease are often left with alopecia, which significantly impairs their self-esteem and interferes with their personal and professional lives. This situation is often not adequately recognized, and withdrawal from social and work functions often leads to or augments long-standing depression in the patient. Our experience at a major tertiary referral center for the cutaneous manifestations of autoimmune disease suggests that once the systemic autoimmune disease is in remission, it is prudent to recognize the importance of alopecia in the patient's overall sense of well-being and QOL clinical outcome.

LUPUS

Hair loss is one of the most common cutaneous signs of systemic lupus erythematosus (SLE) and is present in more than half the patients at some time during the course of their illness.[1] Alopecia can be the presenting manifestation of SLE and may affect the scalp, eyebrows, eyelashes, beard hair, or body hair.[2] Alopecia may be associated with active disease and can also occur or be aggravated because of the medications used to treat lupus. Alopecia in lupus can be scarring, associated with chronic discoid lupus, or nonscarring, as is often seen in acute lupus. Overlapping components are frequently identified. The Systemic Lupus International Collaborating Clinics (SLICC) has recently recommended revision of the current American College of Rheumatology SLE classification criteria.[3] Discoid lupus had always been present in the most widely used classification criteria for SLE, including the SLICC classification criteria. However, nonscarring alopecia is again being suggested to be included in the newest revision as an individual criterion for SLE, as it was in the original 1971 American Rheumatism Association criteria.[4]

Nonscarring Alopecia

Nonscarring alopecia in lupus often develops during flares of acute systemic disease and can occur under multiple scenarios. One is telogen effluvium, which is a reactive process, not specific to lupus, characterized by a diffuse thinning of the scalp and

[a] University of Pittsburgh Medical Center, Pittsburgh, PA, USA; [b] Skin Lupus & Autoimmune Connective Tissue Disease Center; The Ronald O. Perelman Department of Dermatology, New York University School of Medicine, New York, NY 10016, USA
* Corresponding author.
E-mail address: andrew.franks@nyumc.org

Dermatol Clin 31 (2013) 75–91
http://dx.doi.org/10.1016/j.det.2012.08.008
0733-8635/13/$ – see front matter © 2013 Elsevier Inc. All rights reserved.

hair shedding caused by any metabolic or hormonal stress such as high fever, anemia, or pregnancy, as well as the use of various medications such as antimalarials, glucocorticoids, methotrexate, azathioprine, and mycophenolate. Generally, the normal hair grows back within 6 months, when the antecedent cause resolves. With diffuse hair loss, up to 30% of the hair can be lost before it is cosmetically visible, and in some instances, it may not be noted until higher amounts are lost. Therefore, complaints of hair loss should not be discredited in individuals who still have a full head of hair. Another scenario is the so-called "lupus hair" (**Fig. 1**), which is characterized by dry, course hair prominently over the frontal hairline that is brittle and easily damaged. This condition is almost always observed during exacerbations of SLE and may resolve when the disease activity abates.[5] Considerable overlap occurs between lupus hair and telogen effluvium, the latter usually more extensive and trending posteriorly across the scalp. A distinctive form of alopecia in lupus can occur as a wavy bandlike area of hair loss extending across the peripheral temporal and occipital scalp, looking like the hair has been cut around a bowl placed over the head, it may be both nonscarring or scarring.[6] The term ophiasis pattern (**Fig. 2**) gets its name from the Greek word *ophis*, meaning snake, as if a snake was wrapped around the base of the scalp.

Differential diagnosis

Nonscarring alopecia in lupus must be distinguished from other nonscarring alopecias. The differential diagnosis includes alopecia areata, telogen effluvium, traumatic alopecia, traction alopecia, female pattern hair loss (FPHL), and male pattern alopecia (MPA) (**Box 1**).

Alopecia areata Alopecia areata is a chronic inflammatory disease that causes recurrent nonscarring

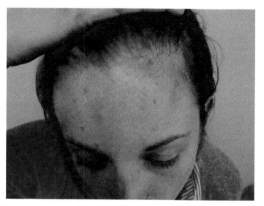

Fig. 1. "Lupus Hair" with recession on frontal scalpline in active SLE.

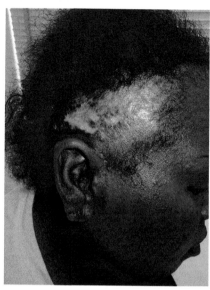

Fig. 2. Lupus ophiasis pattern may be both non-scarring as well as scarring with gradations in between.

alopecia. It is believed to be an autoimmune condition caused by T-cell–mediated immune dysfunction. There is an increased incidence of alopecia areata in patients with other autoimmune conditions such as lupus and discoid lupus erythematosus (DLE).[7] It usually affects the scalp and presents with discrete circular well-delineated smooth patches of complete hair loss, with little or no inflammation. The scalp lesions may be associated with burning sensation and slight erythema. Dermoscopy or 7x loupe magnification can aid in diagnosis and can reveal yellow dots and exclamation-point hairs with a tapering base and a ragged proximal portion, which are diagnostic of the disease. Hairs that grow back are temporarily or permanently hypopigmented. This is another characteristic feature of alopecia areata. Scalp biopsy is useful in equivocal cases.[8,9]

Telogen effluvium Telogen effluvium is a nonscarring alopecia in which a physiologic stressor causes an increased number of hairs going into resting phase (telogen phase). The hair loss in telogen effluvium occurs in a diffuse pattern. A hair-pull test can result in many hairs (more than 2 hairs on a group of 50 hairs) coming out easily from their roots, with an elongated hair bulb visible to the naked eye. The scalp appears nonerythematous and unremarkable. Metabolic testing, including complete blood count, ferritin and other iron studies, thyroid function tests, vitamin D levels, serum chemistries, and liver enzymes, should be considered in the search for systemic causes of telogen effluvium. A complete medication history should be obtained as well, because statins and β-blockers among many other

---

Box 1
Differential diagnosis of nonscarring alopecia in lupus

Alopecia areata	Look for discrete, circular, well-delineated, smooth patches of complete hair loss. Hairs that grow back are temporarily or permanently hypopigmented. Exclamation-point hairs with a tapering base and a ragged proximal portion that can be seen under dermoscopy are diagnostic of the disease
Tellogen effluvium	Look for the history of a stressor or new medication, diffuse pattern of hair loss, and unremarkable examination of the scalp. A positive hair test with elongated hair bulbs is suggestive
Traction alopecia	Look for the history of long-term friction. The location of the hair loss at the temporal and frontal margins of the scalp, with broken fine vellus hairs at different stages, is suggestive
Traumatic alopecia (other than traction alopecia)	Trichotillomania: look for patches of alopecia with angulated and irregular borders and hairs that are broken off at varying lengths
FPHL	Look for progressive thinning of hair in the central portion of the scalp, with hairs of various lengths and diameter and retention of the frontal hair line. The loss is gradual. A family history is suggestive
MPA	Look for progressive thinning of hair in an M-shaped pattern in the frontal hairline, with bitemporal recession. The hair loss is gradual. A family history is suggestive

---

medications may also play a role in the hair loss. Scalp biopsy is usually not necessary.[10,11]

Traction alopecia Traction alopecia is a form of traumatic alopecia that occurs as a result of chronic and excessive tension on the hair follicles. Severe cases of traction alopecia caused by chronic long-term friction can be associated with follicular atrophy and permanent nonscarring alopecia. Obtaining a thorough history including the styling techniques and products used is necessary. The location of the hair loss at the temporal and frontal margins of the scalp, with broken fine vellus hairs at different stages, is a distinctive clinical feature of traction alopecia. The scalp appears normal, without evidence of scarring. Scalp biopsy can be helpful in some cases that are hard to differentiate clinically.[12,13]

Traumatic alopecia (other than traction alopecia) These types of hair loss include trichotillomania and alopecia secondary to physical abuse. Trichotilloma-nia usually occurs in adolescents during times of psychosocial stress. It usually presents with patches of alopecia with angulated and irregular borders and with broken hairs of different lengths, usually located on the frontotemporal or frontoparietal scalp oppo-site the dominant hand. Affected areas are not completely bald. Localized perifollicular erythema or hemorrhage may occur. Scalp biopsy can be helpful in complicated cases. Alopecia caused by physical abuse can be difficult to differentiate from other types of alopecia. If there is concern for abuse, look for historical inconsistencies, signs of trauma

such as scalp hematoma or tenderness, and psychosocial risk factors. Signs of inflammation are absent in all types of traumatic alopecia.[14–16]

FPHL FPHL, also referred to as female androge-netic alopecia, is the most common type of hair loss in adult women.[17] FPHL usually presents with diffuse thinning of the central portion of the scalp, with retention of the frontal hair line. The affected area is usually widened and more obvious. Bitemporal recession as occurs in men is rare. The hair loss in FPHL is gradual, with conversion of pigmented thick terminal hairs to shorter indeterminate hairs and nonpigmented miniaturized vellus hairs. These hairs of various lengths and diameter are classic signs of androge-netic alopecia. A family history of similar hair loss is suggestive of FPHL. A hair-pull test may be helpful (3 or fewer hairs on a group of 20 hairs indicating normal shedding). Follicles are intact. Scalp biopsy may help rule out autoimmune or inflamma-tory disorders.[18,19]

MPA MPA, or androgenetic alopecia, is the most common type of alopecia in adult men.[17] It often affects men before the age of 40 years. MPA usually presents with progressive thinning of hair in an M-shaped pattern in the frontal hairline, with bitem-poral recession that moves posteriorly as the alopecia progresses. Similar to FPHL, the hair loss in MPA is gradual, with hairs undergoing a transition from terminal hairs to indeterminate hairs to vellus hairs. Follicles are intact, without evidence of scar-ring. Taking a family history can be helpful.[18–20]

Scarring Alopecia

Introduction

Scarring alopecia or cicatricial alopecia associated with chronic discoid lupus is categorized as a histologic lupus erythematosus–specific skin disease in the Gilliam classification.[21,22]

Epidemiology and pathogenesis

Scarring alopecia is a frequent complication of DLE (a form of chronic cutaneous lupus erythematosus according to the Gilliam classification[21–24] and has been reported in more than half (34%–56%) of patients with DLE.[25–27] Scalp DLE is present in 4% to 14% of patients with SLE.[28] Scalp DLE can often be the presenting manifestation of systemic lupus erythematosus,[25] and can remain the only manifestation of disease in 11% to 20%.[25,26] It has been shown to correlate with disease chronicity.[25] Scalp DLE affects women more often than men.[25,29,30] Onset of disease is usually between 20 and 30 years of age.[25,30] Onset of disease has been reported to occur less frequently in children and particularly those less than age 10 years.[31,32]

The action of genetic, environmental, immunoregulatory, hormonal, and epigenetic factors involved in the pathogenesis of lupus results in the generation of inflammatory T cells, inflammatory cytokines, autoantibodies, and immune complexes, which may damage various target organs. Progressive replacement of the follicular epithelium by connective tissue and varying degrees of permanent injury to the pluripotent hair follicle stem cell region in the bulge of hair follicles (where the arrector pili muscle connects to the outer root sheath) are similar to other forms of scarring alopecia.[33] Like other variants of cicatricial alopecia, permanent destruction of hair follicles in DLE is frequently associated with a loss of the sebaceous gland.[34] In scalp DLE, the localization of inflammation around the upper, permanent portion of the hair follicle seems to result from antigenic stimulation of the Langerhans cells, which are positioned in the follicular epithelium below the entry of the sebaceous glands into the follicle.[35] These Langerhans cells may then trigger a first-line T-cell–mediated or immune-complex–mediated inflammatory response.[36] This pattern of follicular inflammation is similar to the scarring folliculitides of lichen planopilaris (LPP), allogeneic graft versus host reaction, and atopy. In scalp DLE, the antigenic stimulus affecting the Langerhans cells seems to be ultraviolet light[23,24,35]; however, its role on hair-bearing scalp, a site relatively protected from the sun, needs further study. A study showed that patients with coexisting androgenetic alopecia do not preferentially develop DLE in bald areas.[25] The Koebner phenomenon is associated with DLE. Constant rubbing and scratching can lead to new lesions in affected patients. The proinflammatory cytokines interleukin 17 (IL-17), IL-23, and IL-17–producing cells have been shown to be important in the pathogenesis of lupus and lupus nephritis.[37,38] A recent study of 89 patients with systemic and cutaneous lupus showed that IL-17 isoforms (IL-17A and IL-17F) are implicated not only in SLE but also in DLE immunopathogenesis.[39] Another recent study of 15 patients with lupus suggested that T helper 17 lymphocytes and IL-17 are involved in the immunopathogenesis of both SLE and DLE.[40]

As mentioned earlier, DLE scarring alopecia is considered a primary scarring alopecia, because the target of inflammation seems to be the hair follicle. For primary cicatricial alopecia, several classification systems exist in the literature; however, it is still controversial. In 2001, the North American Hair Research Society developed a provisional classification for primary cicatricial alopecia.[41] This classification scheme is a mechanistic system based on pathologic interpretation of dominant inflammatory cell type existing in and around affected hair follicles in scalp biopsy taken from clinically active lesions. This scheme divides the entities into lymphocytic, neutrophilic, mixed, or unspecific. Alopecia caused by DLE is considered to be the most common primary acquired lymphocytic scarring alopecia.[30]

Clinical manifestations

Early classic lesion presents as a well-circumscribed, erythematous, infiltrative patch with adherent follicular hyperkeratosis. Later, the lesion progresses centrifugally to form a coin-shaped (discoid) white-ivory, atrophic, depressed, smooth plaque with follicular plugging and adherent scale with an elevated, active border (**Fig. 3**). Telangiectasia are usually also present.[29,42–45] The mnemonic PASTE is helpful to describe the lesion: plugging, atrophy, scale, telangiectasia, erythema. Patients may have features

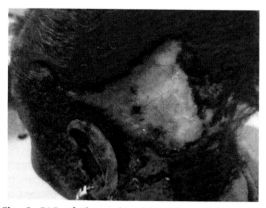

Fig. 3. DLE of the scalp with widespread scarring alopecia. Note the active border with follicular plugging.

of classic discoid lesions elsewhere. Concordance of scalp lesions with ear involvement may approach 50%. In darker-skinned individuals, central hypopigmentation and peripheral hyperpigmentation may occur.[46] The scalp lesions may resemble alopecia areata (**Fig. 4**), LPP, or morphea. Discoid lesions below the neck are associated with a higher incidence of coexistent SLE. Discoid lesions of lupus in the scalp may sometimes be pruritic or tender; however, the condition is often asymptomatic. The patients might report that ultraviolet exposure worsens their symptoms, but because of lag time between exposure and production of an active lesion, this may go unrecognized. Recently, smoking has been found to increase the incidence of facial and scalp DLE and also make it more recalcitrant to treatment.

Diagnosis

The initial approach to the patient with scalp DLE should include examination of the entire scalp, assessing the location and pattern of hair loss and also presence of extracranial cutaneous and systemic features. Scalp biopsy with adjunctive use of direct immunofluorescence is helpful in establishing the diagnosis, evaluating the degree of inflammation, and differentiation of scalp DLE from other primary lymphocytic cicatricial alopecias, respectively. Punch or excisional scalp biopsy specimens should be from the border of early clinically active disease, at least 4 mm in diameter, and extend into the fat. Shave biopsy does not provide the pathologist with what is required to correctly secure the diagnosis. Ideally, 2 biopsy specimens, 1 for standard hematoxylin-eosin sections and 1 for direct immunofluorescence, may be obtained.[42,47] The major histopathologic features include follicular hyperkeratosis, epidermal atrophy, superficial and deep periadnexal lymphocytic infiltrates, thickened basement membrane, and basal vacuolar degeneration at the dermal-epidermal junction. Mucin deposition in the papillary dermis

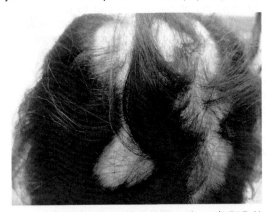

Fig. 4. "Alopecia areata-like" pattern in early DLE. No evident scarring is discernible.

and fibrosis are also often identified. A lumpy-bumpy pattern of granular deposits of C3 and IgG (less commonly IgM) at the dermal-epidermal junction or the junction of the follicular epithelium and dermis is typical in active lesions. Some of these histopathologic aspects can resemble those found in LPP, another inflammatory scarring alopecia, but the clinical and histopathologic distinctions are usually clear.[43]

Differential diagnosis

DLE scarring alopecia must be distinguished from other conditions that cause alopecia. The differential diagnosis of scalp DLE includes LPP, radiation-induced alopecia, central centrifugal cicatricial alopecia (CCCA), sarcoidosis, morphea, psoriasis, burn scar, and squamous cell carcinoma. In addition, a variety of other scalp conditions such as tinea capitis can be inflammatory and must also be considered. Less commonly, nonscarring alopecia can be confused for scalp DLE (**Box 2**).

LPP LPP, also known as follicular lichen planus, can cause scarring alopecia over time. As in lichen planus, LPP is an autoimmune condition, which is most likely caused by cell-mediated immune dysfunction. Similar to the pattern of follicular inflammation in scalp DLE, T lymphocytes targeted at follicular antigens are involved. LPP occurs more frequently in women than in men. Patient with lighter skin are more commonly affected than dark-skinned individuals. There are 3 variants of LPP: classic LPP, frontal fibrosing alopecia, and Graham-Little syndrome. Classic LPP is characterized by perifollicular erythema and patches of alopecia with surrounding keratotic plugs. Frontal fibrosing alopecia presents with bandlike scarring alopecia of the frontal hairline, which commonly affects women. Graham-Little syndrome is characterized by scarring alopecia of the scalp, nonscarring alopecia of the pubic and axillary areas, and a lichenoid follicular eruption. In contrast to scalp DLE, erythema is confined to perifollicular areas in LPP. Also, dyspigmentation is less commonly seen. Complaints of persistent and burning pruritus are more common than in lupus. Dermoscopy or 7x loupe magnification can aid in revealing the perifollicular erythema and loss of follicular orifices. A hair-pull test may reveal increased number of anagen hairs. Scalp biopsy performed at the margin of alopecia from the most active area of disease is the most useful test for the diagnosis. Histologic features of LPP include a lichenoid interface inflammation around the infundibulum and isthmus, sparing the hair bulb. Hyperkeratosis, acanthosis, and hypergranulosis can also be seen. In advanced disease, significant perifollicular lamellar fibrosis can be seen. Direct immunofluorescence is nonspecific

---

Box 2
Differential diagnosis of scarring alopecia associated with discoid lupus

LPP	Look for erythema that is confined to perifollicular areas (in contrast to scalp DLE) and keratotic plugs surrounding the patches of alopecia. Loss of follicular orifices can be viewed under dermoscopy. Dyspigmentation, compared with scalp DLE, is less common
CCCA	Look for shiny scarring alopecia, usually seen from the vertex forward. The presence of a burning sensation or pruritus in the area of hair loss can help. Premature desquamation of the inner root sheath in scalp biopsy is suggestive
Radiation-induced alopecia	Look for the history of radiation exposure, and regular and sharp borders. Decreased number of follicular units with fibrosis of adjacent collagen in scalp biopsy is suggestive
Squamous cell carcinoma	Look for long-standing hyperkeratotic or ulcerated lesions and scars. Biopsy is needed to confirm the diagnosis
Tinea capitis	Look for signs of inflammation in the scalp, including erythema, and scaling. Positive fungal culture and examination of plucked hairs with potassium hydroxide are diagnostic

---

and may show colloid body staining with IgM. These histopathologic features can sometimes resemble those found in scalp DLE.[48–50]

CCCA Formerly known as follicular degeneration syndrome, CCCA is a slowly progressive scarring alopecia, which usually occurs in women. CCCA usually presents with increased follicular spacing and circle-shaped, shiny flesh-colored, smooth scarring alopecia. In contrast to scalp DLE, CCCA usually involves the crown or vertex and expands centrifugally. The presence of burning sensation or pruritus in the area of hair loss can also help to distinguish CCCA from other types of scarring alopecia. A characteristic histologic feature of CCCA on scalp biopsy is premature desquamation of the inner root sheath.[12,51]

Radiation-induced alopecia Radiation-induced alopecia commonly occurs after therapeutic radiation for head and neck cancers or inadvertent overdose. Low radiation dose leads to reversible alopecia. Higher doses can result in severe erythema weeks after the radiation exposure followed by poikilodermatous changes and irreversible scarring alopecia. In contrast to scalp DLE, radiation-induced alopecia often has regular and sharp borders. Radiation-induced alopecia is localized to the treatment zone, and the shape and pattern of the alopecia are relevant to the radiation delivery window. Histopathologic features of radiation-induced alopecia include decreased number of follicular units with fibrosis or hyalinization of adjacent collagen.[52,53]

Squamous cell carcinoma DLE lesions and particularly long-standing hyperkeratotic lesions and scars of chronic DLE are believed to be a predisposing factor for squamous cell carcinoma, with a high rate of local recurrence and metastasis.[54,55] Close observation of every alopecic area is mandatory to determine ulcerated or hyperkeratotic lesions, all of which should be biopsied.[23,24]

Tinea capitis Tinea capitis (trichophyton tonsurans infection of the scalp) is usually associated with signs of inflammation, including erythema and scaling. Cervical adenopathy can be present. Positive fungal culture and examination of plucked hairs with potassium hydroxide are diagnostic for tinea capitis.

Therapy and prognosis
DLE-related alopecia is usually irreversible if not treated early to prevent and mediate the inflammation that affects the upper portion of the hair follicle, including critical elements within the midfollicle in the region of the bulb required for follicular reconstruction. In contradistinction, nonscarring alopecia, such as alopecia areata that affects the lower portion of the hair follicle and not the midfollicle area of the stem-cell–containing bulb, has the potential for regrowth of the hair.[30] DLE scarring alopecia can lead to considerable societal costs and reduced QOL. A recent study by Ferraz and colleagues[56] showed that patients with lupus with alopecia had lower QOL. In contrast, diffuse nonscarring alopecia in lupus is usually responsive to treatment of the lupus; however, it can occasionally be persistent, particularly in individuals with persistent active systemic disease.[1] **Table 1** shows the therapeutic algorithm from New York University (NYU) Skin Lupus and Autoimmune Connective Tissue Disease Center.

DERMATOMYOSITIS

Dermatomyositis (DM) is a systemic autoimmune connective tissue disease that is classified as an

Table 1

Systemic Autoimmune Disease	Therapy

Cutaneous Lupus including Scarring Alopecia	Systemic therapy:
	1st line:
	    Antimalarials:
	      - Hydroxycholoroquine sulfate: usually the first to be started.
	      - Initial blood tests: G6PD, CBC with differential, LFT's.
	      - Eye exam within the first month and annually thereafter.
	      - Induction dose (1st week): 200 mg M-W-F.
	      - 2nd wk: 200 mg daily with dinner.
	      - 200 mg daily or BID (maximum dose 6.5 mg/kg/d to avoid retinopathy.
	      - May require 8–16 wk for therapeutic onset.
	      - Chloroquine phosphate: alternative to hydroxycholoroquine.
	      - May be useful when sulfate allergy precludes use of hydroxycholoroquine.
	      - May be useful if patients do not respond to hydroxycholoroquine sulfate. Do not combine with hydroxycholoroquine.
	      - 250 mg daily or BID (maximum dose 3.0 mg/kg/d to avoid retinopathy.
	      - Quinacrine: may be added to either hydroxycholoroquine or chloroquine for increased response; or used alone as a single agent.
	      - Useful as single agent in patients with higher risk for retinopathy, e.g, diabetic or hypertensive patients. Risk of retinopathy very low.
	      - Single agent dose: 50–200 mg/d. Doses above 100 mg/day will cause considerable hyperpigmentation.
	      - When added to either hydroxycholoroquine or, chloroquine, doses of 50–100 mg every other day to daily may be used.
	    Most (75%) of cutaneous LE patients respond well to antimalarials whether single agent or combined with quinacrine.
	    Smoking inhibits antimalarial activity and requires, not require smoking cessation for therapeutic responses, particularly of the face and scalp.
	      - Dapsone may be useful in those patients with a neutrophilic infiltrate such as acute bullous LE, and may also be tried in patients who are intolerant to the antimalarials.
	      - Baseline G6PD, CBC w diff, and LFT's and careful follow-up as dose titration is attempted.
	      - Dose range: start with 25 mg/d and maximum doses between at about 150 mg. If no response higher doses are generally no more effective but increase the potential for hemolysis and leucopenia.
	      - Oral steroids may be utilized in the acute induction phase in those patients with severe disease as well as high potential for scarring while the maintenance drugs are not yet in full therapeutic efficacy range.

(continued on next page)

Table 1
(continued)

Systemic Autoimmune Disease	Therapy
	2nd line:

Mycophenolate mofetil:
- Generally well-tolerated. Less drug-related hair loss in most patients than with azathioprine or methotrexate. Large therapeutic window usually 1–3 g/d for cutaneous disease. Used for initial Rx and maintenance in lupus nephritis.
- May have fewer side effects in lower dose range.
- Long-term induction and remission studies are ongoing.

Azathioprine:
- May be useful in patients resistant or intolerant of anti malarials or mycophenalate.
- Acetylation status useful in predicting tolerability.
- Low doses may be effective for DLE of scalp, as well as other forms of cutaneous lupus.
- 25–50 mg/d and up to 100 mg/d.
- GI intolerance, increase in LFT's and decreased WBC's.

Methotrexate:
- May be used in recalcitrant DLE but drug-related hair loss may be significant.
- Folic acid replacement useful on days not taking mtx
- R/o Hep B,C Watch LFT's and WBCs.
- Oral single dosing up to 15–25 mg. Older q12 dosing only useful if gi intolerance. Older cell cycle data no longer valid.
- IM dosing reduces GI intolerance more than SC.
- Watch LFT's, WBCs & idiosynchratic pulmonary infiltrates, heralded by chronic cough.

Thalidomide:
- Rapid clinical response: within 2–3 wk.
- Full response in 2–3 mo.
- Effective in 75% of patients who are refractory to antimalarials alone.
- Induction dose: 50–100 mg t.i.w. to daily.
- May be used in combination with antimalarials.
- Maintenance dose 25–100 mg q 3 days to daily.
  - Not a DMARD: Discontinuation may lead to rapid clinical relapse.
  - Peripheral neuropathy, thrombophilia (do not use on patients with lupus anticoagulants or ACAs), and hypotension.

Cyclosporine:
- Used in recalcitrant DLE.
- Low doses may be effective; eg, 25–100 mg/d.
- Watch LFTs and WBC's, and serum creatinine.
- Gingival hyperplasia may occur.

Tacrolimus:
- Use over 1 year not recommended because of cumulative effect on renal function.
- Similar use and toxicity as cyclosporine.

(continued on next page)

Table 1
(continued)

Systemic Autoimmune Disease	Therapy
	3rd line: TNF alpha inhibitors: - Anti-TNF antibodies: Infliximab, adalimumab. - TNF soluble receptor: etanercept. - Improve photosensitive rash and resolve recalcitrant DLE including lupus profundus. - May provoke autoantibody production such as anti-dsDNA, Ro, ANA. - May provoke reactivation of underlying, previously stable SLE or cause lupus-like syndrome during therapy. - Patients with continued scarring, especially of the face and scalp, who are recalcitrant to more conventional treatment may benefit. Monitor clinically and serologically for evidence of increased systemic activity. Rituximab: - Chimeric monoclonal antibody. - Targets the CD-20 antigen on B-cell precursors and mature B-cells. - Depletes B-cells and turns down production of autoantibodies. - Autoimmune disease dosing is usually 500 mg–1000 g IV × 2 doses two weeks apart. Pre-infusion steroids used due to frequent allergic infusion reactions. Onset of action may take weeks to months. Remissions may last for one year or more. Belimumab: - Acts by restoring potential for autoantibody-producing B-cells to undergo normal process of cell death. - FDA approved for use in patient with SLE who have active serology. - Good therapeutic effect on the cutaneous disease & hair loss. - Minimal infusion issues or side effects. - Well tolerated in multiple clinical scenarios. Retinoids: - Both isotretinoin and acitretin may benefit some patients, especially hypertrophic DLE as well as SCLE. Topical thrapy: - Topical steroids, intralesional steroids, calcineurin inhibitors (pimecrolimus or tacrolimus). - Custom formulated higher strengths of tacrolimus (up to 0.3% [not 0.03%]) in alcohol and lotion base may be useful in recalcitrant scalp lesions.

idiopathic inflammatory myopathy.[57] Recent data suggest a trimodal incidence, but it can affect any age group. There is a female predominance (female/male, 2:1).[58] Its association with malignancy, particularly in patients aged 50 years and older, is well documented. DM is associated with striking hallmark skin findings, including Gottron sign and papules over the distal interphalangeal, proximal interphalangeal, and metacarpophalangeal joints. Also, a component of Gottron may include the elbows, knees, and ankles, with similar erythematous and scaling plaques, sometimes mimicking psoriasis. The heliotrope rash affects the eyelids, with a lilac to violaceous rash with or without edema, and is prone to ulcerate. Early in its course, it may mimic contact dermatitis, seborrheic dermatitis, or ocular rosacea. The shawl sign occurs on the nape of the neck, extending out along the shoulders. The V sign affects the area on the lower anterior neck to upper chest. Linear extensor erythema may run down the arms and legs, with sharp cutoffs on the edges, and extend down the hand over the extensor tendons, sometimes obscuring the Gottron papules. The pocket or holster sign occurs, generally symmetrically, on the upper outer thighs near the trochanteric bursae, and if this is the only cutaneous finding, it may elude clinical diagnosis because of its peculiar location. The periungual capillaries reveal corkscrewing, microthrombi and dropout, are often found with cuticular disarray, and are often associated with Raynaud phenomenon. This zone is easily evaluated with a dermatoscope, and when these typical changes are shown, it can greatly expedite the diagnosis, particularly in amyopathic patients who may complain only of scalp involvement. Mechanic's hand is another classic feature, with fissuring suggestive of a contact dermatitis. Typically, the fissures are on the lateral sides of the fingers and extend to the thenar eminence. The poikiloderma (hypopigmentation and hyperpigmentation, telangiectasia, and epidermal atrophy) is a later manifestation, and localizes commonly to the V-area of the neck, as well as the shawl distributed zone along the shoulders and upper back. Calcinosis cutis is usually also a later manifestation and can be severe, painful, and disabling. Extension of the calcium into the muscle is not uncommon, particularly in younger patients, leading to flexion contractures as well as large, recalcitrant ulceration. Involvement of the scalp manifested as diffuse, confluent, atrophic, violaceous, scaly plaques, is commonly seen in DM and can be its presenting manifestation (**Fig. 5**). Contact dermatitis, seborrheic dermatitis, and psoriasis are the usual first clinical impressions, and may elude therapy until a scalp biopsy reveals the true nature of the process. Alopecia tends to be generalized to the entire scalp (**Fig. 6**), but is

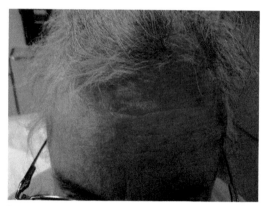

Fig. 6. Generalized non-scarring alopecia in DMS. Scale may be prevalent, mimicking seborrhea or psoriasis.

often more subtle than in lupus, In a case series of 17 patients with DM, scalp involvement was noted in 14, with alopecia present in 6 of the 14 patients.[59] Adult-onset classic DM and clinically amyopathic DM can be associated with scaly scalp and nonscarring, diffuse alopecia, which often follows a flare of the systemic disease.[60–63] This diffuse, violaceous, scaly, nonscarring alopecia is one of the characteristic cutaneous features of DM, despite not being pathognomonic.[61,62] Nonscarring alopecia has also been reported in juvenile-onset DM.[64] Although DM may rarely cause cicatricial alopecia,[65] it may frequently overlap with the scarring alopecia of other connective tissue diseases, particularly scleroderma and lupus.[66] The clinical features that can help to distinguish DM from lupus include the often-striking violaceous color of the rash in contrast to the pinkish-red hue more often seen in lupus. In addition, severe, often intractable burning pruritus of the scalp is a frequent complaint in DM, and less common in lupus. The histopathologic features include epidermal atrophy, basement membrane degeneration, vacuolar changes in the basal keratinocyte layer, and a perivascular lymphocytic infiltrate, which is sparser and more superficial than in lupus. However, the changes may be difficult to distinguish from those seen in lupus on light microscopy. As in lupus, the dermis may be pale as a result of the accumulation of mucin usually confined solely to the papillary zone. Immunofluorescence microscopy frequently reveals deposition of immunoglobulin at the dermal-epidermal junction, but of less intensity than seen in lupus. Complement deposition, particularly the terminal components C5 to C9, are a signature feature of DM, specifically when found in the superficial dermal perivascular zone as opposed to the dermal-epidermal junction alone.[67]

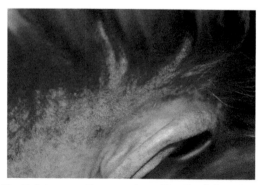

Fig. 5. Intense erythema, scale and localized alopecia in DMS. Burning pain is common.

Several serologic studies may be unique to DM. Anti-Jo antibody and, more recently, MDA-5 antibody as well as anti-Ku antibody may be associated with increased cardiopulmonary involvement. MDA-5 is also associated with increase scalp involvement and hair loss.[68] P140/155 may be associated with an increased risk of malignancy in older patients. Electromyographic, radiographic and muscle biopsy may be necessary depending on the clinical circumstance. A combination of type 2 muscle fiber atrophy and lymphocytic infiltrate in both a perifascicular and a perivascular distribution is considered classic for DM.[69] **Table 2** shows the therapeutic algorithm from NYU.

SCLERODERMA

Scleroderma is a divided into generalized and localized forms. The generalized form, also called systemic sclerosis (SSc) with characteristic internal organ involvement, is further subdivided into diffuse and limited types. Renal disease is more common in the diffuse form, and cardiopulmonary disease in the limited form. The localized form is not associated with internal involvement and is also called morphea.

Generalized scleroderma is more common in women, and the peak age of onset is between 30 and 50 years. The disease involves autoantibodies to characteristic cellular antigens, which are associated with sclerotic changes of the skin. Scleroderma is different from other autoimmune diseases involving skin (lupus, DM), because epithelial injury does not occur.[70] The sclerotic changes can affect the connective tissue of any organ. As stated, there are 2 major subsets of generalized scleroderma or SSc based on the degree of cutaneous involvement: limited

Table 2	
Systemic Autoimmune Disease	Therapy

Dermatomyositis	Targeted therapy depends on the presence of muscle disease or other organ involvement.
	DM/PM:
	- Glucocorticoids (standard if myositis present).
	  - 0.5–2 mg/kg/d of prednisone as induction until CPK and/or aldolase begins to fall.
	  - Taper as muscle enzymes fall to avoid cumulative toxicity.
	- Steroid-sparing agents:
	  - 2nd line therapy. Usually added to glucocorticoids for maintenance control and in cases of rapid deterioration, vasculitis, or presence of anti-synthetase antibodies.
	- Methotrexate:
	  - Most often used agent after or with glucocorticoids.
	  - Starting dose: 7.5 mg/wk; increase by 2.5 mg weekly to maximum dose: 25 mg/wk. Administered orally or intramuscularly.
	- Azathioprine:
	  - Starting dose: 25–50 mg/d, maximum dose: 300 mg/d.
	  - Dose of glucocorticoids should be reduced.
	- Mycophenolate mofetil.
	  - Starting dose 500–1000 mg/d, maximum dose 2–3 gms/d.
	  - Dose of glucocorticoids should be reduced.
	- Plaquenil and other antimalarials should be used with caution because some patients will have idiosyncratic flare targeting the zones of cutaneous activity.
	- IVIG may be effective especially in those patients who are prone to or already are infected. Doses from 1 g/kg to 3 g/kg in divided doses with frequency dependent on disease activity.
	- Rituximab has been utilized in refractory patients. Autoimmune dosing is 750–1000 mg IV q 2 weeks × 2 doses only.
	- Topical Rx: as in cutaneous lupus. For scalp involvement, topical tacrolimus is especially useful.

cutaneous SSc, previously called CREST syndrome, and diffuse cutaneous SSc. SSc is characterized by typical cutaneous changes (**Fig. 7**), including variable extent and severity of skin thickening, shiny and wrinkleless skin, diffuse hyperpigmentation, and depigmentation with sparing of perifollicular skin, leading to a salt-and-pepper appearance, and flat, polygonal telangiectasias, the last most common in the limited form. SSc usually affects the fingers, hands, and face. Autoantibodies, including antinuclear antibodies with a nucleolar pattern as well as anti-Scl-70 antibody in the diffuse form, and anti-centromere antibodies in the limited form, assist in the diagnosis.[70,71] Cyclophosphamide, the prototypic alkylating and immunosuppressant agent that has been used to treat systemic scleroderma renal disease, is associated with alopecia.[72]

The localized form of scleroderma is also known as morphea. Morphea has many etiologies and may occur at any age, but most frequently affects young adults and children. There is a female/male predominance of about 3:1, and the condition is less common in blacks.[73,74] Like SSc, morphea is also characterized by spontaneous sclerosis of the skin, but lacks internal organ involvement, as well as Raynaud phenomenon and sclerodactyly. It involves transition from an early inflammatory stage to sclerosis and subsequent atrophy after 2 to 3 years. It usually presents with shiny, oval, 10 cm or greater in diameter, firm, indurated plaques with surrounding erythema as well as central reticulated telangiectasias. The surrounding red or violaceous rim and the reticulated telangiectasias may fade and change to hypopigmentation or hyperpigmentation with time. Hair follicles and sweat glands are absent in well-developed lesions. The lesions usually affect the trunk and extremities.[73–75] The most common forms of morphea

are plaque, generalized, and linear variants.[76] A form of linear morphea that affects the face or scalp, usually the midline or paramedian forehead, is known as en coup de sabre (**Fig. 8**) because the lesion is reminiscent of a cut from a sword. It usually presents as a unilateral, shiny, hypopigmented or hyperpigmented, atrophic, linear plaque.[77] It can present with more than 1 lesion, typically following Blashcko lines, extend onto the scalp, and cause permanent cicatricial alopecia secondary to loss of hair follicles.[78] The diagnosis is usually made clinically but can be confirmed with a skin biopsy. Biopsies at early stages reveal an intense inflammatory infiltrate at the margin, and biopsies at later stages reveal waning inflammatory infiltrate, with infiltration of lymphocytes and plasma cells at the border and central fibrosis in the lower two-thirds of the dermis and upper subcutaneous tissue and eventually disappearance of pilosebaceous units and eccrine sweat glands, and effacement of the rete ridges (similar to the changes seen in SSc).[77] Ultrasonography can be used to assess skin thickness, which correlates with disease severity,[79] but a Rodnan skin score can also be used on individual lesions to assess sclerosis. Although no drugs are currently approved or adequately shown by clinical study to modify the course of scleroderma, current research has focused on specific organ system involvement as well as global reversal of the disease. Early phases of the disease may benefit from antiinflammatory protocols and later phases from antifibrotic therapy. **Table 3** shows the NYU protocol for cutaneous involvement.

FIBROMYALGIA

Primary fibromyalgia must be distinguished from secondary fibromyalgia, which is a soft tissue

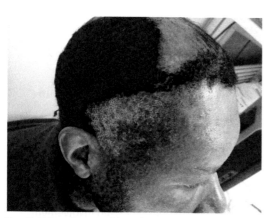

Fig. 7. Scleroderma with ophiasis pattern of alopecia with residual "salt & pepper" appearance.

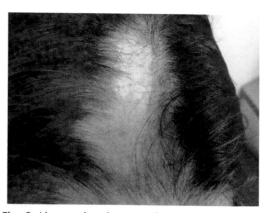

Fig. 8. Linear scleroderma with atrophic plaque of scarring alopecia extending into scalp.

Table 3

Systemic Autoimmune Disease	Therapy

Localized Scleroderma (Morphea) including related hair loss	NYU Rx protocol for Morphea:
	Because of the varied etiology of morphea: infectious, autoimmune, heavy metal, initial assessment includes a Western Blot (WB) for Borrelia which is prevalent in our area. Our definition of WB+ for the purposes of this protocol is that which is suggestive of exposure, but not necessarily meeting CDC criteria for Lyme Disease per se. Autoimmune serology (AISer) including ANA by IFA, ssDNA, Rheumatoid Factor, anti-centromere, anti-Sc-70, as well as a screen for heavy metals including inorganic mercury and cadmium.
	   - If WB + and AISer–then we treat with four three week cycles of doxycycline with one week off between cycles to avoid cumulative bowel toxicity.
	   - If WB + and AISer + then we treat with 3 wk of antibiotics and assess for systemic scleroderma or other autoimmune disease.
	   - If WB – and AISer – then we treat with 3 wk of antibiotics and follow with anti-inflammatory, antifibrotic, and/or phototherapy.
	   - If WB – and AISer + then we assess for systemic scleroderma or other autoimmune disease.
	After the above initial protocol, we then may choose any of the modalities below with the understanding that treatment in early disease (active borders, reticulated central erythema) may be directed at decreasing inflammation while anti-fibrotic modalities are necessary in older lesions.
	Topical as well as intra-lesional corticosteroids may be used to reduce inflammation in early lesions but should be avoid in lichen sclerosus atrophicus variants.
	Vitamin D analogues have been shown to inhibit fibroblast activity and TGF-beta production as well as having anti-inflammatory effects.
	Calcipotriene or calcitriol topicals may have both anti-inflammatory as well as anti-fibrotic mechanisms.
	Topical calcineurin inhibitors may also be utilized to reduce inflammation but have not been shown to have anti-fibrotic potential.
	Oral calcitriol may also be utilized as an anti-fibrotic agent in doses of 25–50 micrograms/day. Watch serum calcium levels.
	Methotrexate is used in early and progressive lesions for its anti-inflammatory effect and has little benefit to late lesions as it is actually pro-fibrotic due to its effect on the adensosine receptor. Both oral and intramuscular doses range up to 25 mg/weekly.
	Antimalarial therapy may be useful in early lesions or when autoimmune disease is coexistent.
	Colchicine modulates matrix metalloproteins which are increased in fibrotic skin and also decreases pro-collagen synthesis and may be utilized in low doses of 0.6–1.2 mg/d.
	The tetracycline family of antibiotics such as doxycycline are modulators of inflammation and also have an effect on matrix metalloproteins. Because of this dual effect, they may be useful in both in patients with or without Borrelia infection in doses of 50–100 mg bid.
	Phototherapy with broadband UVA, narrowband UVA (UVA1), or psoralen plus UVA (oral or bath) may soften the skin.
	Narrowband UVB therapy also has been shown to soften plaques of morphea. Combining UV therapy with topical corticosteroids, vitamin D analogues or calcineurin inhibitors may also increase effectiveness. Intense pulse light (IPL) has also been effective in many of our patients, especially for residual PIH.

inflammatory component of many autoimmune diseases. Primary fibromyalgia is believed to be a functional somatic syndrome caused by alterations in central nervous system pain processing. It is characterized by chronic generalized musculoskeletal pain, fatigue, and multiple tender points at specific soft tissue locations. There is typically no evidence of joint or muscle inflammation on physical examination or laboratory testing.[80,81] Fibromyalgia is currently considered to be the most common cause of widespread, musculoskeletal pain in women between 20 and 55 years of age. The prevalence is approximately 2% and increases with age.[82,83] As stated, secondary fibromyalgia may coexist with other inflammatory rheumatic diseases, such as SLE, which can cause nonscarring or scarring alopecia.[84] The medications that are used in the treatment of fibromyalgia can also cause alopecia. Tricyclic antidepressants, including amitriptyline and desipramine, can be associated with alopecia. Serotonin reuptake inhibitors, particularly fluoxetine and citalopram, can rarely (<1%) cause alopecia.

ALOPECIA CAUSED BY MEDICATIONS USED TO TREAT SYSTEMIC AUTOIMMUNE DISEASE AND FIBROMYALGIA

Many drugs that are currently used to treat systemic autoimmune disease have been reported to cause alopecia (**Box 3**). The medication-induced hair loss is usually diffuse, nonscarring, and limited to the scalp. Women are more commonly affected than men.

Box 3
Alopecia caused by medications used to treat systemic autoimmune disease and fibromyalgia

Associated medications

Citalopram[85]

Cyclophosphamide[86]

Danazol[87]

Fluoxetine[88]

Fluvoxamine[89]

Gold[90]

Interferon α[91]

Intravenous immunoglobulin[92]

Leflunomide[93]

Methotrexate[94]

Mycophenolate mofetil[95]

Phenytoin[96]

Tacrolimus[11]

Venlafaxine[97]

REFERENCES

1. Wysenbeek AJ, Leibovici L, Amit M, et al. Alopecia in systemic lupus erythematosus. Relation to disease manifestations. J Rheumatol 1991;18(8):1185–6.
2. McCauliffe DP, Sontheimer RD. Cutaneous lupus erythematosus. In: Schur PH, editor. The clinical management of systemic lupus erythematosus. 2nd edition. Philadelphia: Lippincott; 1996.
3. Petri M, Orbai A, Alarcón G, et al. Derivation and validation of Systemic Lupus International Collaborating Clinics classification criteria for systemic lupus erythematosus. Arthritis Rheum 2012;64(8): 2677–86.
4. Cohen AS, Reynolds WE, Franklin EC, et al. Preliminary criteria for the classification of systemic lupus erythematosus. Bull Rheum Dis 1971;21:643–8.
5. Alarcon-Segovia D, Cetina JA. Lupus hair. Am J Med Sci 1974;267(4):241–2.
6. Ahmed I, Nasreen S, Bhatti R. Alopecia areata in children. J Coll Physicians Surg Pak 2007;17(10): 587–90.
7. Werth VP, White WL, Sanchez MR, et al. Incidence of alopecia areata in lupus erythematosus. Arch Dermatol 1992;128(3):368–71.
8. Alkhalifah A, Alsantali A, Wang E, et al. Alopecia areata update: part I. Clinical picture, histopathology, and pathogenesis. J Am Acad Dermatol 2010;62(2):177–88.
9. Alkhalifah A, Alsantali A, Wang E, et al. Alopecia areata update: part II. Treatment. J Am Acad Dermatol 2010;62(2):191–202.
10. Harrison S, Sinclair R. Telogen effluvium. Clin Exp Dermatol 2002;27(5):389–5.
11. Tosti A, Pazzaglia M. Drug reactions affecting hair: diagnosis. Dermatol Clin 2007;25(2):223–31.
12. Borovicka JH, Thomas L, Prince C, et al. Scarring alopecia: clinical and pathologic study of 54 African-American women. Int J Dermatol 2009;48(8):840–5.
13. Khumalo NP, Jessop S, Gumedze F, et al. Determinants of marginal traction alopecia in African girls and women. J Am Acad Dermatol 2008;59(3): 432–8.
14. Saraswat A. Child abuse and trichotillomania. BMJ 2005;330(7482):83–4.
15. Papadopoulos AJ, Janniger CK, Chodynicki MP, et al. Trichotillomania. Int J Dermatol 2003;42(5):330–4.
16. Whiting DA. Traumatic alopecia. Int J Dermatol 1999;38(Suppl 1):34–44.
17. Olsen EA. Androgenetic alopecia. In: Olsen EA, editor. Disorders of hair growth: diagnosis and treatment. New York: McGraw-Hill; 1994. p. 257–83.

18. Price VH. Treatment of hair loss. N Engl J Med 1999; 341(13):964–73.

19. Olsen EA, Messenger AG, Shapiro J, et al. Evaluation and treatment of male and female pattern hair loss. J Am Acad Dermatol 2005;52(2):301–11.

20. Sinclair R. Male pattern androgenetic alopecia. BMJ 1998;317(7162):865–9.

21. Gilliam JN, Sontheimer RD. Distinctive cutaneous subsets in the spectrum of lupus erythematosus. J Am Acad Dermatol 1981;4(4):471–5.

22. Gilliam JN, Sontheimer RD. Skin manifestations of SLE. Clin Rheum Dis 1982;8(1):207–18.

23. Ross EK, Tan E, Shapiro J. Update on primary cicatricial alopecias [Erratum in: J Am Acad Dermatol. 2005;53(3):496] [review]. J Am Acad Dermatol 2005;53(1):1–37 [quiz: 38–40].

24. Otberg N, Wu WY, McElwee KJ, et al. Diagnosis and management of primary cicatricial alopecia: part I. Skinmed 2008;7(1):19–26.

25. Wilson CL, Burge SM, Dean D, et al. Scarring alopecia in discoid lupus erythematosus. Br J Dermatol 1992;126(4):307–14.

26. Callen JP. Chronic cutaneous lupus erythematosus. Clinical, laboratory, therapeutic, and prognostic examination of 62 patients. Arch Dermatol 1982; 118(6):412–6.

27. de Berker D, Dissaneyeka M, Burge S. The sequelae of chronic cutaneous lupus erythematosus. Lupus 1992;1(3):181–6.

28. Yell JA, Mbuagbaw J, Burge SM. Cutaneous manifestations of systemic lupus erythematosus. Br J Dermatol 1996;135(3):355–62.

29. Whiting DA. Cicatricial alopecia: clinico-pathological findings and treatment. Clin Dermatol 2001;19(2): 211–25.

30. Tan E, Martinka M, Ball N, et al. Primary cicatricial alopecias: clinicopathology of 112 cases. J Am Acad Dermatol 2004;50(1):25–32.

31. George PM, Tunnessen WW Jr. Childhood discoid lupus erythematosus. Arch Dermatol 1993;129(5): 613–7.

32. Moises-Alfaro C, Berrón-Pérez R, Carrasco-Daza D, et al. Discoid lupus erythematosus in children: clinical, histopathologic, and follow-up features in 27 cases. Pediatr Dermatol 2003;20(2):103–7.

33. Cotsarelis G, Sun TT, Lavker RM. Label-retaining cells reside in the bulge area of pilosebaceous unit: implications for follicular stem cells, hair cycle, and skin carcinogenesis. Cell 1990;61(7):1329–37.

34. Sellheyer K, Bergfeld WF. Histopathologic evaluation of alopecias. Am J Dermatopathol 2006;28(3):236–59.

35. Moresi JM, Horn TD. Distribution of Langerhans cells in human hair follicle. J Cutan Pathol 1997;24(10): 636–40.

36. Dutz JP, Sontheimer RD. Pathomechanisms of cutaneous lupus erythematosus. In: Wallace DJ, Hahn BH, editors. Dubois' lupus erythematosus. 6th edition. Philadelphia: Lippincott Williams & Wilkins; 2002. p. 549–71.

37. Crispín JC, Oukka M, Bayliss G, et al. Expanded double negative T cells in patients with systemic lupus erythematosus produce IL-17 and infiltrate the kidneys. J Immunol 2008;181(12):8761–6.

38. Zhang Z, Kyttaris VC, Tsokos GC. The role of IL-23/IL-17 axis in lupus nephritis. J Immunol 2009;183(5): 3160–9.

39. Tanasescu C, Balanescu E, Balanescu P, et al. IL-17 in cutaneous lupus erythematosus. Eur J Intern Med 2010;21(3):202–7.

40. Bălănescu P, Bălănescu E, Tănăsescu C, et al. T helper 17 cell population in lupus erythematosus. Rom J Intern Med 2010;48(3):255–9.

41. Olsen EA, Bergfeld WF, Cotsarelis G, et al. Workshop on Cicatricial Alopecia. Summary of North American Hair Research Society (NAHRS)-sponsored Workshop on Cicatricial Alopecia, Duke University Medical Center, February 10 and 11, 2001. J Am Acad Dermatol 2003;48(1):103–10.

42. Shapiro J. Cicatricial (scarring) alopecias. In: Shapiro J, editor. Hair loss: principles of diagnosis and management of alopecia. London: Martin Dunitz; 2002. p. 155–74.

43. Fabbri P, Amato L, Chiarini C, et al. Scarring alopecia in discoid lupus erythematosus: a clinical, histopathologic and immunopathologic study. Lupus 2004;13(6):455–62.

44. Donnelly AM, Halbert AR, Rohr JB. Discoid lupus erythematosus [review]. Australas J Dermatol 1995; 36(1):3–10 [quiz: 11–2].

45. Headington JT. Cicatricial alopecia. Dermatol Clin 1996;14(4):773–82.

46. Sontheimer RD, McCauliffe DP. Cutaneous manifestations of lupus erythematosus. In: Wallace DJ, Hahn BH, editors. Dubois' lupus erythematosus. 6th edition. Philadelphia: Lippincott Williams & Wilkins; 2002. p. 573–618.

47. Elston DM, McCollough ML, Angeloni VL. Vertical and transverse sections of alopecia biopsy specimens: combining the two to maximize diagnostic yield. J Am Acad Dermatol 1995;32(3):454–7.

48. Assouly P, Reygagne P. Lichen planopilaris: update on diagnosis and treatment. Semin Cutan Med Surg 2009;28(1):3–10.

49. Kang H, Alzolibani AA, Otberg N, et al. Lichen planopilaris. Dermatol Ther 2008;21(4):249–56.

50. Chieregato C, Zini A, Barba A, et al. Lichen planopilaris: report of 30 cases and review of the literature. Int J Dermatol 2003;42(5):342–5.

51. Gathers RC, Lim HW. Central centrifugal cicatricial alopecia: past, present, and future. J Am Acad Dermatol 2009;60(4):660–8.

52. Al-Mohanna H, Al-Khenaizan S. Permanent alopecia following cranial irradiation in a child. J Cutan Med Surg 2010;14(3):141–3.

53. Severs GA, Griffin T, Werner-Wasik M. Cicatricial alopecia secondary to radiation therapy: case report and review of the literature. Cutis 2008;81(2):147–53.

54. Garrett AB. Multiple squamous cell carcinomas in lesions of discoid lupus erythematosus. Cutis 1985;36(4):313–4, 316.

55. Sulica VI, Kao GF. Squamous-cell carcinoma of the scalp arising in lesions of discoid lupus erythematosus. Am J Dermatopathol 1988;10(2):137–41.

56. Ferraz LB, Almeida FA, Vasconcellos MR, et al. The impact of lupus erythematosus cutaneous on the quality of life: the Brazilian-Portuguese version of DLQI. Qual Life Res 2006;15(3):565–70.

57. Dalakas MC, Hohlfeld R. Polymyositis and dermatomyositis. Lancet 2003;362(9388):971–82.

58. Tymms KE, Webb J. Dermatopolymyositis and other connective tissue diseases: a review of 105 cases. J Rheumatol 1985;12(6):1140–8.

59. Kasteler JS, Callen JP. Scalp involvement in dermatomyositis. Often overlooked or misdiagnosed. JAMA 1994;272(24):1939–41.

60. Euwer RL, Sonthheimer RD. Dermatomyositis. In: Sontheimer RD, Provost TT, editors. Cutaneous manifestations of rheumatic disease. Baltimore (MD): Williams & Wilkins; 1996. p. 73.

61. Callen JP, Wortmann RL. Dermatomyositis. Clin Dermatol 2006;24(5):363–73.

62. Callen JP. Dermatomyositis. Lancet 2000;355(9197): 53–7.

63. Santmyire-Rosenberger B, Dugan EM. Skin involvement in dermatomyositis. Curr Opin Rheumatol 2003;15(6):714–22.

64. Palero TM, Miller OF, Hahn TF, et al. Juvenile dermatomyositis: a retrospective review of a 30-year-experience. J Am Acad Dermatol 2001;45(1):28–34.

65. Oremović L, Lugović L, Vucić M, et al. Cicatricial alopecia as a manifestation of different dermatoses. Acta Dermatovenerol Croat 2006;14(4):246–52.

66. Dawkins MA, Jorizzo JL, Walker FO, et al. Dermatomyositis: a dermatology-based case series. J Am Acad Dermatol 1998;38(3):397–404.

67. Magro CM, Crowson AN. The immunofluorescent profile of dermatomyositis: a comparative study with lupus erythematosus. J Cutan Pathol 1997; 24(9):543–52.

68. Fiorentino D, Chung L, Zwerner J, et al. The mucocutaneous and systemic phenotype of dermatomyositis patients with antibodies to MDA5 (CADM-140): a retrospective study. J Am Acad Dermatol 2011; 65(1):25–34.

69. Schwarz HA, Slavin G, Ward P, et al. Muscle biopsy in polymyositis and dermatomyositis: a clinicopathological study. Ann Rheum Dis 1980;39(5):500–7.

70. Gilliam AC. Scleroderma. Curr Dir Autoimmun 2008; 10:258–79.

71. Chung L, Lin J, Furst DE, et al. Systemic and localized scleroderma. Clin Dermatol 2006;24(5):374–92.

72. Furst D, Pope J, Clements P. Systemic sclerosis. In: Tugwell P, et al, editors. Evidence-based rheumatology. London: BMJ Books; 2004. p. 443–83.

73. Christen-Zaech S, Hakim MD, Afsar FS, et al. Pediatric morphea (localized scleroderma): review of 136 patients. J Am Acad Dermatol 2008;59(3):385–96.

74. Leitenberger JJ, Cayce RL, Haley RW, et al. Distinct autoimmune syndromes in morphea: a review of 245 adult and pediatric cases. Arch Dermatol 2009; 145(5):545–50.

75. Rochen M, Ghoreschi. Morphea and lichen sclerosus. In: Bolognia J, Jorizzo JL, Rapini RP, editors. Dermatology. 2nd edition. St Louis (MO): Mosby/ Elsevier; 2008. p. 1469–76.

76. Marzano AV, Menni S, Parodi A, et al. Localized scleroderma in adults and children. Clinical and laboratory investigations on 239 cases. Eur J Dermatol 2003;13(2):171–6.

77. Peterson L, Nelson A, Su W. Classification of morphea (localized scleroderma). Mayo Clin Proc 1995;70:1068–76.

78. Soma Y, Fujimoto M. Frontoparietal scleroderma (en coup de sabre) following Blaschko's lines. J Am Acad Dermatol 1998;38(2 Pt 2):366–8.

79. Hesselstrand R, Scheja A, Wildt M, et al. High-frequency ultrasound of skin involvement in systemic sclerosis reflects oedema, extension and severity in early disease. Rheumatology (Oxford) 2008;47(1):84–7.

80. Bennett RM. Clinical manifestations and diagnosis of fibromyalgia. Rheum Dis Clin North Am 2009;35(2): 215–32.

81. Goldenberg DL. Fibromyalgia syndrome a decade later: what have we learned? Arch Intern Med 1999;159(8):777–85.

82. Bannwarth B, Blotman F, Roué-Le Lay K, et al. Fibromyalgia syndrome in the general population of France: a prevalence study. Joint Bone Spine 2009;76(2):184–7.

83. Weir PT, Harlan GA, Nkoy FL, et al. The incidence of fibromyalgia and its associated comorbidities: a population-based retrospective cohort study based on International Classification of Diseases, 9th Revision codes. J Clin Rheumatol 2006;12(3):124–8.

84. Gräfe A, Wollina U, Tebbe B, et al. Fibromyalgia in lupus erythematosus. Acta Derm Venereol 1999; 79(1):62–4.

85. Gupta S, Masand PS. Citalopram and hair loss. Prim Care Companion J Clin Psychiatry 2000; 2(2):61–2.

86. Trüeb RM. Chemotherapy-induced alopecia. Semin Cutan Med Surg 2009;28(1):11–4.

87. Duff P, Mayer AR. Generalized alopecia: an unusual complication of danazol therapy. Am J Obstet Gynecol 1981;141(3):349–50.

88. Ogilvie AD. Hair loss during fluoxetine treatment. Lancet 1993;342(8884):1423.

89. Parameshwar E. Hair loss associated with fluvoxamine use. Am J Psychiatry 1996;153(4):581–2.

90. Burrows NP, Grant JW, Crisp AJ, et al. Scarring alopecia following gold therapy. Acta Derm Venereol 1994;74(6):486.

91. Descamps V. Cutaneous side effects of alpha interferon. Presse Med 2005;34(21):1668–72 [in French].

92. Orbach H, Katz U, Sherer Y, et al. Intravenous immunoglobulin: adverse effects and safe administration. Clin Rev Allergy Immunol 2005;29(3):173–84.

93. van Riel PL, Smolen JS, Emery P, et al. Leflunomide: a manageable safety profile. J Rheumatol Suppl 2004;71:21–4.

94. Susser WS, Whitaker-Worth DL, Grant-Kels JM. Mucocutaneous reactions to chemotherapy. J Am Acad Dermatol 1999;40(3):367–98.

95. Aalamian Z. Reducing adverse effects of immunosuppressive agents in kidney transplant recipients. Prog Transplant 2001;11(4):271–82.

96. Mangalvedhekar SS, Gogtay NJ, Manjula S, et al. Phenytoin associated alopecia: drug induced lupus. J Assoc Physicians India 2001; 49:929–30.

97. Pereira CE, Goldman-Levine JD. Extended-release venlafaxine-induced alopecia. Ann Pharmacother 2007;41(6):1084.

Alopecia Areata Update

Abdullah Alkhalifah, MD

KEYWORDS

- Alopecia areata • Totalis • Universalis • Autoimmune • Corticosteroids • Intralesional
- Contact immunotherapy • Phototherapy

KEY POINTS

- Alopecia areata (AA) is a common nonscarring autoimmune condition that has no race or gender predilection.
- Although most AA patches are asymptomatic, few patients may complain of itching or burning sensation.
- Diagnosis is usually straightforward and routine blood testing is not generally indicated.
- Treatment is tailored according to the age of the patient and the extent of the disease.
- The most important poor prognostic factor is extensive disease presentation.

EPIDEMIOLOGY

Alopecia areata (AA) is a common nonscarring hair condition responsible for 0.7% to 3.8% of dermatology clinics visits.[1] The lifetime risk in the United States was estimated at 1.7%.[2] The 2 sexes are equally affected.[3] When it comes to age distribution, children constitute approximately 20% of patients with AA,[4] and as many as 60% present with their first patch before the age of 20.[5] Only 20% of patients are older than 40.[6]

CLINICAL PICTURE

AA is most commonly noticed incidentally by the patient, a family member, or hairdresser. The disease is asymptomatic although some patients may report pruritus, burning sensation, or pain.[7]

Typical lesions are sharply demarcated, round to oval, skin-colored patches of nonscarring alopecia (Fig. 1).[6] Less commonly, the color of the lesions can be peachy or reddened (Fig. 2).[1] Hairs that are tapered proximally and wider distally ("exclamation mark hairs") are characteristic findings within or at the periphery of the lesions (Fig. 3A, B).[3] The hair pull test can be positive at the periphery of active lesions.[1] Although any hair-bearing area can be affected, the scalp is involved in 90% of the cases.[3] In patients with graying hair, AA initially spares the white hairs.[8] Eventually, these hairs will be involved as the disease progresses. Initial hair regrowth can also be hypopigmented, but it usually restores the color with time.[1]

AA can be classified according to the extent or the pattern of hair loss (Table 1).[1] Based on the extent of hair loss, the disease is clinically classified as follows: patchy AA (see Fig. 1), in which there is a partial loss of scalp hair; alopecia totalis (AT) (Fig. 4), in which 100% of scalp hair is lost; or alopecia universalis (AU) (Fig. 5), in which there is a 100% loss of all scalp and body hair. Patchy AA is seen in up to 75% of patients and is the most common pattern.[6] Other patterns include reticular pattern; ophiasis type (Fig. 6), bandlike hair loss in parieto-temporo-occipital area; ophiasis inversus (sisapho), very rare bandlike hair loss in the fronto-parieto-temporal area; and a diffuse thinning over part of or the entire scalp.

A recently described, distinct clinical variant is acute diffuse and total alopecia.[9,10] This new variant is characterized by its rapid progression and extensive involvement, along with a favorable prognosis.

Disclosures: I have no conflict of interest.
Riyadh Military Hospital, PO Box 92525, Riyadh 11663, Saudi Arabia
E-mail address: dralkhalifah@hotmail.com

Dermatol Clin 31 (2013) 93–108
http://dx.doi.org/10.1016/j.det.2012.08.010

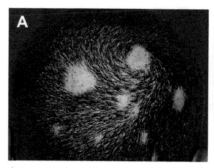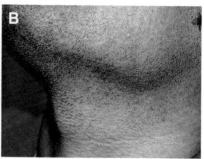

Fig. 1. (A) Patchy AA involving the scalp. (B) Patchy AA involving the beard.

Dermoscopic features that are seen in AA include yellow dots, black dots, broken hairs, short vellus hairs, and tapered hairs (see **Fig. 3**B).[11–13] These findings are not specific for AA but can be very helpful when the diagnosis is uncertain.

Nail pitting is the most common nail abnormality observed in AA.[14,15] Other reported nail abnormalities include trachyonychia, beau lines, onychorhexis, thinning or thickening, onychomadesis, koilonychia, punctuate or transverse leukonychia, and red spotted lunulae.[1] The reported frequency of nail abnormalities ranges from 7% to 66%.[14]

ASSOCIATED ABNORMALITIES

Autoimmune thyroid disease is the most common abnormality associated with AA with an incidence between 8% and 28%.[16] The presence of thyroid autoantibodies has no clinical correlation with AA severity.[17] Vitiligo occurs in 3% to 8% of AA patients compared with 1% in the general US population.[18] Atopy is twice as common in AA patients as it is in the general population.[18]

Other diseases and genetic disorders reported to be associated with AA include Down syndrome, Addison disease, autosomal recessive autoimmune polyglandular syndrome (APS-1) (chronic hypoparathyroidism-mucocutaneous candidiasis-autoimmune adrenal insufficiency), pernicious anemia, psoriasis, lupus, Sjögren syndrome, intermediate uveitis, rheumatoid arthritis, celiac disease, ulcerative colitis, myasthenia gravis, and multiple sclerosis.[19–21] These less common autoimmune diseases are more likely to be associated with AT/AU.[19]

There may be an increased risk of type 1 diabetes in family members of AA patients; in contrast, the patients themselves may have a reduced incidence compared with the general population.[22] There may be a high psychiatric morbidity in AA, especially anxiety and mood disturbance.[23] Ophthalmologic findings such as asymptomatic lens opacities and fundus changes occurred in 51% and 41% of patients with AA, respectively.[24]

DIFFERENTIAL DIAGNOSIS

In children, AA should be differentiated from tineacapitis and trichotillomania. Tineacapitis can be associated with inflammation and scaling, which are typically not seen in AA. Trichotillomania is usually bizarre shaped and has broken hairs with varying length. In children with a single congenital patch of hair loss on the temporal area, temporal triangular alopecia should be considered in the differential diagnosis. If AA involves the frontal and temporal hair line, frontal fibrosing alopecia (FFA) should be ruled out. FFA is a scarring hair condition primarily affecting postmenopausal women. FFA may have perifollicular erythema and scales, which are not present in AA. Diffuse AA can be challenging and may require a biopsy to differentiate it from telogen effluvium. If the clinical context is suspicious for syphilis or lupus, serologic examination is indicated to rule out this possibility.

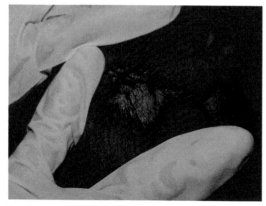

Fig. 2. Unusual red color of patchy AA.

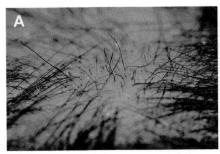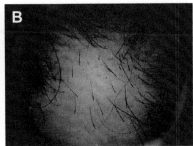

Fig. 3. (A) Close-up view of exclamation mark hairs. (B) Dermoscopic examination of AA showing exclamation mark hairs and black dots. (Original magnification ×10.)

ETIOPATHOGENESIS

Many etiologic factors have been suggested to contribute to the development of AA. These include stress,[25] infectious agents,[26] vaccinations,[27] hormonal factors,[28] and genetics.[29,30] The exact cause is still unknown. The disease onset and severity are probably determined by multiple factors.

Most of the recent literature supports autoimmunity as the major pathogenic process in AA.[1,31] Several observations support this hypothesis. These include the presence of lesional inflammatory cells, hair follicle–specific autoantibodies in the blood of patients with AA, the response to treatment with immunosuppressive medications, and the association of AA with other autoimmune diseases.

The follicular infiltrate is mainly composed of CD4[+] and CD8[+] T cells.[31] This leads to disruption of the normal hair cycle. Inflammation can maintain hair follicles in dystrophic anagen state, force them into premature telogen, or –in chronic cases–keep them in prolonged telogen state.

Recently, genomewide association study in AA has identified at least 8 regions in the genome with evidence for association with AA.[30] This may have significant implications on the way this common disease is treated.

PROGNOSIS

The most important factors indicating a poor prognosis are the extent of hair loss presentation (extensive AA/AT/AU)[32] or an ophiasis pattern of hair loss.[9] Other factors associated with a poor prognosis include a long duration of hair loss,[9] atopy, a positive family history, the presence of other autoimmune diseases, nail involvement, and young age at first onset.[7]

The course of AA is unpredictable. Up to 50% of patients will recover within 1 year even without treatment.[1] However, 85% of patients will have more than 1 episode of hair loss.[33] In patients with AA before puberty, the chance of AT is 50%.[33] In AT/AU, the chance of full recovery is less than 10%.[1]

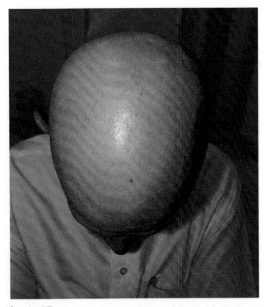

Fig. 4. AT.

Table 1
Classification of AA

Classification by Extent	Classification by Pattern
Patchy AA	Patchy AA
AT	Ophiasis
AU	Ophiasis inversus
	Reticular
	Diffuse

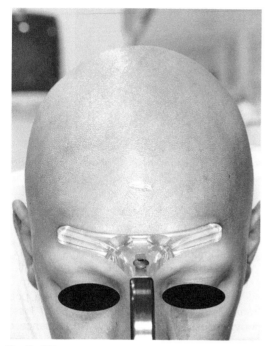

Fig. 5. AU.

INVESTIGATIONS

Routine blood testing in AA is not generally indicated because of insufficient clinical evidence.[34] Potassium hydroxide, fungal culture, lupus serology, syphilitic screening, and a scalp biopsy may be necessary if the diagnosis is in question. However, most AA cases are straight forward and don't require investigations.

HISTOPATHOLOGY

The histologic picture of AA varies according to the duration of the disease.[1] In acute stage, anagen follicles are targeted by lymphocytic infiltrate

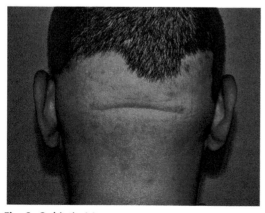

Fig. 6. Ophiatic AA.

"swarm of bees" composed of CD4[+] and CD8[+] T cells.[35] Other cells that can be found include Langerhans cells, eosinophils, mast cells, and plasma cells.[36] Edema, microvesiculation, apoptosis, necrosis, macrophages, and foreign body giant cells can be seen in and around the affected hair follicles.[37]

In the subacute stage, there is marked increase in the catagen, followed by telogen hair. Some inflammation may still present around fibrous streamers as the follicles ascend higher in the dermis.[37] Significant hair follicle miniaturization with little or no inflammation characterizes chronic AA.[37]

TREATMENT

There are no Food and Drug Administration–approved treatments for AA. Many therapeutic options exist, but none are curative or preventive. For many reasons, it is difficult to assess treatment options for AA. There is high rate of spontaneous remission in patchy AA. There is also paucity of randomized-controlled trials investigating treatment efficacy. Long-term follow-up is not addressed in many of the published reports. Another important drawback is the great variation in treatment outcome evaluation. To overcome this issue in particular, the Severity of Alopecia Tool score seems to be ideal.[38]

In this section, localized and systemic agents used in the treatment of AA will be discussed. At the end, approach to treatment is suggested based on age of the patient and extent of the disease.

LOCALIZED THERAPIES
Intralesional Corticosteroids

Since 1958,[39,40] intralesional corticosteroids (ILCS) have been used widely for the treatment of AA. Despite their common use, there are no randomized controlled trials.[40,41] The most commonly used drug is triamcinolone acetonide. Hair regrowth has been reported in 71% of patients with subtotal AA treated by triamcinolone acetonide injections 3 times every 2 weeks and in 7% of control subjects injected with isotonic saline.[42] Porter and Burton showed that hair regrowth was possible in 64% and 97% of AA sites treated by intralesional injections of triamcinolone acetonide and its less soluble derivative, triamicinolone hexacetonide, respectively.[43] Using monthly intralesional triamcinolone acetonide, 40 of 62 patients with AA (63%) showed complete regrowth in 4 months.[44] In this uncontrolled trial, response was better in patients with fewer patches (<5), shorter duration of disease (<1 month), and smaller patches diameter (<3 cm). In another report, 6 of 10 patients with extensive AA responded to intralesional triamcinolone acetonide.[45]

For adult patients with limited involvement, ILCS (preferably triamicinolone acetonide) are considered first-line therapy. Triamicinolone acetonide is injected in the deep dermal/upper subcutaneous plane using a ½-inch-long 30-gauge needle (**Fig. 7**); 0.1 mL is injected at 0.5- to 1-cm intervals every 4 to 6 weeks. Various concentrations (2.5–10 mg/mL) are used but 5 mg/mL and 2.5 mg/mL are the preferred concentrations used by the author for the scalp and face, respectively. The maximum dose per session was suggested to be 20 mg of triamcinolone acetonide.[46] Topical anesthetic cream can be applied before treatment to minimize pain, especially if treating younger patients. Treatment should be stopped if there is no improvement after 6 months. The decreased expression of thioredoxin reductase 1 in the outer root sheath may be the cause for glucocorticoid resistance in some patients with AA.[47]

Side effects include transient atrophy and telangiectasia, which can be prevented by the use of smaller concentrations and volumes, minimizing the number of injections per site, and avoiding injecting too superficially.

Topical Corticosteroids

Midpotent and potent topical corticosteroids are widely used in the treatment of AA. The evidence for their efficacy is limited. A double-blind half-head placebo-controlled study compared 0.2% fluocinolone acetonide cream twice a day with base vehicle and showed unilateral regrowth in 54% in the treatment arm compared with 0% in the vehicle group.[48] A multicenter prospective, randomized, controlled, investigator-blinded trial in patients with less than 26% hair loss showed a greater than 75% hair regrowth rate in 61% of patients using 0.1% betamethasone valerate foam in comparison with 27% in the 0.05% betamethasone dipropionate lotion group.[49] In a study of

unilateral application of 0.05% clobetasol propionate ointment under occlusion in patients with AT/AU, Tosti and colleagues[50] showed that 28.5% of patients had almost complete hair regrowth and 17.8% of patient had long-term benefit on the treated side. In another randomized, double-blind, placebo-controlled trial, 47% of 0.05% clobetasol propionate foam–treated patients had greater than 25% hair regrowth, and 25% of participants had hair regrowth greater than 50%.[51] No significant modifications in cortisol and adrenocorticotropic hormone blood levels were observed during this trial. On the other hand, in another randomized, double-blinded, placebo-controlled trial using desoximetasone cream 0.25%, the complete regrowth rates in the active and control groups were 57.6% and 39.2%, respectively. These results were not statistically significant compared with placebo.[52]

Side effects include folliculitis (more with ointment compared with foam formulations) and rarely skin atrophy and telangiectasia. The relapse rate varies from 37% to 63% after topical corticosteroid treatment has stopped and even with continuation of therapy.[48,50]

Minoxidil

Minoxidil was initially used as antihypertensive therapy. Although it has been used to promote hair growth for more than 20 years, its mechanism of action is not fully understood. Vasodilatation,[53,54] angiogenesis,[55] enhanced cell proliferation,[56,57] and potassium channel opening[58,59] have been all proposed.

In a double-blind placebo-controlled trial on extensive AA, 3% minoxidil under occlusion with petrolatum resulted in hair regrowth in 63.6% compared with 35.7% in the placebo arm.[60] Only 27.3% of minoxidil-treated patients had cosmetically acceptable hair growth. A dose-response efficacy was shown in a study comparing 1% and 5% topical minoxidil in the treatment of patients with extensive AA. The response rates were 38% and 81% with 1% and 5% topical minoxidil, respectively.[61,62]

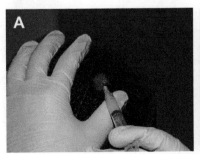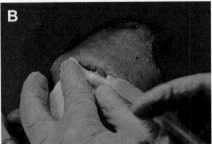

Fig. 7. (A) ILCS injection into the scalp. (B) ILCS injection into the eyebrow.

Minoxidil 5% solution twice daily is used as adjuvant treatment to conventional AA therapy (mainly topical corticosteroids or ILCS). Contact dermatitis and hypertrichosis are the most common side effects.[63,64] Contact dermatitis can be minimized by using minoxidil foam, which does not contain propylene glycol.[65]

Anthralin

There are a few uncontrolled case series assessing anthralin efficacy in the treatment of AA. Response rates of 75% in patients with patchy AA and 25% in patients with AT have been reported (**Fig. 8**).[66] Anthralin cream 0.5% to 1.0% was used to treat 68 patients with severe AA. Cosmetic response was seen in 25% of the patients.[67]

In mice, anthralin has been shown to decrease the expression of tumor necrosis factor (TNF)-α and -β in the treated area in comparison to vehicle-treated sites.[68] Its mechanism of action in AA treatment is unknown.

Anthralin 1% cream can be used as short-contact therapy. It is applied daily for 15 to 20 minutes initially then washed. The contact time is increased by 5 minutes weekly up to 1 hour or until low-grade dermatitis develops. The contact time is then fixed and continued daily for at least 3 months before judging the response to treatment. Anthralin should produce a mild irritant reaction to be effective.[34] Side effects include severe irritation, folliculitis, regional lymphadenopathy, and staining of skin (**Fig. 9**), clothes, and fair hair.[66,69,70] Patients should avoid eye contact with this chemical and the treated area should be protected from the sun.

Topical Immunotherapy

The mechanism of action of topical sensitizers is poorly understood. Many theories have been suggested including antigenic competition,[71] perifollicular lymphocytes apoptosis,[72] changes in the peribular CD4/CD8 lymphocyte ratio,[73,74] and interleukin (IL)-10 secretion after diphenylcyclopropenone (DPCP) application.[75]

Dinitrochlorobenzene was the first topical sensitizer to be used in the treatment of extensive AA since 1976, but it has been discontinued because it has been shown to be mutagenic in the Ames test.[76,77] Squaric acid dibutylester (SADBE) and DPCP are the 2 compounds still in use today. DPCP is preferred because it is cheaper and is more stable in acetone.[78,79]

Although no randomized controlled trials have evaluated the effectiveness of topical immunotherapy in AA, observational studies have used the half-head method to control for spontaneous regrowth of hair. A comprehensive review of published topical immunotherapy studies (SABDE = 13 trials; DPCP = 17 trials) found little difference between the 2 agents.[80,81] The success rate of DPCP and SADBE is about 50% to 60% with a wide range of 9% to 87%.[81] The largest reported series of DPCP treatment found that cosmetically acceptable regrowth was achieved in 17.4% of patients with AT/AU, 60.3% with 75% to 99% AA, 88.1% with 50% to 74% AA, and 100% with 25% to 49% AA. A lag of 3 months was present between initiation of therapy and development of significant hair regrowth in the first responders. Relapse after achieving significant regrowth developed in 62.6% of patients with median time to relapse being 2½ years.[82] Although contact immunotherapy has been used mainly for adults, there are reports of success in the pediatric population.[83,84]

In a recent study of 20 patients treated with DPCP, neoangiogenesis seen with videocapillaroscopy was significantly correlated with a better clinical response.[85] The most important negative prognostic factors in the treatment of AA with DPCP are disease severity, duration of AA before therapy, and presence of nail changes.[82,86] Other

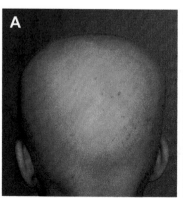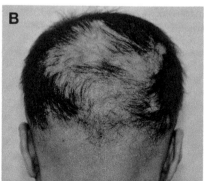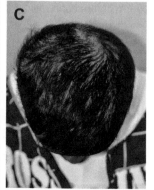

Fig. 8. (*A*) AT before anthralin treatment. (*B, C*) AT after 4 months of treatment with anthralin 1% short-contact therapy.

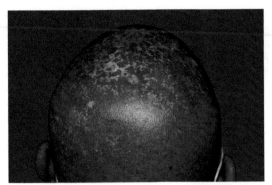

Fig. 9. Scalp hyperpigmentation secondary to anthralin 1% cream.

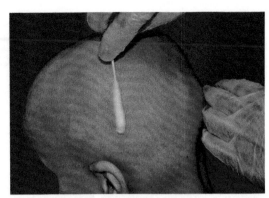

Fig. 11. One side of the scalp is painted with 2 DPCP coatings (anteroposterior and lateral).

factors include age at onset, atopy, and a family history of AA.[32,87–89] It was also suggested that if patients with AT or AU are suffering with hyperpigmentation from the sensitizer, these patients will show poor response to contact immunotherapy.[90]

Because DPCP is very light sensitive, it should be stored in amber bottles to protect it from exposure to ultraviolet light (Fig. 10).[78] DPCP 2% is applied using a cotton swab to a 4-cm circular area on the scalp to sensitize the patient. Two weeks later, a 0.001% DPCP solution is applied to the same half of the scalp (Fig. 11). The concentration of DPCP is increased gradually each week until a mild dermatitis reaction is obtained. The goal is to achieve a low-grade erythema and mild pruritus on the treated area for 24 to 36 hours after application.[91]

After establishing the appropriate concentration for the patient, therapy should be continued on a weekly basis. DPCP should be left on the scalp for 48 hours and then washed off. Patients should not expose the treated area to the sun during this

time. Treatment of both sides is recommended only after achieving a trichogenic response on the treated side (Fig. 12). If there is no improvement at 6 months, DPCP is less likely to be successful. If the patient does not develop an allergic reaction to 2% DPCP, SADBE can be tried.[83,92]

A vesicular or bullous reaction is one of the undesired adverse effects of topical sensitizers. If this reaction develops, the patient should wash off the contact sensitizer and a topical corticosteroid should be applied to the affected area. Other adverse effects include cervical and occipital lymphadenopathy,[89,93] facial and scalp edema, contact urticaria,[94–96] flulike symptoms, erythema multiforme-like reactions,[89,97] and pigmentary disturbances (hyperpigmentation, hypopigmentation, dyschromia in confetti, and even vitiligo) (Fig. 13).[93,98,99]

Prostaglandin Analogs

Latanoprost, a prostaglandin F2α analog, and bimatoprost, a synthetic prostamide F2α analog, are used in the treatment of open angle glaucoma patients.[100] Hypertrichosis of the eyelashes and vellus hair on the malar area is one of the reported side effects.[101–104] Prostaglandin F2α and its analogs showed stimulatory effects on murine hair follicles and follicular melanocytes in both the telogen and anagen stages and stimulated conversion from the telogen to the anagen phase.[105] Bimatoprost (Lattisse; Allergan, Inc, Irvine, CA) received approval from the Food and Drug Administration for the treatment of hypotrichosis of the eyelashes.

Latanoprost and bimatoprost failed to induce regrowth in a blinded randomized controlled trial on 11 patients with extensive (>50%) eyelash AA.[106] Another 16-week randomized, right-left, investigator-blinded study of 8 patients with severe eyebrow AA showed the same result.[107]

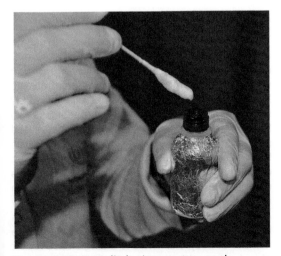

Fig. 10. DPCP is applied using a cotton swab.

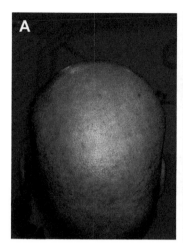
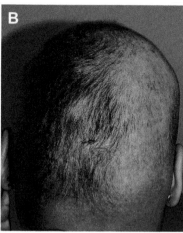

Fig. 12. (*A*) AT before DPCP treatment. (*B*) Trichogenic response on the DPCP-treated side.

In a larger trial, 26 patients with symmetric eyelash and eyebrow AA were treated during 4 months with topical latanoprost for one side. This trial also failed to show a difference between the treated and the untreated sides.[108] On the other hand, a recent nonblinded, nonrandomized trial showed a cosmetically acceptable response in 45% of the latanoprost-treated group compared with none of the control group.[109] Complete eyelashes regrowth was noted in 24% of 37 patients of AU using 0.03% bimatoprost to the eyelid margin once a day during the course of 1 year.[110] Patients with less extensive eyelash loss caused by AA may benefit from treatment with instilled bimatoprost.[111] This attractive area of AA therapy needs further evaluation with blinded prospective right-left controlled trials to confirm either of the conflicting evidence available so far. The treatment is usually well tolerated. Side effects include transient mild eye irritation or hyperemia.[111]

Phototherapy

Randomized controlled trials for phototherapy with oral or topical psoralen plus ultraviolet A light are lacking. Two large retrospective studies showed that the response rate is no better than the spontaneous remission rate.[112,113] Insufficient evidence and the risk of cutaneous malignancies with psoralen plus ultraviolet A make it a less-favored treatment option. Narrow band ultraviolet B was not effective in a retrospective analysis of 25 patients with AA.[114] A few case series have shown successful results with 308-nm excimer laser in treating patchy AA.[115–119] The initial fluences were 50 mJ/cm^2 less than the minimal erythema dose. Fluences were then increased by 50 mJ/cm^2 every 2 sessions. Each patch was treated twice a week for a maximum of 24 sessions. Hair regrowth has been shown in 41.5% of patches.[118]

Potential Topical and Localized Treatments

There are several treatment modalities that can be administered locally and have shown some efficacy. Indeed, these require further testing and evaluation. Bexarotene 1% gel treatment on half head was evaluated in a single blinded study involving 42 patients with AA. Five patients (12%) had 50% or more partial regrowth on the treated side, and 6 patients (14%) had a response on both sides. 73% of the subjects had some degree of dermal irritation.[120] Capsaicin ointment was comparable to clobetasol 0.05% ointment in a nonblinded study of 50 subjects with patchy AA.[121] This finding should be supported with blinded randomized controlled trials with large number of subjects. There is a single case report of refractory AA that responded to fractional

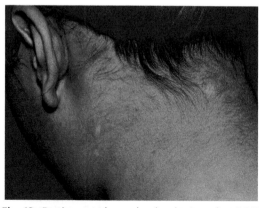

Fig. 13. Depigmented macules developing after DPCP immunotherapy.

Er:glass laser.[122] One animal study demonstrated the efficacy of 655-nm laser comb in a C3H/HeJ mouse model for AA.[123]

SYSTEMIC THERAPIES
Corticosteroids

Systemic corticosteroids have been used for decades in patients with extensive AA. Several regimens have been used with varying success. The only randomized placebo-controlled study on oral prednisolone was published in 2005.[124] Forty-three patients with extensive AA were randomized to receive prednisolone 200 mg weekly or placebo. The treatment period was 3 months followed by 3 months of observation time. Significant hair regrowth was noted in 35% of patients in the treatment group compared with none in the placebo group. The relapse rate was 25% during the observation period. Significant hair regrowth was noted in 28 of 34 patients (82%) with extensive AA treated with prednisolone 300 mg once monthly for 3 to 6 months.[125] Poor response was associated with presence of other autoimmune abnormality, nail involvement, and universalis form. Only 15% of the patients had side effects in that report.

Other systemic corticosteroids regimens include prednisolone 40 mg daily tapered over 6 weeks,[126,127] dexamethasone 5 mg on 2 consecutive days weekly,[128] intravenous methylprednisolone 250 mg twice daily on 3 consecutive days monthly,[129] dexamethasone 0.5 mg daily for 6 months, intramuscular triamcinolone acetonide 40 mg monthly, and prednisolone 80 mg daily on 3 consecutive days every 3 months.[130]

The side effects of systemic steroids include hyperglycemia, osteoporosis, cataracts, immunosuppression, mood changes, obesity, dysmenorrhea, acne, and Cushing syndrome.[130–132] The reported relapse rate is 14% to 100%.[133] The addition of 2% topical minoxidil 3 times daily may alleviate poststeroid relapse.[126] Systemic steroids used in AA is less-favored option because of the side effect profile and high relapse rate.

Cyclosporine

Cyclosporine is an immunosuppressant agent that inhibits helper T-cell activation and suppresses interferon-γ production. Cyclosporine alone or in conjunction with systemic steroids was tried with variable results.[134–137] The success rate ranges from 25%[136] to 76.7%.[135] Notably, however, AA has been reported in several organ transplant patients who were taking cyclosporine.[138–141] One report suggested that increased serum soluble IL-2 receptor level and lower IL-18 level at baseline was associated with a poor response to a combination of cyclosporine and methylprednisolone.[142]

Cyclosporine is not a preferred option in AA because of high side effect profile and relapse rate. Side effects include nephrotoxicity, immune suppression, hypertension, and hypertrichosis of body hair.[143]

Although no beneficial response has been observed by using topical cyclosporine in humans,[144,145] Verma and colleagues[146] showed good hair regrowth and reduced inflammation in the Dundee experimental bald rat model using cyclosporine specially formulated in lipid vesicles. No response was noted in the Dundee experimental bald rat group treated with cyclosporine in ethanol, but further studies in humans are needed to assess the efficacy and safety of this specific formulation.

Sulfasalazine

Sulfasalazine has both immunomodulatory and immunosuppressive actions, including inhibition of T-cell proliferation, natural killer cell activity, and antibody production. Sulfasalazine also inhibits the T-cell cytokines IL-2 and interferon-γ and the monocyte/macrophage cytokines IL-1, TNF- α, and IL-6.[147]

In a retrospective study, cosmetically acceptable hair regrowth was noted in 23% of patients with severe AA.[148] In another open-label study done on patients with severe AA, complete hair regrowth was achieved in 27.3% of patients.[149] Sulfasalazine was started at 0.5 g twice daily for 1 month, 1 g twice daily for 1 month, and then 1.5 g twice daily for 4 months. The relapse rate was 45.5%. Thirty-two percent of patients suffered from adverse effects, which included gastrointestinal distress, rash, headache, and laboratory abnormalities. A similar response rate (25.6%) was shown in another uncontrolled trial of 39 patients with AA.[150]

Methotrexate

Methotrexate (15–25 mg/wk) alone or in conjunction with 10 to 20 mg/d of prednisone resulted in complete regrowth in 57% and 63% of patients, respectively.[151] The onset of hair regrowth was noted after a median delay of 3 months. Relapsed rate was 80% (16 of 20 responders). Seven patients (21%) experienced adverse events consisting of transient elevated transaminases, persistent nausea, and lymphocytopenia. Using the same regimens, complete hair regrowth was achieved in 64% of 22 patients with AT/AU.[152] In a retrospective study including 14 children with severe AA treated with methotrexate (mean dose of 18.9 mg/wk), the response rate was 38%.[153]

Azathioprine

Azathioprine is a cytotoxic and immunosuppressive drug that has been used in the treatment of autoimmune diseases for more than 50 years. It seems to impair T-cell function and IL-2; it seems to be more selective for T lymphocyte than for B lymphocytes.[143] Azathioprine was used on 20 patients with extensive AA in an open-label uncontrolled study.[154] With use of azathioprine 2 mg/kg/d for 6 months, the mean hair regrowth was 52%. Azathioprine had its onset of action after 3 months of therapy. Side effects included gastrointestinal symptoms, mild leukopenia, and elevated liver enzymes.

Psychosocial Support

AA is associated with high psychiatric comorbidities (mainly adjustment disorder, generalized anxiety disorder, and depressive disorders).[23] The efficacy of antidepressants in AA treatment has not been evaluated by large-scale randomized controlled trials. In a small trial of 8 patients with AA treated with 20 mg paroxetine, a selective serotonin reuptake inhibitor, and 5 patients with placebo for 3 months, complete hair regrowth was observed in 2 patients in the paroxetine group versus 1 patient in the placebo arm. Four patients in the paroxetine group showed partial hair regrowth.[155] Willemsen and colleagues[156] showed 75% to 100% hair regrowth in 12 of 21 patients with extensive AA after 3 to 8 sessions of hypnotherapy. In the follow-up period (ranging from 4 months to 4 years), the relapse rate was 42%. The small sample size and less than optimum hair regrowth assessment make the evaluation of some trials of antidepressants difficult.

Support groups that involve regular meetings of patients with AA and family members can be an invaluable resource for them. Patients can derive emotional support and information that can help them develop positive coping strategies, overall improved quality of life, and increased treatment compliance. The National Alopecia Areata Foundation (www.naaf.org) provides patients and physicians with brochures, research updates, bimonthly newsletters, a pen pal program, sources for scalp prostheses, and many patient conferences. Also, the National Alopecia Areata Foundation supports research and research workshops that add to the scientific knowledge about AA.

Treatment Failures

Topical tacrolimus and pimecrolimus have been tried in several case series in the treatment of AA, but the results have not been encouraging.[157–161] Imiquimod was tried on patchy and extensive AA but failed to show positive results.[162,163] Photodynamic therapy was shown to be ineffective in the treatment of patients with AA.[164,165] There are a few reported cases that have shown either development of AA or complete failure to respond to different TNF-α antibodies, including adalimumab,[166–169] infliximab,[170,171] and etanercept.[172–174]

Management Plan

At the patient's first visit, a careful medical history and a good physical examination should be conducted, including an examination of all hair-bearing areas and nails. Full information about his or her disease including the relapsing nature of AA, prognosis, and risk/benefit ratio of treatment options should be provided. No routine testing is required for patients with AA. Because of the possibility of spontaneous remission in 34% to 50% of patients within 1 year,[34] some patchy AA patients can just be followed without active intervention. If the patient opted for active treatment, options would be offered according to the patient's age and extent of the disease (Fig. 14).

For children younger than 10 years, a combination of 5% minoxidil solution twice daily with a mid-potent topical corticosteroid is the first line of therapy. If there is no response after 6 months, short-contact anthralin can be tried. For patients older than 10 years with less than 50% scalp involvement, intralesional injections of triamcinolone acetonide is the author's first option for therapy. If there is no improvement after 6 months, other therapeutic options can be offered, including 5% topical minoxidil twice a day, potent topical corticosteroid under occlusion at night, and short-contact anthralin.

For those with greater than 50% scalp involvement, topical immunotherapy with DPCP is the treatment of choice. For those patients who have only a partial responce, intralesional triamcinolone acetonide injections are used to treat the resistant alopecic patches. DPCP may be discontinued if there is no response by 6 months of treatment. Alternative remedies include 5% minoxidil solution, topical clobetasol propionate nightly under occlusion, or short-contact anthralin. Systemic agents can be offered if this fails; minoxidil 5% solution with or without intralesional injections of triamcinolone acetonide 2.5 mg/mL (maximum, 1 mL) can be administered to AA of the eyebrows.

Dermatography or medical tattooing of the eyebrows may be suggested to patients with AA

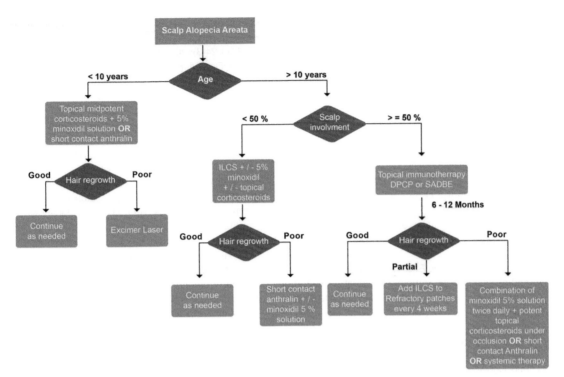

Fig. 14. Treatment algorithm for AA involving the scalp.

who have prolonged eyebrow loss. Scalp prostheses, such as wigs, hairpieces, or other scalp coverings may be valuable options for patients with AA during treatment or when treatment fails.

REFERENCES

1. Alkhalifah A, Alsantali A, Wang E, et al. Alopecia areata update: part I. Clinical picture, histopathology, and pathogenesis. J Am Acad Dermatol 2010;62(2):177–88 [quiz: 189–90].
2. Safavi KH, Muller SA, Suman VJ, et al. Incidence of alopecia areata in Olmsted County, Minnesota, 1975 through 1989. Mayo Clin Proc 1995;70(7): 628–33.
3. Wasserman D, Guzman-Sanchez DA, Scott K, et al. Alopecia areata. Int J Dermatol 2007;46(2): 121–31.
4. Nanda A, Al-Fouzan AS, Al-Hasawi F. Alopecia areata in children: a clinical profile. Pediatr Dermatol 2002;19(6):482–5.
5. Price VH. Alopecia areata: clinical aspects. J Invest Dermatol 1991;96(5):68S.
6. Lu W, Shapiro J, Yu M, et al. Alopecia areata: pathogenesis and potential for therapy. Expert Rev Mol Med 2006;8(14):1–19.
7. Madani S, Shapiro J. Alopecia areata update. J Am Acad Dermatol 2000;42(4):549–66 [quiz: 567–70].
8. Tan C, Zhu WY, Min ZS. A case of patchy alopecia areata sparing lesional greying hairs. Int J Dermatol 2008;47(8):864–5.
9. Lew BL, Shin MK, Sim WY. Acute diffuse and total alopecia: a new subtype of alopecia areata with a favorable prognosis. J Am Acad Dermatol 2009;60(1):85–93.
10. Sato-Kawamura M, Aiba S, Tagami H. Acute diffuse and total alopecia of the female scalp. A new subtype of diffuse alopecia areata that has a favorable prognosis. Dermatology 2002;205(4):367–73.
11. Mane M, Nath AK, Thappa DM. Utility of dermoscopy in alopecia areata. Indian J Dermatol 2011; 56(4):407–11.
12. Ross EK, Vincenzi C, Tosti A. Videodermoscopy in the evaluation of hair and scalp disorders. J Am Acad Dermatol 2006;55(5):799–806.
13. Tosti A, Whiting D, Iorizzo M, et al. The role of scalp dermoscopy in the diagnosis of alopecia areata incognita. J Am Acad Dermatol 2008;59(1):64–7.
14. Gandhi V, Baruah MC, Bhattacharaya SN. Nail changes in alopecia areata: incidence and pattern. Indian J Dermatol Venereol Leprol 2003;69(2):114–5.
15. Kasumagic-Halilovic E, Prohic A. Nail changes in alopecia areata: frequency and clinical presentation. J Eur Acad Dermatol Venereol 2009;23(2): 240–1.
16. Seyrafi H, Akhiani M, Abbasi H, et al. Evaluation of the profile of alopecia areata and the prevalence of

thyroid function test abnormalities and serum auto-antibodies in Iranian patients. BMC Dermatol 2005; 5:11.

17. Kasumagic-Halilovic E. Thyroid autoimmunity in patients with alopecia areata. Acta Dermatovenerol Croat 2008;16(3):123–5.

18. Hordinsky M, Ericson M. Autoimmunity: alopecia areata. J Investig Dermatol Symp Proc 2004;9(1): 73–8.

19. Goh C, Finkel M, Christos PJ, et al. Profile of 513 patients with alopecia areata: associations of disease subtypes with atopy, autoimmune disease and positive family history. J Eur Acad Dermatol Venereol 2006;20(9):1055–60.

20. Rosenstein ED, Warshauer BL. Alopecia areata and autoimmunity. J Am Acad Dermatol 2010; 62(6):1065.

21. Ayuso VK, Pott JW, de Boer JH. Intermediate uveitis and alopecia areata: is there a relationship? Report of 3 pediatric cases. Pediatrics 2011;128(4):e1013–8.

22. Wang SJ, Shohat T, Vadheim C, et al. Increased risk for type I (insulin-dependent) diabetes in relatives of patients with alopecia areata (AA). Am J Med Genet 1994;51(3):234–9.

23. Ruiz-Doblado S, Carrizosa A, Garcia-Hernandez MJ. Alopecia areata: psychiatric comorbidity and adjustment to illness. Int J Dermatol 2003;42(6):434–7.

24. Recupero SM, Abdolrahimzadeh S, De Dominicis M, et al. Ocular alterations in alopecia areata. Eye (Lond) 1999;13(Pt 5):643–6.

25. Elenkov IJ, Chrousos GP. Stress hormones, proinflammatory and antiinflammatory cytokines, and autoimmunity. Ann N Y Acad Sci 2002;966:290–303.

26. Rodriguez TA, Duvic M. Onset of alopecia areata after Epstein-Barr virus infectious mononucleosis. J Am Acad Dermatol 2008;59(1):137–9.

27. Ikeda T. Produced alopecia areata based on the focal infection theory and mental motive theory. Dermatologica 1967;134(1):1–11.

28. McElwee KJ, Silva K, Beamer WG, et al. Melanocyte and gonad activity as potential severity modifying factors in C3H/HeJ mouse alopecia areata. Exp Dermatol 2001;10(6):420–9.

29. McElwee K, Freyschmidt-Paul P, Ziegler A, et al. Genetic susceptibility and severity of alopecia areata in human and animal models. Eur J Dermatol 2001;11(1):11–6.

30. Petukhova L, Cabral RM, Mackay-Wiggan J, et al. The genetics of alopecia areata: what's new and how will it help our patients? Dermatol Ther 2011; 24(3):326–36.

31. Wang E, McElwee KJ. Etiopathogenesis of alopecia areata: why do our patients get it? Dermatol Ther 2011;24(3):337–47.

32. Tosti A, Bellavista S, Iorizzo M. Alopecia areata: a long term follow-up study of 191 patients. J Am Acad Dermatol 2006;55(3):438–41.

33. Finner AM. Alopecia areata: clinical presentation, diagnosis, and unusual cases. Dermatol Ther 2011;24(3):348–54.

34. MacDonald Hull SP, Wood ML, Hutchinson PE, et al. Guidelines for the management of alopecia areata. Br J Dermatol 2003;149(4):692–9.

35. Todes-Taylor N, Turner R, Wood GS, et al. T cell subpopulations in alopecia areata. J Am Acad Dermatol 1984;11(2 Pt 1):216–23.

36. Dy LC, Whiting DA. Histopathology of alopecia areata, acute and chronic: why is it important to the clinician? Dermatol Ther 2011;24(3):369–74.

37. Whiting DA. Histopathologic features of alopecia areata: a new look. Arch Dermatol 2003;139(12): 1555–9.

38. Olsen EA, Hordinsky MK, Price VH, et al. Alopecia areata investigational assessment guidelines–Part II. National Alopecia Areata Foundation. J Am Acad Dermatol 2004;51(3):440–7.

39. Kalkoff KW, Macher E. Growing of hair in alopecia areata & maligna after intracutaneous hydrocortisone injection. Hautarzt 1958;9(10):441–51 [in German].

40. Garg S, Messenger AG. Alopecia areata: evidence-based treatments. Semin Cutan Med Surg 2009; 28(1):15–8.

41. Delamere FM, Sladden MM, Dobbins HM, et al. Interventions for alopecia areata. Cochrane Database Syst Rev 2008;(2):CD004413.

42. Abell E, Munro DD. Intralesional treatment of alopecia areata with triamcinolone acetonide by jet injector. Br J Dermatol 1973;88(1):55–9.

43. Porter D, Burton JL. A comparison of intra-lesional triamcinolone hexacetonide and triamcinolone acetonide in alopecia areata. Br J Dermatol 1971; 85(3):272–3.

44. Kubeyinje EP. Intralesional triamcinolone acetonide in alopecia areata amongst 62 Saudi Arabs. East Afr Med J 1994;71(10):674–5.

45. Chang KH, Rojhirunsakool S, Goldberg LJ. Treatment of severe alopecia areata with intralesional steroid injections. J Drugs Dermatol 2009;8(10): 909–12.

46. Shapiro J, Price VH. Hair regrowth. Therapeutic agents. Dermatol Clin 1998;16(2):341–56.

47. Sohn KC, Jang S, Choi DK, et al. Effect of thioredoxin reductase 1 on glucocorticoid receptor activity in human outer root sheath cells. Biochem Biophys Res Commun 2007;356(3):810–5.

48. Pascher F, Kurtin S, Andrade R. Assay of 0.2 percent fluocinolone acetonide cream for alopecia areata and totalis. Efficacy and side effects including histologic study of the ensuing localized acneform response. Dermatologica 1970;141(3): 193–202.

49. Mancuso G, Balducci A, Casadio C, et al. Efficacy of betamethasone valerate foam formulation in

comparison with betamethasone dipropionate lotion in the treatment of mild-to-moderate alopecia areata: a multicenter, prospective, randomized, controlled, investigator-blinded trial. Int J Dermatol 2003;42(7):572–5.

50. Tosti A, Piraccini BM, Pazzaglia M, et al. Clobetasol propionate 0.05% under occlusion in the treatment of alopecia totalis/universalis. J Am Acad Dermatol 2003;49(1):96–8.

51. Tosti A, Iorizzo M, Botta GL, et al. Efficacy and safety of a new clobetasol propionate 0.05% foam in alopecia areata: a randomized, double-blind placebo-controlled trial. J Eur Acad Dermatol Venereol 2006;20(10):1243–7.

52. Charuwichitratana S, Wattanakrai P, Tanrattanakorn S. Randomized double-blind placebo-controlled trial in the treatment of alopecia areata with 0.25% desoximetasone cream. Arch Dermatol 2000;136(10):1276–7.

53. Bunker CB, Dowd PM. Alterations in scalp blood flow after the epicutaneous application of 3% minoxidil and 0.1% hexyl nicotinate in alopecia. Br J Dermatol 1987;117(5):668–9.

54. Wester RC, Maibach HI, Guy RH, et al. Minoxidil stimulates cutaneous blood flow in human balding scalps: pharmacodynamics measured by laser Doppler velocimetry and photopulse plethysmography. J Invest Dermatol 1984;82(5):515–7.

55. Lachgar S, Charveron M, Gall Y, et al. Minoxidil up-regulates the expression of vascular endothelial growth factor in human hair dermal papilla cells. Br J Dermatol 1998;138(3):407–11.

56. Mori O, Uno H. The effect of topical minoxidil on hair follicular cycles of rats. J Dermatol 1990;17(5):276–81.

57. Uno H, Cappas A, Brigham P. Action of topical minoxidil in the bald stump-tailed macaque. J Am Acad Dermatol 1987;16(3 Pt 2):657–68.

58. Buhl AE, Waldon DJ, Conrad SJ, et al. Potassium channel conductance: a mechanism affecting hair growth both in vitro and in vivo. J Invest Dermatol 1992;98(3):315–9.

59. Messenger AG, Rundegren J. Minoxidil: mechanisms of action on hair growth. Br J Dermatol 2004;150(2):186–94.

60. Price VH. Double-blind, placebo-controlled evaluation of topical minoxidil in extensive alopecia areata. J Am Acad Dermatol 1987;16(3 Pt 2):730–6.

61. Fiedler-Weiss VC. Topical minoxidil solution (1% and 5%) in the treatment of alopecia areata. J Am Acad Dermatol 1987;16(3 Pt 2):745–8.

62. Fiedler-Weiss VC, West DP, Buys CM, et al. Topical minoxidil dose-response effect in alopecia areata. Arch Dermatol 1986;122(2):180–2.

63. Lucky AW, Piacquadio DJ, Ditre CM, et al. A randomized, placebo-controlled trial of 5% and 2% topical minoxidil solutions in the treatment of female pattern hair loss. J Am Acad Dermatol 2004;50(4):541–53.

64. Olsen EA, Dunlap FE, Funicella T, et al. A randomized clinical trial of 5% topical minoxidil versus 2% topical minoxidil and placebo in the treatment of androgenetic alopecia in men. J Am Acad Dermatol 2002;47(3):377–85.

65. Olsen EA, Whiting D, Bergfeld W, et al. A multicenter, randomized, placebo-controlled, double-blind clinical trial of a novel formulation of 5% minoxidil topical foam versus placebo in the treatment of androgenetic alopecia in men. J Am Acad Dermatol 2007;57(5):767–74.

66. Schmoeckel C, Weissmann I, Plewig G, et al. Treatment of alopecia areata by anthralin-induced dermatitis. Arch Dermatol 1979;115(10):1254–5.

67. Fiedler-Weiss VC, Buys CM. Evaluation of anthralin in the treatment of alopecia areata. Arch Dermatol 1987;123(11):1491–3.

68. Tang L, Cao L, Sundberg JP, et al. Restoration of hair growth in mice with an alopecia areata-like disease using topical anthralin. Exp Dermatol 2004;13(1):5–10.

69. Fiedler VC, Wendrow A, Szpunar GJ, et al. Treatment-resistant alopecia areata. Response to combination therapy with minoxidil plus anthralin. Arch Dermatol 1990;126(6):756–9.

70. Sasmaz S, Arican O. Comparison of azelaic acid and anthralin for the therapy of patchy alopecia areata: a pilot study. Am J Clin Dermatol 2005;6(6):403–6.

71. Happle R. Antigenic competition as a therapeutic concept for alopecia areata. Arch Dermatol Res 1980;267(1):109–14.

72. Herbst V, Zoller M, Kissling S, et al. Diphenylcyclopropenone treatment of alopecia areata induces apoptosis of perifollicular lymphocytes. Eur J Dermatol 2006;16(5):537–42.

73. Happle R, Klein HM, Macher E. Topical immunotherapy changes the composition of the peribulbar infiltrate in alopecia areata. Arch Dermatol Res 1986;278(3):214–8.

74. Wasylyszyn T, Kozlowski W, Zabielski SL. Changes in distribution pattern of CD8 lymphocytes in the scalp in alopecia areata during treatment with diphencyprone. Arch Dermatol Res 2007;299(5–6):231–7.

75. Hoffmann R, Wenzel E, Huth A, et al. Cytokine mRNA levels in alopecia areata before and after treatment with the contact allergen diphenylcyclopropenone. J Invest Dermatol 1994;103(4):530–3.

76. Strobel R, Rohrborn G. Mutagenic and cell transforming activities of 1-chlor-2,4-dinitrobenzene (DNCB) and squaric-acid-dibutylester (SADBE). Arch Toxicol 1980;45(4):307–14.

77. Summer KH, Goggelmann W. 1-Chloro-2,4-dinitrobenzene depletes glutathione in rat skin and is

mutagenic in Salmonella typhimurium. Mutat Res 1980;77(1):91–3.

78. Wilkerson MG, Henkin J, Wilkin JK. Diphenylcyclopro- penone: examination for potential contaminants, mechanisms of sensitization, and photochemical stability. J Am Acad Dermatol 1984;11(5 Pt 1):802–7.

79. Wilkerson MG, Henkin J, Wilkin JK, et al. Squaric acid and esters: analysis for contaminants and stability in solvents. J Am Acad Dermatol 1985; 13(2 Pt 1):229–34.

80. Harries MJ, Sun J, Paus R, et al. Management of alopecia areata. BMJ 2010;341:c3671.

81. Rokhsar CK, Shupack JL, Vafai JJ, et al. Efficacy of topical sensitizers in the treatment of alopecia area- ta. J Am Acad Dermatol 1998;39(5 Pt 1):751–61.

82. Wiseman MC, Shapiro J, MacDonald N, et al. Predictive model for immunotherapy of alopecia areata with diphencyprone. Arch Dermatol 2001; 137(8):1063–8.

83. Orecchia G, Malagoli P, Santagostino L. Treatment of severe alopecia areata with squaric acid dibuty- lester in pediatric patients. Pediatr Dermatol 1994; 11(1):65–8.

84. Orecchia G, Malagoli P. Topical immunotherapy in children with alopecia areata. J Invest Dermatol 1995;104(Suppl 5):35S–6S.

85. Ganzetti G, Campanati A, Simonetti O, et al. Video- capillaroscopic pattern of alopecia areata before and after diphenylciclopropenone treatment. Int J Immunopathol Pharmacol 2011;24(4):1087–91.

86. van der Steen PH, van Baar HM, Happle R, et al. Prognostic factors in the treatment of alopecia areata with diphenylcyclopropenone. J Am Acad Dermatol 1991;24(2 Pt 1):227–30.

87. Weise K, Kretzschmar L, John SM, et al. Topical immunotherapy in alopecia areata: anamnestic and clinical criteria of prognostic significance. Dermatology 1996;192(2):129–33.

88. Galadari I, Rubaie S, Alkaabi J, et al. Diphenylcy- clopropenone (diphencyprone, DPCP) in the treat- ment of chronic severe alopecia areata (AA). Eur Ann Allergy Clin Immunol 2003;35(10):397–401.

89. Gordon PM, Aldrige RD, McVittie E, et al. Topical diphencyprone for alopecia areata: evaluation of 48 cases after 30 months' follow-up. Br J Dermatol 1996;134(5):869–71.

90. Ito T. Advances in the management of alopecia areata. J Dermatol 2012;39(1):11–7.

91. Orecchia G, Perfetti L. Alopecia areata and topical sensitizers: allergic response is necessary but irri- tation is not. Br J Dermatol 1991;124(5):509.

92. Dall'oglio F, Nasca MR, Musumeci ML, et al. Topical immunomodulator therapy with squaric acid dibu- tylester (SADBE) is effective treatment for severe alopecia areata (AA): results of an open-label, paired-comparison, clinical trial. J Dermatolog Treat 2005;16(1):10–4.

93. Sotiriadis D, Patsatsi A, Lazaridou E, et al. Topical immunotherapy with diphenylcyclopropenone in the treatment of chronic extensive alopecia areata. Clin Exp Dermatol 2007;32(1):48–51.

94. Francomano M, Seidenari S. Urticaria after topical immunotherapy with diphenylcyclopropenone. Contact Dermatitis 2002;47(5):310–1.

95. Alam M, Gross EA, Savin RC. Severe urticarial reac- tion to diphenylcyclopropenone therapy for alopecia areata. J Am Acad Dermatol 1999;40(1):110–2.

96. Tosti A, Guerra L, Bardazzi F. Contact urticaria during topical immunotherapy. Contact Dermatitis 1989;21(3):196–7.

97. Perret CM, Steijlen PM, Zaun H, et al. Erythema multiforme-like eruptions: a rare side effect of topical immunotherapy with diphenylcycloprope- none. Dermatologica 1990;180(1):5–7.

98. Pan JY, Theng C, Lee J, et al. Vitiligo as an adverse reaction to topical diphencyprone. Ann Acad Med Singapore 2009;38(3):276–7.

99. Henderson CA, Ilchyshyn A. Vitiligo complicating diphencyprone sensitization therapy for alopecia universalis. Br J Dermatol 1995;133(3):496–7.

100. Alkhalifah A. Topical and intralesional therapies for alopecia areata. Dermatol Ther 2011;24(3):355–63.

101. Bearden W, Anderson R. Trichiasis associated with prostaglandin analog use. Ophthal Plast Reconstr Surg 2004;20(4):320–2.

102. Tosti A, Pazzaglia M, Voudouris S, et al. Hypertri- chosis of the eyelashes caused by bimatoprost. J Am Acad Dermatol 2004;51(Suppl 5):S149–50.

103. Hart J, Shafranov G. Hypertrichosis of vellus hairs of the malar region after unilateral treatment with bi- matoprost. Am J Ophthalmol 2004;137(4):756–7.

104. Herane MI, Urbina F. Acquired trichomegaly of the eyelashes and hypertrichosis induced by bimato- prost. J Eur Acad Dermatol Venereol 2004;18(5): 644–5.

105. Sasaki S, Hozumi Y, Kondo S. Influence of prosta- glandin F2alpha and its analogues on hair regrowth and follicular melanogenesis in a murine model. Exp Dermatol 2005;14(5):323–8.

106. Roseborough I, Lee H, Chwalek J, et al. Lack of efficacy of topical latanoprost and bimatoprost ophthalmic solutions in promoting eyelash growth in patients with alopecia areata. J Am Acad Derma- tol 2009;60(4):705–6.

107. Ross EK, Bolduc C, Lui H, et al. Lack of efficacy of topical latanoprost in the treatment of eyebrow alopecia areata. J Am Acad Dermatol 2005;53(6): 1095–6.

108. Faghihi G, Andalib F, Asilian A. The efficacy of lata- noprost in the treatment of alopecia areata of eyelashes and eyebrows. Eur J Dermatol 2009; 19(6):586–7.

109. Coronel-Perez IM, Rodriguez-Rey EM, Camacho- Martinez FM. Latanoprost in the treatment of

eyelash alopecia in alopecia areata universalis. J Eur Acad Dermatol Venereol 2010;24(4):481–5.

110. Vila TO, Camacho Martinez FM. Bimatoprost in the treatment of eyelash universalis alopecia areata. Int J Trichol 2010;2(2):86–8.

111. Ochoa BE, Sah D, Wang G, et al. Instilled bimatoprost ophthalmic solution in patients with eyelash alopecia areata. J Am Acad Dermatol 2009;61(3): 530–2.

112. Taylor CR, Hawk JL. PUVA treatment of alopecia areata partialis, totalis and universalis: audit of 10 years' experience at St John's Institute of Dermatology. Br J Dermatol 1995;133(6):914–8.

113. Healy E, Rogers S. PUVA treatment for alopecia areata–does it work? A retrospective review of 102 cases. Br J Dermatol 1993;129(1):42–4.

114. Bayramgurler D, Demirsoy EO, Akturk AS, et al. Narrowband ultraviolet B phototherapy for alopecia areata. Photodermatol Photoimmunol Photomed 2011;27(6):325–7.

115. Zakaria W, Passeron T, Ostovari N, et al. 308-nm excimer laser therapy in alopecia areata. J Am Acad Dermatol 2004;51(5):837–8.

116. Raulin C, Gundogan C, Greve B, et al. Excimer laser therapy of alopecia areata–side-by-side evaluation of a representative area. J Dtsch Dermatol Ges 2005;3(7):524–6 [in German].

117. Gundogan C, Greve B, Raulin C. Treatment of alopecia areata with the 308-nm xenon chloride excimer laser: case report of two successful treatments with the excimer laser. Lasers Surg Med 2004;34(2):86–90.

118. Al-Mutairi N. 308-nm Excimer laser for the treatment of alopecia areata. Dermatol Surg 2007; 33(12):1483–7.

119. Al-Mutairi N. 308-nm Excimer laser for the treatment of alopecia areata in children. Pediatr Dermatol 2009;26(5):547–50.

120. Talpur R, Vu J, Bassett R, et al. Phase I/II randomized bilateral half-head comparison of topical bexarotene 1% gel for alopecia areata. J Am Acad Dermatol 2009;61(4):592.e1–9.

121. Ehsani AH, Toosi S, Seirafi H, et al. Capsaicin vs. clobetasol for the treatment of localized alopecia areata. J Eur Acad Dermatol Venereol 2009; 23(12):1451–3.

122. Yoo KH, Kim MN, Kim BJ, et al. Treatment of alopecia areata with fractional photothermolysis laser. Int J Dermatol 2010;49(7):845–7.

123. Wikramanayake TC, Rodriguez R, Choudhary S, et al. Effects of the Lexington LaserComb on hair regrowth in the C3H/HeJ mouse model of alopecia areata. Lasers Med Sci 2012;27(2):431–6.

124. Kar BR, Handa S, Dogra S, et al. Placebo-controlled oral pulse prednisolone therapy in alopecia areata. J Am Acad Dermatol 2005;52(2): 287–90.

125. Ait Ourhroui M, Hassam B, Khoudri I. Treatment of alopecia areata with prednisone in a once-monthly oral pulse. Ann Dermatol Venereol 2010;137(8–9): 514–8.

126. Olsen EA, Carson SC, Turney EA. Systemic steroids with or without 2% topical minoxidil in the treatment of alopecia areata. Arch Dermatol 1992; 128(11):1467–73.

127. Price VH. Treatment of hair loss. N Engl J Med 1999;341(13):964–73.

128. Sharma VK, Gupta S. Twice weekly 5 mg dexamethasone oral pulse in the treatment of extensive alopecia areata. J Dermatol 1999;26(9):562–5.

129. Friedli A, Labarthe MP, Engelhardt E, et al. Pulse methylprednisolone therapy for severe alopecia areata: an open prospective study of 45 patients. J Am Acad Dermatol 1998;39(4 Pt 1):597–602.

130. Kurosawa M, Nakagawa S, Mizuashi M, et al. A comparison of the efficacy, relapse rate and side effects among three modalities of systemic corticosteroid therapy for alopecia areata. Dermatology 2006;212(4):361–5.

131. Alkhalifah A, Alsantali A, Wang E, et al. Alopecia areata update: part II. Treatment. J Am Acad Dermatol 2010;62(2):191–202 [quiz: 203–4].

132. Lester RS, Knowles SR, Shear NH. The risks of systemic corticosteroid use. Dermatol Clin 1998; 16(2):277–88.

133. Alsantali A. Alopecia areata: a new treatment plan. Clin Cosmet Investig Dermatol 2011;4:107–15.

134. Gupta AK, Ellis CN, Cooper KD, et al. Oral cyclosporine for the treatment of alopecia areata. A clinical and immunohistochemical analysis. J Am Acad Dermatol 1990;22(2 Pt 1):242–50.

135. Kim BJ, Min SU, Park KY, et al. Combination therapy of cyclosporine and methylprednisolone on severe alopecia areata. J Dermatolog Treat 2008;19(4):216–20.

136. Shapiro J, Lui H, Tron V, et al. Systemic cyclosporine and low-dose prednisone in the treatment of chronic severe alopecia areata: a clinical and immunopathologic evaluation. J Am Acad Dermatol 1997;36(1):114–7.

137. Shaheedi-Dadras M, Karami A, Mollaei F, et al. The effect of methylprednisolone pulse-therapy plus oral cyclosporine in the treatment of alopecia totalis and universalis. Arch Iran Med 2008;11(1):90–3.

138. Cerottini JP, Panizzon RG, de Viragh PA. Multifocal alopecia areata during systemic cyclosporine A therapy. Dermatology 1999;198(4):415–7.

139. Dyall-Smith D. Alopecia areata in a renal transplant recipient on cyclosporin. Australas J Dermatol 1996;37(4):226–7.

140. Phillips MA, Graves JE, Nunley JR. Alopecia areata presenting in 2 kidney-pancreas transplant recipients taking cyclosporine. J Am Acad Dermatol 2005;53(5 Suppl 1):S252–5.

141. Davies MG, Bowers PW. Alopecia areata arising in patients receiving cyclosporin immunosuppression. Br J Dermatol 1995;132(5):835–6.

142. Lee D, Hong SK, Park SW, et al. Serum levels of IL-18 and sIL-2R in patients with alopecia areata receiving combined therapy with oral cyclosporine and steroids. Exp Dermatol 2010;19(2):145–7.

143. Otberg N. Systemic treatment for alopecia areata. Dermatol Ther 2011;24(3):320–5.

144. Gilhar A, Pillar T, Etzioni A. Topical cyclosporin A in alopecia areata. Acta Derm Venereol 1989;69(3):252–3.

145. Mauduit G, Lenvers P, Barthelemy H, et al. Treatment of severe alopecia areata with topical applications of cyclosporin A. Ann Dermatol Venereol 1987;114(4):507–10 [in French].

146. Verma DD, Verma S, McElwee KJ, et al. Treatment of alopecia areata in the DEBR model using cyclosporin A lipid vesicles. Eur J Dermatol 2004;14(5):332–8.

147. Ranganath VK, Furst DE. Disease-modifying antirheumatic drug use in the elderly rheumatoid arthritis patient. Rheum Dis Clin North Am 2007;33(1):197–217.

148. Ellis CN, Brown MF, Voorhees JJ. Sulfasalazine for alopecia areata. J Am Acad Dermatol 2002;46(4):541–4.

149. Aghaei S. An uncontrolled, open label study of sulfasalazine in severe alopecia areata. Indian J Dermatol Venereol Leprol 2008;74(6):611–3.

150. Rashidi T, Mahd AA. Treatment of persistent alopecia areata with sulfasalazine. Int J Dermatol 2008;47(8):850–2.

151. Chartaux E, Joly P. Long-term follow-up of the efficacy of methotrexate alone or in combination with low doses of oral corticosteroids in the treatment of alopecia areata totalis or universalis. Ann Dermatol Venereol 2010;137(8–9):507–13 [in French].

152. Joly P. The use of methotrexate alone or in combination with low doses of oral corticosteroids in the treatment of alopecia totalis or universalis. J Am Acad Dermatol 2006;55(4):632–6.

153. Royer M, Bodemer C, Vabres P, et al. Efficacy and tolerability of methotrexate in severe childhood alopecia areata. Br J Dermatol 2011;165(2):407–10.

154. Farshi S, Mansouri P, Safar F, et al. Could azathioprine be considered as a therapeutic alternative in the treatment of alopecia areata? A pilot study. Int J Dermatol 2010;49(10):1188–93.

155. Cipriani R, Perini GI, Rampinelli S. Paroxetine in alopecia areata. Int J Dermatol 2001;40(9):600–1.

156. Willemsen R, Vanderlinden J, Deconinck A, et al. Hypnotherapeutic management of alopecia areata. J Am Acad Dermatol 2006;55(2):233–7.

157. Price VH, Willey A, Chen BK. Topical tacrolimus in alopecia areata. J Am Acad Dermatol 2005;52(1):138–9.

158. Thiers BH. Topical tacrolimus: treatment failure in a patient with alopecia areata. Arch Dermatol 2000;136(1):124.

159. Rigopoulos D, Gregoriou S, Korfitis C, et al. Lack of response of alopecia areata to pimecrolimus cream. Clin Exp Dermatol 2007;32(4):456–7.

160. Feldmann KA, Kunte C, Wollenberg A, et al. Is topical tacrolimus effective in alopecia areata universalis? Br J Dermatol 2002;147(5):1031–2.

161. Park SW, Kim JW, Wang HY. Topical tacrolimus (FK506): treatment failure in four cases of alopecia universalis. Acta Derm Venereol 2002;82(5):387–8.

162. Koc E, Tunca M, Akar A, et al. Lack of efficacy of topical imiquimod in the treatment of patchy alopecia areata. Int J Dermatol 2008;47(10):1088–9.

163. D'Ovidio R, Claudatus J, Di Prima T. Ineffectiveness of imiquimod therapy for alopecia totalis/universalis. J Eur Acad Dermatol Venereol 2002;16(4):416–7.

164. Bissonnette R, Shapiro J, Zeng H, et al. Topical photodynamic therapy with 5-aminolaevulinic acid does not induce hair regrowth in patients with extensive alopecia areata. Br J Dermatol 2000;143(5):1032–5.

165. Fernandez-Guarino M, Harto A, Garcia-Morales I, et al. Failure to treat alopecia areata with photodynamic therapy. Clin Exp Dermatol 2008;33(5):585–7.

166. Garcia Bartels N, Lee HH, Worm M, et al. Development of alopecia areata universalis in a patient receiving adalimumab. Arch Dermatol 2006;142(12):1654–5.

167. Kirshen C, Kanigsberg N. Alopecia areata following adalimumab. J Cutan Med Surg 2009;13(1):48–50.

168. Chaves Y, Duarte G, Ben-Said B, et al. Alopecia areata universalis during treatment of rheumatoid arthritis with anti-TNF-alpha antibody (adalimumab). Dermatology 2008;217(4):380.

169. Pelivani N, Hassan AS, Braathen LR, et al. Alopecia areata universalis elicited during treatment with adalimumab. Dermatology 2008;216(4):320–3.

170. Ettefagh L, Nedorost S, Mirmirani P. Alopecia areata in a patient using infliximab: new insights into the role of tumor necrosis factor on human hair follicles. Arch Dermatol 2004;140(8):1012.

171. Fabre C, Dereure O. Worsening alopecia areata and de novo occurrence of multiple halo nevi in a patient receiving infliximab. Dermatology 2008;216(2):185–6.

172. Posten W, Swan J. Recurrence of alopecia areata in a patient receiving etanercept injections. Arch Dermatol 2005;141(6):759–60.

173. Abramovits W, Losornio M. Failure of two TNF-alpha blockers to influence the course of alopecia areata. Skinmed 2006;5(4):177–81.

174. Pan Y, Rao NA. Alopecia areata during etanercept therapy. Ocul Immunol Inflamm 2009;17(2):127–9.

Genetic Basis of Alopecia Areata
A Roadmap for Translational Research

Ali Jabbari, MD, PhD[a], Lynn Petukhova, MS[a,b],
Rita M. Cabral, PhD[a], Raphael Clynes, MD, PhD[a,c,d],
Angela M. Christiano, PhD[a,e,*]

KEYWORDS

- Alopecia areata • Autoimmune disease • Genetic • Translational research

KEY POINTS

- Alopecia areata is a relatively common cause of nonscarring alopecia that lacks targeted treatments.
- Genetic studies have identified several immune-related as well as end-organ target specific genes associated with AA including CTLA4, ULBP3/6, IL2/21 and IL2RA.
- The association of immune related genes and AA support the common cause hypothesis of autoimmune diseases.
- Identified genes offer the hope of designing specific targeted treatments for AA.

ALOPECIA AREATA: A COMMON AUTOIMMUNE DISEASE
Epidemiology of Alopecia Areata

Alopecia areata (AA) is a frequent autoimmune disease with a lifetime risk of about 1.7% in the general population, including males and females across all ethnic groups.[1] The prevalence of AA is 0.1% to 0.2% worldwide, as well as in the United States, and is responsible for 0.7% to 3.0% of patients seen by dermatologists.[2,3] The peak incidence of AA seems to occur among 15- to 29-year-old individuals, with as many as 44% of people having onset of the disease before their 20s and less than 30% of patients having onset after their 40s. The clinical course of AA is highly unpredictable, and it can occur at any age from birth to the late decades of life.

Clinical Findings and Cause

AA is a nonscarring type of hair loss that usually manifests suddenly as 1 or more well-defined circumscribed areas that can occur anywhere in the body, although they are most frequently seen on the scalp (90% of cases).[3–5] The disease can then remit spontaneously or, alternatively, the initial patches can coalesce and progress to cover the scalp (alopecia totalis) or even the entire body surface (alopecia universalis). The clinical heterogeneity and unpredictable course of AA is a major source of distress for affected individuals.

[a] Department of Dermatology, Russ Berrie Medical Science Pavilion, Columbia University, 1150 Saint Nicholas Avenue, New York, NY 10032, USA; [b] Department of Epidemiology, Russ Berrie Medical Science Pavilion, Columbia University, 1150 Saint Nicholas Avenue, New York, NY 10032, USA; [c] Department of Medicine, Russ Berrie Medical Science Pavilion, Columbia University, 1150 Saint Nicholas Avenue, New York, NY 10032, USA; [d] Department of Pathology, Russ Berrie Medical Science Pavilion, Columbia University, 1150 Saint Nicholas Avenue, New York, NY 10032, USA; [e] Department of Genetics & Development, Russ Berrie Medical Science Pavilion, Columbia University, 1150 Saint Nicholas Avenue, New York, NY 10032, USA
* Corresponding author. Department of Dermatology, Russ Berrie Medical Science Pavilion, Columbia University, 1150 Saint Nicholas Avenue, New York, NY 10032.
E-mail address: amc65@columbia.edu

Dermatol Clin 31 (2013) 109–117
http://dx.doi.org/10.1016/j.det.2012.08.014
0733-8635/13/$ – see front matter © 2013 Elsevier Inc. All rights reserved.

Epidemiologic studies in AA have demonstrated that a history of autoimmune disease increases the risk of AA.[6] Specific reported associations include AA with thyroid disease,[4,7–11] celiac disease (CeD),[12] rheumatoid arthritis (RA),[7,8,13] vitiligo,[4,7–9,14,15] and type 1 diabetes (T1D).[7,10,13,16] Although the exact pathophysiology of AA is not clear, AA is a T-lymphocyte mediated autoimmune condition that occurs in genetically susceptible individuals.[17] Histopathologic findings have revealed inflammatory perifollicular infiltrates of T cells around anagen (growth phase) hair follicles ("swarm of bees"), which consist of both CD4+ and CD8+ T cells.[18,19] The focus of the attack by the infiltrating lymphocytes is the base of the hair follicle, such that the stem cell compartment, is spared from destruction and, therefore, hair regrowth remains possible. Increased levels of autoantibodies, cytokine abnormalities, and increased prevalence of autoimmune comorbidities have been described in patients with AA.[20,21] An acute onset of disease has been documented in affected individuals at times of profound stress, grief, or fear,[22] indicating that besides the autoimmune and genetic components, environmental (nongenetic) factors may contribute to the manifestation of this disease, thus supporting the multifactorial cause of AA.

Lack of Cure or Preventive Treatment of AA

AA can cause tremendous emotional and psychosocial distress in affected individuals and their families. Patients can experience profound feelings and frustrations, such as loneliness, isolation, anger, depression, and embarrassment, among many others. However, despite the high prevalence and extreme psychosocial burden of AA, there are no evidence-based treatments as yet, and treatment of AA is symptomatic and directed toward halting disease activity.[23] A comprehensive Cochrane analysis assessment of 17 randomized control trials (RCTs) involving a total of 540 participants found no proven treatment of AA.[24] These trials included 6 to 85 individuals each; treatments included topical and oral corticosteroids, topical cyclosporine, photodynamic therapy, and topical minoxidil. Even though topical corticosteroids and minoxidil have been widely used to reduce inflammation and/or stimulate hair growth, respectively, and seem to be safe, there is no convincing evidence that they are beneficial in the long term. Most trials have been poorly reported and/or are small and underpowered, resulting in inconclusive results.[17] No RCTs were found on the use of other drugs that are also commonly used for the treatment of AA, such as diphencyprone, dinitrochlorobenzene, dithranol, or intralesional corticosteroids.

Because of this lack of evidence-based treatment of AA and because of the high rate of spontaneous remission, particularly in individuals with a recent onset and small patches of hair loss, the initial approach typically includes topical or intralesional steroids or observation. However, approximately 20% to 30% of cases fail to resolve using these strategies, and only one-third of all cases achieve complete recovery for about 10 to 15 years.[25]

THE IMPACT OF GENETIC STUDIES IN AA RESEARCH
Candidate Gene and Linkage Studies

Genetics and disease gene discovery are promising and robust strategies to gain critical insights into pathogenic mechanisms in general. In the case of AA, initial evidence supporting a complex, polygenic basis for the disease was supported by multiple studies revealing (1) positive family history,[26–28] (2) twin concordance,[29,30] (3) familial aggregation,[26] (4) HLA associations,[31,32] and (5) studies in animal models.[33] The first genetic studies in AA were candidate gene association studies. In these studies, a single gene is chosen base on a previous hypothesis about its function (usually in another autoimmune disease) and then tested for association in a small sample of cases and controls. These studies were fruitful because they identified associations to genes residing in the HLA region (HLA-DQB1, HLA-DRB1, HLA-A, HLA-B, HLA-C, NOTCH4, MICA) and also outside of this region (PTPN22, AIRE).[34]

More recently, it became possible to survey the entire genome in a nonbiased way for evidence of genetic contributions to the disease using genome-wide genetic studies. These studies, which identify genes based on their position in the genome (as opposed to their function), are very powerful to uncover disease mechanisms when not much is known about the disease cause. Strong evidence for linkage is one of the most reliable evidences that a disease has a genetic component, although these studies usually result in the association of large regions of the genome, each containing many genes, and do not allow identification of particular causal variants. The authors previously performed a genome-wide linkage study and found several regions that cosegregate with AA among families, providing compelling evidence that the disease is, in fact, polygenic.[35]

Genome-Wide Association Studies and AA

In recent years, the identification of genetic markers for which an allele exists at a higher frequency among a group of unrelated cases, relative to a group of unrelated controls, has become possible with genome-wide association studies (GWAS). This technique, which most frequently uses single-nucleotide polymorphism (SNP) markers, can identify much smaller regions or linkage disequilibrium (LD) blocks compared with linkage studies. GWAS can survey between 500 000 and 1 million genetic markers among hundreds or thousands of people, counting alleles at each SNP, to identify regions in the genome where the distribution of alleles is skewed in the presence of disease.

The authors recently completed the first GWAS in AA interrogating allele frequencies across 500,000 SNPs between a group of 1054 unrelated patients with AA and 3278 population-based controls.[17] The authors identified several 139 SNPs that exceeded genome-wide significance ($P<5 \times 10^{-7}$), which clustered in 8 regions across the genome and implicated genes of the immune system as well as genes that are unique to the hair follicle: (1) 2q33.2 containing the CTLA4 gene; (2) 4q27 containing the IL2/IL21 locus; (3) 6p21.32 containing the HLA class II region; (4) 6q25.1, which harbors the ULBP gene cluster; (5) 9q31.1 containing syntaxin 17; (6) 10p15.1 containing IL2RA; (7) 11q13 containing peroxiredoxin 5 (PRDX5); and (8) 12q13 containing Eos. Several risk loci identified in the authors' GWAS were shared with other forms of autoimmunity, such as RA, T1D, CeD, systemic lupus erythematosus (SLE), multiple sclerosis (MS), and psoriasis, in particular CTLA4, IL2/IL2RA, IL21, NKG2D ligands and genes critical to the function of regulatory T cells. Importantly, all of the authors' loci have been replicated.[36]

Immune Genes Associated with AA

CTLA4 on chromosome 2q33.2

Extensive previous evidence arising from genetic studies exists for the involvement of CTLA4 in at least 30 different autoimmune diseases, including T1D, MS, Graves disease (GD), RA, CeD, and SLE. Independent evidence supporting these findings is the association of CTLA4 with 4 different autoimmune diseases, which have been found in 6 independent GWAS according to the National Institutes of Health database of GWAS (http://www.genome.gov/gwastudies). These studies associated CTLA4 with AA (the authors' study),[17,37] RA,[38,39] T1D,[40,41] and CeD.[42] Importantly, the authors' GWAS findings regarding the association of CTLA4 with AA have been replicated for the first time in an independent cohort.[37] This group genotyped 22 SNPs across the CTLA4 locus in about 1200 cases and 1200 controls and demonstrated a statistically significant association of 6 SNPs. One of these SNPs, rs231775, occurs in the coding region of CTLA4 and results in an amino acid substitution. The biologic function of CTLA4 is described later.

IL2/IL21 on chromosome 4q27

Interleukin 2 (IL-2) and IL-21 are 2 closely related cytokines and their encoded genes are adjacent, with similar exon/intron structures, which suggests that they might have arisen by gene duplication.[43,44] Although both cytokines are known to promote the function of effector CD8+ T cells, an antagonistic relationship between the actions of IL-2 and IL-21 on the differentiation of CD8+ T cells has been demonstrated.[45]

Many of the immunosuppressive drugs commonly used to treat autoimmune diseases function either by inhibiting the production of IL-2 by antigen-activated T cells (corticosteroids, cyclosporine, tacrolimus, sirolimus) or by blocking IL-2 receptor signaling. Cyclosporine, tacrolimus, and sirolimus have antiproliferative properties by inhibiting the response to IL-2, thereby preventing expansion and function of antigen-selected T cells.

HLA on chromosome 6p21.32

The HLA super locus, residing on chromosome 6, contains a large number of genes related to the immune system, including genes encoding cell-surface antigen-presenting proteins, among many others. The HLA class II region contains genes responsible for foreign antigen presentation to T cells, which specifically stimulate proliferation of helper T cells, which later stimulate antibody production by B cells or the activation of other immune cells. There are different HLA types, which are inherited, some of which have been overwhelmingly associated with autoimmune diseases. Several candidate gene studies have also previously demonstrated HLA associations with AA.[34]

In the authors' GWAS, they found the strongest association between the HLA class II locus and AA. One hundred five of the 139 SNPs that exceeded statistical significance reside in the HLA and genome wide, both the most significant SNP, rs9275572 ($P = 1.38 \times 10^{-35}$), and the SNP with the greatest magnitude of effect, rs11752643 (odds ratio: 5.56; 95% confidence interval: 3.03–10.00), were found here.

ULBP3/ULBP6 on chromosome 6q25.1

The authors' GWAS was the first to identify the cytomegalovirus UL16-binding protein (ULBP) gene cluster in association with an autoimmune disease. This gene cluster encodes activating ligands for the natural killer (NK) cell receptor NKG2D that have not been previously implicated in any autoimmune disease and, therefore, had been missed from candidate gene studies.

NKG2D is a homodimeric activating receptor that is expressed on the surface of not only all NK cells but also most NKT cells, all human CD8+ cytotoxic T cells, activated mouse CD8+ T cells, subsets of gamma-delta T cells, and under certain circumstances, such as in patients with RA, CD4+ T cells. Although NKG2D is expressed constitutively on human and mouse NK cells, cytokines, such as IL-15, IL-2, and interferon-gamma, upregulate its expression on human NK cells.[46] The NKG2D receptor is remarkable in that it can bind to a wide range of different ligands, which are distantly related homologs of the major histocompatibility complex class I proteins.

The authors' GWAS results point to the specific LD block containing ULBP3 and ULBP6 as being strongly implicated in AA. Although their data show, for the first time, the involvement of the ULBP family of NKG2D ligands (NKG2DLs) in the pathogenesis of an autoimmune disease,[17] other NKG2DLs have been associated with various autoimmune disorders.[47] For example, specific MHC class I polypeptide-related sequence A (MICA) alleles are overrepresented in RA, inflammatory bowel disease, and patients with T1D, implicating a role in disease pathogenesis.[48,49] Likewise, MHC class I polypeptide-related sequence B (MICB) polymorphisms are also associated with CeD, ulcerative colitis, and MS.[50–52] By probing the role of ULBP3 in disease pathogenesis, the authors also showed that its expression in lesional scalp from patients with AA is markedly upregulated in the hair follicle dermal sheath during active disease.

IL2RA on chromosome 10p15.1

The IL-2-receptor α (IL2RA or CD25) is an important regulatory T cell marker; genetic polymorphisms of the IL2RA gene are associated with several autoimmune diseases, such as T1D, MS, GD, SLE, RA, systemic sclerosis, and now AA.[17,53–57] Regulatory T cells function to maintain the immune tolerance and have been reported to have an important role in several autoimmune diseases.

Genetic variants in the IL2RA locus differentially confer risk to MS and T1D, demonstrating genetic heterogeneity of the associated polymorphisms and risk alleles between MS and T1D.[56,58] Additionally, several independent genetic variants of IL2RA correlate with the levels of a soluble form of the IL-2 receptor (sIL2RA) in human serum. High concentrations of sIL2RA are found in sera from healthy individuals and have been reported to be increased in patients with autoimmune disease, inflammation, and infection.[59–61] However, T1D susceptibility genotypes of IL2RA have been associated with reduced circulating levels of sIL2RA, suggesting that an inherited lower immune responsiveness predisposes to this autoimmune disease.[55] These results suggest some discordance between sIL2RA levels and disease susceptibility, and further studies addressing the causality of sIL2RA in autoimmune disease will be needed. Independent biologic pathways contributing to disease susceptibility may include IL2RA transcriptional regulation, cell surface expression levels of IL2RA, and serum sIL2RA levels.[56]

One of the most remarkable findings in the authors' GWAS in AA was the presence of the association at both the IL-2 locus and its receptor IL2RA, suggesting a prominent role for this signaling pathway in AA disease pathogenesis.

EOS/ERBB3 on chromosome 12q13

The Eos locus in chromosome 12q13 has been previously associated with T1D, placing this locus among the shared autoimmune loci.[41] The authors also identified a significant GWAS association on a haplotype block on chromosome 12q13, which contains several genes, with AA. Among these, Eos emerged as a plausible candidate gene, given its know function in CD4+ regulatory T cells. These cells are known to maintain immunologic self-tolerance and immune homeostasis by suppressing aberrant immune responses, a process that depends on the transcription factor Foxp3-dependent gene activation.[62] Recently, the zinc-finger transcription factor of the Ikaros family, Eos, was identified as a critical mediator of Foxp3-dependent gene silencing in regulatory T cells.[63] Eos silencing in these cells causes them to lose their ability to suppress immune responses, demonstrating the crucial role of Eos for regulatory T-cell specification and function.[63]

Despite this recent evidence making Eos a compelling candidate gene at this locus, ERBB3 has also been previously implicated as a plausible candidate gene at this locus for autoimmune diseases.[41] It is possible that the underlying susceptibility alleles may influence both Eos and ERBB3 transcripts.

IL13 on chromosome 5q31 and CLEC16A on 16p13.13

As mentioned earlier, all loci from the authors' initial GWAS have been corroborated by independent studies.[35–37,64] The most recent of these studies further identified IL-13 and CLEC16A as 2 additional gene associations that showed a nominal signal in their GWAS and have now surpassed the genome-wide significance threshold in a meta-analysis.[36]

IL-13 is a cytokine classically associated with CD4 T helper 2 responses, although other cell types, including innatelike T cells, can also express this cytokine. As such, it is thought to be important in the pathogenesis of allergic responses and associated diseases. Indeed, IL-13–proximal SNPs have been associated with asthma[65,66] as well as with other autoimmune diseases, including psoriasis.[67,68]

CLEC16A encodes a protein with unknown function. CLEC16A contains a putative C-type lectin domain and a likely immunoreceptor tyrosine-based activation motif. C-type lectins are receptors that bind carbohydrates and function as adhesion receptors and pathogen recognition receptors[69]; CLEC16A may, therefore, be important in engendering or modulating immune responses. Interestingly, CLEC16A has been associated with MS[70,71] and T1D,[72,73] further supporting its role as a modulator of the immune response.

Hair Follicle–Specific Genes

PRDX5 on chromosome 11q13
Reactive oxygen species are a potentially deleterious byproduct of mitochondrial respiration that can damage DNA, proteins, and organelle membranes. Peroxiredoxins (PRDXs) are a family of enzymes responsible for quenching reactive oxygen species. PRDX5 is expressed in many tissues, including the hair follicle, and is induced under conditions of cellular stress. Upregulation of PRDX5 may confer an antiapoptotic phenotype and may ultimately enable survival of aberrant cells, which harbor danger signals, leading to the presentation of damaged self-antigens to the immune system and, subsequently, autoimmune disease.[74,75] In a mouse model of diabetes, overexpression of a PRDX in islet cells protected against hyperglycemia and hypoinsulinemia, illustrating the protective function of PRDXs in an end-organ immune target.[76] A GWAS meta-analysis for Crohn disease demonstrated a statistically significant association for the same allele that the authors identified in AA.[77]

STX17 on chromosome 9q31.1
STX17 belongs to a family of molecules called syntaxins, which belong to the Soluble NSF Attachment Protein Receptor (SNARE) superfamily. SNARE complexes are involved in vesicular trafficking and membrane fusion. No other human disease associations with STX17 to date have been identified. However, an insertion with enhancerlike activity in an intronic segment of STX17 was found to be responsible for the gray hair phenotype in horses.[78,79] This finding is intriguing because AA is known to preferentially affect pigmented hair follicles and to spare gray hairs.

AUTOIMMUNE DISEASES: COMMON CAUSE, COMMON TREATMENT

It has been suspected that autoimmune diseases affecting different end organs in fact share common disease mechanisms. First, through epidemiologic studies and later using genetic studies, researchers have demonstrated certain similarities at the molecular level (ie, susceptibility regions on the chromosomes or the involvement of common genes).[80] Although the cause of autoimmune diseases is still unclear, these advances have contributed to the development of a common cause theory of autoimmunity.

In accordance with the common cause hypothesis of autoimmune diseases, the authors have uncovered several risk loci in common with other forms of autoimmunity, such as RA, T1D, CeD, Crohn disease/colitis, SLE, MS, and psoriasis, in particular CTLA4, IL2/IL2RA, IL-21, and genes that are crucial for the homeostasis of regulatory T cells. The genetic commonality with RA, T1D, and CeD is especially noteworthy in light of the pathogenic significance of the expression of an NK ligand in the end organ (synovial fluid, islets, gut, respectively, and hair follicle for AA), and the involvement of the NKG2DL/NKG2D pathway in the pathogenesis of each of these 3 diseases.

The recent successes of GWAS studies have identified susceptibility alleles in specific genes that underlie sets of autoimmune diseases; importantly, most of these shared genes can be mapped onto a discrete set of immunologic molecular pathways. These discoveries have made possible the identification of important pathologic processes and general mechanisms that dysregulate immune tolerance and might be common to several autoimmune diseases. Furthermore, these advances have important implications for translational research in autoimmune diseases. Firstly, the identification of particular drug targets that are common to multiple diseases will allow us to establish a rationale for using a drug that gained approval for treatment of one autoimmune disorder to treat others. Secondly, the goal of personalized medicine might allow us, in the future, to tailor therapeutic approaches based on their susceptibility genes as opposed to the inefficient process of trial and error.

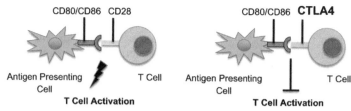

Fig. 1. Proposed mode of action of CTLA4. The costimulatory receptor CD28 present on the surface of T cells interacts with its ligands, CD80/CD86, that are present on the surface of antigen-presenting cells (including macrophages, dendritic cells, and B cells), driving initial T-cell activation. Endogenous CTLA4 and the therapeutic CTLA4-Ig binds CD80/86 with higher affinity than CD28, effectively competing away costimulatory drive. Ig, immunoglobulin; APS, antigen-presenting cell.

Pursuing CTLA4 as a drugable target serves as a potential example of realizing this approach. Before GWAS studies, several genetic studies had implicated the costimulatory locus, which includes CTLA4, in several autoimmune diseases. CTLA4 effectively turns off immune responses (**Fig. 1**) and is thought to prevent excessive, unnecessary bystander damage and autoimmune disease by an untempered immune system. A soluble CTLA4-Ig recombinant fusion molecule can serve the same purpose, and this molecule demonstrated inhibition of naive CD4+ T cell activation and proliferation[81,82] and prevention of autoimmunity and inhibition of graft rejection in animal models.[83–87] Abatacept, a CTLA4 immunoglobulin (Ig) approved for use in humans, has been shown to be efficacious in the treatment of RA and psoriasis.[88,89] Moreover, approximately 54 clinical trials are currently underway to test this drug (or a similar drug, belatacept) in several other autoimmune diseases as well as in organ transplantations (**Table 1**). Interestingly, in AA, preclinical studies using CTLA4-Ig have shown efficacy in preventing alopecia in the C3H/HeJ mouse model of disease.[90] Collectively, the authors' genetic evidence, taken together with the efficacy data in the AA mouse model, as well as the safety and efficacy of abatacept in RA and other autoimmune diseases, make a strong case for the testing of this drug in AA clinical trials.[91]

SUMMARY

The great advances that genetics has brought into the study of autoimmune diseases in general, and AA in particular, have paved the way for an exciting new era of translational research that we are about to enter. The continuous discovery of molecular and signaling pathways that overlap between different autoimmune diseases greatly helps to illuminate pathologically important disease processes, arguing for unifying/general mechanisms that dysregulate immune tolerance at one of several multiple end-organ sites.

The authors' GWAS findings in AA, together with other studies, have already opened new avenues for the exploration of therapeutic strategies based on the actual underlying mechanisms of the disease, with a focus on T cells as well as cells that express the NKG2D receptor. Taking advantage of the common molecular pathways and of the fact that several drugs and biologics are currently being used or tested for the treatment of other autoimmune diseases, the authors anticipate that new therapies for AA will be available in the near future.

Table 1
Abatacept or belatacept clinical trials for autoimmune diseases

Disease	Number of Studies
Rheumatoid arthritis	23
Renal transplant	10
Type I diabetes mellitus	5
Lupus nephritis	3
Solid organ transplant	1
Acute graft-versus-host disease	1
Takayasu Arteritis; Giant Cell Arteritis	1
Urticaria	1
Wegener granulomatosis	1
Polymyositis, dermatomyositis	1
Alopecia totalis/universalis	1
Uveitis	1
Multiple sclerosis, relapsing-remitting	1
Ankylosing spondylitis	1
Relapsing polychondritis	1
Allergic asthma	1
Juvenile idiopathic arthritis	1
Total	54

Data from: http://www.clinicaltrials.gov. Accessed July 1, 2012.

REFERENCES

1. Hon KL, Leung AK. Alopecia areata. Recent Pat Inflamm Allergy Drug Discov 2011;5:98.
2. Safavi K. Prevalence of alopecia areata in the First National Health and Nutrition Examination Survey. Arch Dermatol 1992;128:702.
3. Safavi KH, Muller SA, Suman VJ, et al. Incidence of alopecia areata in Olmsted County, Minnesota, 1975 through 1989. Mayo Clin Proc 1995;70:628.
4. Tan E, Tay YK, Goh CL, et al. The pattern and profile of alopecia areata in Singapore–a study of 219 Asians. Int J Dermatol 2002;41:748.
5. Tan E, Tay YK, Giam YC. A clinical study of childhood alopecia areata in Singapore. Pediatr Dermatol 2002;19:298.
6. Barahmani N, Schabath MB, Duvic M. History of atopy or autoimmunity increases risk of alopecia areata. J Am Acad Dermatol 2009;61:581.
7. Muller SA, Winkelmann RK. Alopecia areata. An evaluation of 736 patients. Arch Dermatol 1963;88:290.
8. Shellow WV, Edwards JE, Koo JY. Profile of alopecia areata: a questionnaire analysis of patient and family. Int J Dermatol 1992;31:186.
9. Wang SJ, Shohat T, Vadheim C, et al. Increased risk for type I (insulin-dependent) diabetes in relatives of patients with alopecia areata (AA). Am J Med Genet 1994;51:234.
10. Friedmann PS. Alopecia areata and auto-immunity. Br J Dermatol 1981;105:153.
11. Cunliffe WJ, Hall R, Stevenson CJ, et al. Alopecia areata, thyroid disease and autoimmunity. Br J Dermatol 1969;81:877.
12. Corazza GR, Andreani ML, Venturo N, et al. Celiac disease and alopecia areata: report of a new association. Gastroenterology 1995;109:1333.
13. Rzhetsky A, Wajngurt D, Park N, et al. Probing genetic overlap among complex human phenotypes. Proc Natl Acad Sci U S A 2007;104:11694.
14. Cunliffe WJ, Hall R, Newell DJ, et al. Vitiligo, thyroid disease and autoimmunity. Br J Dermatol 1968;80:135.
15. Narita T, Oiso N, Fukai K, et al. Generalized vitiligo and associated autoimmune diseases in Japanese patients and their families. Allergol Int 2011;60(4):505–8.
16. Sipetic S, Vlajinac H, Kocev N, et al. Family history and risk of type 1 diabetes mellitus. Acta Diabetol 2002;39:111.
17. Petukhova L, Duvic M, Hordinsky M, et al. Genomewide association study in alopecia areata implicates both innate and adaptive immunity. Nature 2010;466:113.
18. Ghersetich I, Campanile G, Lotti T. Alopecia areata: immunohistochemistry and ultrastructure of infiltrate and identification of adhesion molecule receptors. Int J Dermatol 1996;35:28.
19. Todes-Taylor N, Turner R, Wood GS, et al. T cell subpopulations in alopecia areata. J Am Acad Dermatol 1984;11:216.
20. Gregoriou S, Papafragkaki D, Kontochristopoulos G, et al. Cytokines and other mediators in alopecia areata. Mediators Inflamm 2010;2010:928030.
21. Brajac I, Kastelan M, Perisa D, et al. Treatment of alopecia areata: modern principles and perspectives. Lijec Vjesn 2010;132:365 [in Croatian].
22. Jelinek JE. Sudden whitening of the hair. Bull N Y Acad Med 1972;48:1003.
23. Wasserman D, Guzman-Sanchez DA, Scott K, et al. Alopecia areata. Int J Dermatol 2007;46:121.
24. Delamere FM, Sladden MM, Dobbins HM, et al. Interventions for alopecia areata. Cochrane Database Syst Rev 2008;(2):CD004413.
25. Mitchell AJ, Balle MR. Alopecia areata. Dermatol Clin 1987;5:553.
26. Blaumeiser B, van der Goot I, Fimmers R, et al. Familial aggregation of alopecia areata. J Am Acad Dermatol 2006;54:627.
27. McDonagh AJ, Tazi-Ahnini R. Epidemiology and genetics of alopecia areata. Clin Exp Dermatol 2002;27:405.
28. van der Steen P, Traupe H, Happle R, et al. The genetic risk for alopecia areata in first degree relatives of severely affected patients. An estimate. Acta Derm Venereol 1992;72:373.
29. Jackow C, Puffer N, Hordinsky M, et al. Alopecia areata and cytomegalovirus infection in twins: genes versus environment? J Am Acad Dermatol 1998;38:418.
30. Scerri L, Pace JL. Identical twins with identical alopecia areata. J Am Acad Dermatol 1992;27:766.
31. Colombe BW, Lou CD, Price VH. The genetic basis of alopecia areata: HLA associations with patchy alopecia areata versus alopecia totalis and alopecia universalis. J Investig Dermatol Symp Proc 1999;4:216.
32. de Andrade M, Jackow CM, Dahm N, et al. Alopecia areata in families: association with the HLA locus. J Investig Dermatol Symp Proc 1999;4:220.
33. Sundberg JP, Silva KA, Li R, et al. Adult-onset alopecia areata is a complex polygenic trait in the C3H/HeJ mouse model. J Invest Dermatol 2004;123:294.
34. Gilhar A, Paus R, Kalish RS. Lymphocytes, neuropeptides, and genes involved in alopecia areata. J Clin Invest 2007;117:2019.
35. Martinez-Mir A, Zlotogorski A, Gordon D, et al. Genomewide scan for linkage reveals evidence of several susceptibility loci for alopecia areata. Am J Hum Genet 2007;80:316.
36. Jagielska D, Redler S, Brockschmidt FF, et al. Follow-up study of the first genome-wide association scan in alopecia areata: IL13 and KIAA0350 as susceptibility loci supported with genome-wide significance. J Invest Dermatol 2012;132(9):2192–7.

37. John KK, Brockschmidt FF, Redler S, et al. Genetic variants in CTLA4 are strongly associated with alopecia areata. J Invest Dermatol 2011;131:1169.

38. Gregersen PK, Amos CI, Lee AT, et al. REL, encoding a member of the NF-kappaB family of transcription factors, is a newly defined risk locus for rheumatoid arthritis. Nat Genet 2009;41:820.

39. Stahl EA, Raychaudhuri S, Remmers EF, et al. Genome-wide association study meta-analysis identifies seven new rheumatoid arthritis risk loci. Nat Genet 2010;42:508.

40. Barrett JC, Clayton DG, Concannon P, et al. Genome-wide association study and meta-analysis find that over 40 loci affect risk of type 1 diabetes. Nat Genet 2009;41:703.

41. Cooper JD, Smyth DJ, Smiles AM, et al. Meta-analysis of genome-wide association study data identifies additional type 1 diabetes risk loci. Nat Genet 2008;40:1399.

42. Dubois PC, Trynka G, Franke L, et al. Multiple common variants for celiac disease influencing immune gene expression. Nat Genet 2010;42:295.

43. Parrish-Novak J, Dillon SR, Nelson A, et al. Interleukin 21 and its receptor are involved in NK cell expansion and regulation of lymphocyte function. Nature 2000;408:57.

44. Parrish-Novak J, Foster DC, Holly RD, et al. Interleukin-21 and the IL-21 receptor: novel effectors of NK and T cell responses. J Leukoc Biol 2002; 72:856.

45. Hinrichs CS, Spolski R, Paulos CM, et al. IL-2 and IL-21 confer opposing differentiation programs to CD8+ T cells for adoptive immunotherapy. Blood 2008;111:5326.

46. Champsaur M, Lanier LL. Effect of NKG2D ligand expression on host immune responses. Immunol Rev 2010;235:267.

47. Ito T, Ito N, Saatoff M, et al. Maintenance of hair follicle immune privilege is linked to prevention of NK cell attack. J Invest Dermatol 2008;128:1196.

48. Gambelunghe G, Brozzetti A, Ghaderi M, et al. MICA gene polymorphism in the pathogenesis of type 1 diabetes. Ann N Y Acad Sci 2007;1110:92.

49. Kirsten H, Petit-Teixeira E, Scholz M, et al. Association of MICA with rheumatoid arthritis independent of known HLA-DRB1 risk alleles in a family-based and a case control study. Arthritis Res Ther 2009;11:R60.

50. Fernandez-Morera JL, Rodriguez-Rodero S, Tunon A, et al. Genetic influence of the nonclassical major histocompatibility complex class I molecule MICB in multiple sclerosis susceptibility. Tissue Antigens 2008;72:54.

51. Li Y, Xia B, Lu M, et al. MICB0106 gene polymorphism is associated with ulcerative colitis in central China. Int J Colorectal Dis 2010;25:153.

52. Rodriguez-Rodero S, Rodrigo L, Fdez-Morera JL, et al. MHC class I chain-related gene B promoter polymorphisms and celiac disease. Hum Immunol 2006;67:208.

53. Martin JE, Carmona FD, Broen JC, et al. The autoimmune disease-associated IL2RA locus is involved in the clinical manifestations of systemic sclerosis. Genes Immun 2012;13(2):191–6.

54. Lindner E, Weger M, Steinwender G, et al. IL2RA gene polymorphism rs2104286 A>G seen in multiple sclerosis is associated with intermediate uveitis: possible parallel pathways? Invest Ophthalmol Vis Sci 2011;52:8295.

55. Lowe CE, Cooper JD, Brusko T, et al. Large-scale genetic fine mapping and genotype-phenotype associations implicate polymorphism in the IL2RA region in type 1 diabetes. Nat Genet 2007;39:1074.

56. Maier LM, Anderson DE, Severson CA, et al. Soluble IL-2RA levels in multiple sclerosis subjects and the effect of soluble IL-2RA on immune responses. J Immunol 2009;182:1541.

57. Carr EJ, Clatworthy MR, Lowe CE, et al. Contrasting genetic association of IL2RA with SLE and ANCA-associated vasculitis. BMC Med Genet 2009;10:22.

58. Alcina A, Fedetz M, Ndagire D, et al. IL2RA/CD25 gene polymorphisms: uneven association with multiple sclerosis (MS) and type 1 diabetes (T1D). PLoS One 2009;4:e4137.

59. Makis AC, Galanakis E, Hatzimichael EC, et al. Serum levels of soluble interleukin-2 receptor alpha (sIL-2Ralpha) as a predictor of outcome in brucellosis. J Infect 2005;51:206.

60. Giordano C, Galluzzo A, Marco A, et al. Increased soluble interleukin-2 receptor levels in the sera of type 1 diabetic patients. Diabetes Res 1988;8:135.

61. Greenberg P, Klarnet J, Kern D, et al. Requirements for T cell recognition and elimination of retrovirally-transformed cells. Princess Takamatsu Symp 1988; 19:287.

62. Hill JA, Feuerer M, Tash K, et al. Foxp3 transcription-factor-dependent and -independent regulation of the regulatory T cell transcriptional signature. Immunity 2007;27:786.

63. Pan F, Yu H, Dang EV, et al. Eos mediates Foxp3-dependent gene silencing in CD4+ regulatory T cells. Science 2009;325:1142.

64. Entz P, Blaumeiser B, Betz RC, et al. Investigation of the HLA-DRB1 locus in alopecia areata. Eur J Dermatol 2006;16:363.

65. Elias JA, Lee CG. IL-13 in asthma. The successful integration of lessons from mice and humans. Am J Respir Crit Care Med 2011;183:957.

66. Li X, Howard TD, Zheng SL, et al. Genome-wide association study of asthma identifies RAD50-IL13 and HLA-DR/DQ regions. J Allergy Clin Immunol 2010;125:328.

67. Chang M, Li Y, Yan C, et al. Variants in the 5q31 cytokine gene cluster are associated with psoriasis. Genes Immun 2008;9:176.

68. Nair RP, Duffin KC, Helms C, et al. Genome-wide scan reveals association of psoriasis with IL-23 and NF-kappaB pathways. Nat Genet 2009;41:199.

69. van den Berg LM, Gringhuis SI, Geijtenbeek TB. An evolutionary perspective on C-type lectins in infection and immunity. Ann N Y Acad Sci 2012;1253:149.

70. Barahmani N, Lopez A, Babu D, et al. Serum T helper 1 cytokine levels are greater in patients with alopecia areata regardless of severity or atopy. Clin Exp Dermatol 2010;35(4):409–16.

71. Hafler DA, Compston A, Sawcer S, et al. Risk alleles for multiple sclerosis identified by a genomewide study. N Engl J Med 2007;357:851.

72. Hakonarson H, Grant SF, Bradfield JP, et al. A genome-wide association study identifies KIAA0350 as a type 1 diabetes gene. Nature 2007; 448:591.

73. Wellcome Trust Case Control Consortium. Genome-wide association study of 14,000 cases of seven common diseases and 3,000 shared controls. Nature 2007;447:661.

74. Kropotov A, Serikov V, Suh J, et al. Constitutive expression of the human peroxiredoxin V gene contributes to protection of the genome from oxidative DNA lesions and to suppression of transcription of noncoding DNA. FEBS J 2006;273:2607.

75. Kubo E, Singh DP, Fatma N, et al. TAT-mediated peroxiredoxin 5 and 6 protein transduction protects against high-glucose-induced cytotoxicity in retinal pericytes. Life Sci 2009;84:857.

76. Ding Y, Yamada S, Wang KY, et al. Overexpression of peroxiredoxin 4 protects against high-dose streptozotocin-induced diabetes by suppressing oxidative stress and cytokines in transgenic mice. Antioxid Redox Signal 2010;13:1477.

77. Franke A, McGovern DP, Barrett JC, et al. Genome-wide meta-analysis increases to 71 the number of confirmed Crohn's disease susceptibility loci. Nat Genet 2010;42:1118.

78. Sundstrom E, Komisarczuk AZ, Jiang L, et al. Identification of a melanocyte-specific, microphthalmia-associated transcription factor-dependent regulatory element in the intronic duplication causing hair greying and melanoma in horses. Pigment Cell Melanoma Res 2012;25:28.

79. Rosengren Pielberg G, Golovko A, Sundstrom E, et al. A cis-acting regulatory mutation causes premature hair graying and susceptibility to melanoma in the horse. Nat Genet 2008;40:1004.

80. Karopka T, Fluck J, Mevissen HT, et al. The Autoimmune Disease Database: a dynamically compiled literature-derived database. BMC Bioinformatics 2006;7:325.

81. Linsley PS, Greene JL, Tan P, et al. Coexpression and functional cooperation of CTLA-4 and CD28 on activated T lymphocytes. J Exp Med 1992;176: 1595.

82. Tan R, Teh SJ, Ledbetter JA, et al. B7 costimulates proliferation of CD4-8+ T lymphocytes but is not required for the deletion of immature CD4+8+ thymocytes. J Immunol 1992;149:3217.

83. Knoerzer DB, Karr RW, Schwartz BD, et al. Collagen-induced arthritis in the BB rat. Prevention of disease by treatment with CTLA-4-Ig. J Clin Invest 1995;96:987.

84. Pearson TC, Alexander DZ, Hendrix R, et al. CTLA4-Ig plus bone marrow induces long-term allograft survival and donor specific unresponsiveness in the murine model. Evidence for hematopoietic chimerism. Transplantation 1996;61:997.

85. Ndejembi MP, Teijaro JR, Patke DS, et al. Control of memory CD4 T cell recall by the CD28/B7 costimulatory pathway. J Immunol 2006;177:7698.

86. Finck BK, Linsley PS, Wofsy D. Treatment of murine lupus with CTLA4Ig. Science 1994;265:1225.

87. Khoury SJ, Akalin E, Chandraker A, et al. CD28-B7 costimulatory blockade by CTLA4Ig prevents actively induced experimental autoimmune encephalomyelitis and inhibits Th1 but spares Th2 cytokines in the central nervous system. J Immunol 1995;155: 4521.

88. Kremer JM, Dougados M, Emery P, et al. Treatment of rheumatoid arthritis with the selective costimulation modulator abatacept: twelve-month results of a phase iib, double-blind, randomized, placebo-controlled trial. Arthritis Rheum 2005;52:2263.

89. Abrams JR, Lebwohl MG, Guzzo CA, et al. CTLA4Ig-mediated blockade of T-cell costimulation in patients with psoriasis vulgaris. J Clin Invest 1999;103:1243.

90. Carroll JM, McElwee KJ, E King L, et al. Gene array profiling and immunomodulation studies define a cell-mediated immune response underlying the pathogenesis of alopecia areata in a mouse model and humans. J Invest Dermatol 2002;119:392.

91. Sundberg JP, McElwee KJ, Carroll JM, et al. Hypothesis testing: CTLA4 co-stimulatory pathways critical in the pathogenesis of human and mouse alopecia areata. J Invest Dermatol 2011;131:2323.

Hair: What is New in Diagnosis and Management?
Female Pattern Hair Loss Update: Diagnosis and Treatment

Natasha Atanaskova Mesinkovska, MD, PhD,
Wilma F. Bergfeld, MD*

KEYWORDS

- Alopecia • Pattern hair loss • New • Update • Treatment • Androgenetic

KEY POINTS

- Female pattern hair loss (FPHL) is the most common cause of alopecia in women, and it is characterized by follicular miniaturization.
- Androgens and estrogens are the main hormonal regulators implicated in FPHL.
- Realistic expectations need to be set when treating patients with FPHL.
- All treatments seem to work best when initiated early and when used in combinations.

DEFINITION

Female pattern hair loss (FPHL) is the most common cause of alopecia in women. It affects 6% to 12% of women between the ages of 20 and 30 years, and more than 55% of women older than 70 years.[1] FPHL clinically presents with diffuse nonscarring loss of hair, with prominent thinning over the frontal, central, and parietal scalp. The frontal hairline is characteristically retained. A similar pattern of hair loss with follicular miniaturization is seen in male androgenetic alopecia (AGA). Because the role of androgens on alopecia in women remains uncertain, FPHL has emerged as the preferred term rather than AGA in women.[2]

DIAGNOSIS

The diagnosis of FPHL is made clinically based on the appearance of the scalp. Biopsies are reserved only for situations when the diagnosis is uncertain.

A 4-mm cylindrical punch from the central area of hair loss is preferred. It is recommended to avoid biopsies from the temporal area, because miniaturized hair follicles can be found there even in the absence of FPHL.[3] Preferably vertical and horizontal tissue sections should be processed, and reviewed by a dermatopathologist experienced in interpreting alopecia biopsies.

FPHL is characterized histologically with increased numbers of miniaturized, velluslike hair follicles. In FPHL, the ratio of terminal to velluslike hairs is usually less than 3:1.[4] There is a reduction in follicle size, depth, and hair shaft diameter, with an increased telogen/anagen ratio.[5] Low levels of inflammation can be found as lymphocytic microfolliculitis targeting the hair bulge, with IgM and complement deposits on the basement membrane.[6]

Although most patients with FPHL have normal levels of testosterone, this type of alopecia can be a marker of hyperandrogenism in women.[7] Evaluation of patients with FPHL should include

Department of Dermatology, Dermatology and Plastic Surgery Institute, Cleveland Clinic, A61, 9500 Euclid Avenue, Cleveland, OH 44195, USA
* Corresponding author.
E-mail address: bergfew@ccf.org

Dermatol Clin 31 (2013) 119–127
http://dx.doi.org/10.1016/j.det.2012.08.005
0733-8635/13/$ – see front matter © 2013 Elsevier Inc. All rights reserved.

clinical assessment for hirsutism, menstrual abnormalities, and acne. Hormonal studies should include serum levels of androgens, to evaluate for presence of polycystic ovary syndrome (PCOS), androgen-producing tumors, or congenital adrenal hyperplasia. A referral to an endocrinologist may be helpful in complicated cases. Additional useful laboratory tests include thyroid, iron studies with ferritin, prolactin, and zinc levels.

PATHOGENESIS

Androgens and estrogens are the main hormonal regulators implicated in FPHL. The hair follicle is sensitive to alterations in circulating estrogen and androgen levels; these hormones are also synthesized and metabolized locally.[8] Most of the evidence about the role of androgens comes from studies of male AGA. Androgens have a clearly established role via binding of dihydrotestosterone (DHT) to hair follicle androgen receptors (AR) in male pattern hair loss. In scalp hair follicles, testosterone is converted to DHT by the enzyme 5-α reductase type II. DHT has a 5-fold higher affinity for the AR and is believed to be the more important player in AGA.[9] The 5a reductase inhibitors, finasteride and dutasteride, can be used to block DHT synthesis and arrest hair loss in men. Functional polymorphisms of AR can be a marker for premature AGA in men and can predict treatment response to 5a reductase inhibitors.[10]

In contrast, the role of androgens in FPHL has not been clearly established and it does not seem to be as essential as in AGA. Pattern hair loss has been described in cases with complete androgen insensitivity syndromes, suggesting that mechanisms other than androgens may be involved.[11] Although FPHL can be associated with hyperandrogenic states, the circulating testosterone levels do not differ between patients with FPHL and normal controls.[7] Many women with FPHL have low levels of circulating sex hormone binding globulin (SHBG), which may increase the available free testosterone at the level of the hair follicle.[11] Although it has been postulated that there is an increased peripheral sensitivity to androgens in FPHL, the response to treatment with 5a reductase inhibitors is unpredictable. Also, AR polymorphisms have not been uniformly confirmed and cannot completely explain the mechanism of FPHL.[12]

The observed differences between androgen regulation in FPHL and male AGA may lie in the presence of estrogens. Estrogen signaling can modify androgen metabolism at the hair follicle, by unclear mechanisms. Estrogens may positively affect hair loss through inhibition of 5a reductase.[13] High systemic estrogen levels in pregnancy are implicated in the prolongation of anagen. The sudden loss of estrogen postpartum is believed to lead to shedding, known as telogen gravidarum.[14] Conversely, lower systemic estrogen levels have been implicated in the increase of FPHL after menopause.[15] FPHL has been correlated with low systemic estrogen levels when aromatase inhibitors are used in cancer therapy. Topical estrogen preparations are used to treat FPHL in some countries, but their efficacy is questionable.[16]

Outside the sex hormonal milieu, FPHL may be influenced by insulin resistance, microvascular insufficiency, and inflammatory abnormalities. Insulin resistance has been associated with low circulating levels of SHBG and early onset of AGA in male patients.[17] Patients with FPHL show higher prevalence of carotid atheromatosis, with higher levels of inflammatory markers, such as C-reactive protein, fibrinogen, and D-dimer.[18] Increased systolic blood pressures are found in patients with FPHL in comparison to control individuals.

Genetic Studies

Studies on the genetic base of FPHL show increased frequency of alopecia in both male (54%) and female (21%) first-degree relatives.[19] Based on the experience from AGA, the speculated FPHL genetic link may lie in variations of the AR gene.[20] The AR gene is a nuclear transcription factor located on the X-chromosome. The amino-terminal domain of the AR gene contains a region of CAG repeats, which affects its transcriptional activity.[20] The number of CAG repeats inversely correlates with androgen function. Particular CAG variants in the AR gene are implicated with a risk of developing AGA in men.[10] Variations in the CAG length have been associated with PCOS, hirsutism, and acne in women.[21] These findings led to the development of a screening test for FPHL and AGA, the Hair Genetic Test (http://hairdx.com), which differs for men and women. In women, the Hair Genetic Test measures the length of CAG and GGC repeats within the AR gene. Shorter CAG and GGC repeats are associated with a significant risk of developing FPHL. Short repeat lengths (15 or less) correlate with types of FPHL in 97.3% of patients.[22]

TREATMENT

The goal of treatment of FPHL is to arrest hair loss progression and stimulate hair regrowth. Realistic expectations need to be set, because the efforts to treat FPHL have mixed success and do not accomplish complete regrowth. All treatments seem to work best when initiated early. Combinations of treatments tend to be more efficacious than single products (**Fig. 1**). The treatments for

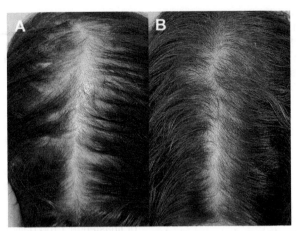

Fig. 1. (*A*) A 41-year-old patient with FPHL at initial visit. (*B*) Improvement with a combination therapy for minoxidil, spironolactone, ketoconazole shampoo, and biotin/zinc supplement after 14 months.

FPHL can be divided into androgen-dependent and androgen-independent (**Table 1**). There is an important adjuvant role for nutritional supplements, light therapy, and hair transplants.

Antiandrogen Therapies

The antiandrogenic agents used in FPHL can be divided into 2 classes: the classic androgen receptor antagonists, which prevent testosterone and DHT from binding to their receptors, and the peripheral antiandrogens, which alter androgen levels at the hair follicle.

Androgen receptor antagonists
Spironolactone
Spironolactone and cyproterone acetate are the most commonly used oral antiandrogens in the

Table 1
Treatments for FPHL

Product	Mechanism of Action	Treatment Recommendations	Pregnancy Category
Spironolactone	Antiandrogen, reduces testosterone levels, and competitive AR blocker	100–200 mg by mouth daily in divided doses	D
Cyproterone acetate	Antiandrogen, competitive AR blocker, decreases testosterone levels by suppressing luteinizing hormone and follicle-stimulating hormone	2 mg cyproterone acetate by mouth daily generally prescribed together with an oral contraceptive, or cyproterone acetate 25–50 mg/d on days 1–10 of menstrual cycle	X
Flutamide	Antiandrogen, competitive AR blocker	62.5 mg–250 mg by mouth once daily	D
Finasteride	5-α reductase inhibitor	0.2–5 mg by mouth once daily	X
Dutasteride	5-α reductase inhibitors	0.25–0.5 mg by mouth daily	X
Minoxidil	Unknown, possible antiandrogenic, vasodilatory, and antiinflammatory effects	2%–5% topical application once or twice daily to scalp	C
Ketoconazole	Decreases DHT levels at the hair follicle	Shampoo scalp every other day as tolerated. Leave on for 5 min and then rinse	C

treatment of FPHL. The effects of these agents are comparable, with 44% of patients with FPHL experiencing regrowth.[23] Spironolactone is a potassium-sparing diuretic, a structural antagonist of aldosterone. It acts as an antiandrogenic by reducing the levels of total testosterone and competitively blocking the androgen receptor in target tissues. It is commonly used to treat hirsutism associated with PCOS.[24] It has been used to treat FPHL off-label in doses of 50 to 200 mg daily, ideally for at least 6 months.[25] Commonly described transient side effects are lethargy, nausea, and menorrhagia, which tend to improve after 3 months of therapy. Low-dose oral contraceptive pills (OCP) can be added to help reduce the menorrhagia.[24] Spironolactone can be associated with hyperkalemia, which warrants monitoring of potassium levels. Topical spironolactone 2% solution exists and has been used in combination with minoxidil with variable success. Spironolactone is pregnancy category D.

Cyproterone acetate

Cyproterone acetate is an oral antiandrogen that can directly block AR and decrease testosterone levels by suppressing luteinizing hormone and follicle-stimulating hormone release.[25] Treatment with cyproterone can improve hair growth in patients with FPHL, alone or in combination with ethinyl estradiol or spironolactone.[26] Cyproterone has shown efficacy in treating patients with FPHL with both increased and normal androgen levels.[27] It is approved for use in Europe and Canada to treat hirsutism, acne, and female alopecia. It can cause feminization of the male fetus, and it is best used in combination with an OCP. It is absolutely contraindicated in patients with liver disease.[25] This medication is not available in the United States.

Flutamide

Flutamide is a potent orally administered antiandrogen that competitively blocks the binding of androgen to its receptor.[28] It is an effective treatment of hirsutism and FPHL in hyperandrogenic women.[29] Flutamide can improve hair growth after only 6 months of treatment, and offers long-term stability in FPHL.[28] Its use is limited because of the risk of severe liver toxicity, which seems to be dose-dependent. The doses that have been shown efficacious in FPHL (62.5 mg/d) are low and well tolerated.[29]

Fluridil

Fluridil is a novel topical antiandrogen. This compound is highly hydrophobic, with high local efficacy and tolerance, but systemically nonresorbable. In men with AGA, application of fluridil for 3 months resulted in increased anagen to telogen rates.[30] In FPHL, fluridil 2% solution prevented progression of

hair loss and increased hair diameter in an open clinical study.[31] Fluridil is being used throughout Europe, but is still awaiting approval from the Food and Drug Administration (FDA) in the United States.

5-α reductase inhibitors

The treatment of male AGA has been revolutionized by the advent of the 5-α reductase inhibitors. These agents work by inhibiting the conversion of testosterone to DHT, and result in increased hair growth and halt progression of hair loss. Their use in women is limited because they are contraindicated in women of childbearing age. Finasteride has not shown the same efficacy in FPHL as seen in male AGA. In postmenopausal women, a 1-year course of finasteride 1 mg daily failed to improve hair loss over placebo.[32] In premenopausal women, finasteride has shown benefit in treating FPHL associated with hyperandrogenism.[33] In normoandrogenic women, it seems to be efficacious when used in higher doses (5 mg) or in combination with drospirenone and ethinyl estradiol OCP.[34,35] The specific subset of women who respond well to finasteride may have excessive activity of the 5-α reductase enzyme. In men with AGA, greater efficacy of finasteride is correlated with shorter CAG repeats of the AR gene, whereas the efficacy in patients with FPHL cannot be predicted with certainty.[36]

Topical preparations of finasteride 0.05% have a potential role in the treatment of male AGA and FPHL.[37] Finasteride is metabolized in the liver, and it should be used with caution in patients with liver abnormalities.[32] It is a pregnancy category X medication, associated with feminization of a male fetus. Women of childbearing age should use strict birth control, and should not handle crushed or broken pills.

Dutasteride

Dutasteride is a 5-α reductase inhibitor with superior antiandrogenic effects to finasteride. It can decrease serum DHT levels by more than 90%.[38] In male patients with AGA, dutasteride can stop the progression of hair loss and increase scalp hair growth in a dose-dependent fashion. Dutasteride is not currently approved by the FDA for the treatment of hair loss. The off- label use of dutasteride (0.25–0.5 mg/d) has led to resolution of FPHL in postmenopausal women.[39] This medication should not be administered to women of reproductive age. Liver function needs to be monitored in all patients.

Fulvestrant

The pure estrogen receptor antagonist, fulvestrant (ICI 182,780), was developed as a treatment of estrogen-sensitive breast cancer. In vitro studies have shown that fulvestrant can increase hair growth in mice, by stimulating telogen hair follicles to re-enter anagen.[40] Topical formulation of fulvestrant was subsequently developed to be used as a potential treatment of AGA. In human studies, topical fulvestrant preparations have not been shown to be superior over control vehicle in the treatment of FPHL.[41]

Androgen-Independent

Minoxidil

Minoxidil is a hair growth stimulator that is the current standard of treatment of hair loss in women. It was originally produced as an oral hypertensive agent, with a peculiar side effect of increased scalp hair growth. This serendipitous discovery led to the production of topical formulations, now available as solution or foam, in 2% or 5% strength. Its mechanisms of action remain unknown, and include proposed enhanced vasodilatory, proliferative, antiandrogenic, and antiinflammatory effects.[26] The efficacy of minoxidil in pattern hair loss has been proved in double-blind, placebo-controlled trials.[42,43] There is also evidence that minoxidil prolongs the anagen stage of the hair cycle and increases hair follicle size. Minoxidil has a significant ability to maintain and thicken preexisting hair. In addition, patients with FPHL treated with minoxidil 2% have 10% to 16% more regrowth compared with controls, with higher concentrations (5%) potentially more effective.[44] Minoxidil has a well-established safety profile. The most frequently associated side effects are facial hypertrychosis, contact dermatitis, pruritus, scale, and dryness.

Ketoconazole

Ketoconazole is an antifungal used in the treatment of seborrheic dermatitis. The use of ketoconazole shampoo, especially in combination with finasteride, results in increased hair growth in FPHL.[45] The mechanism by which it can improve hair growth is unclear. It has antiinflammatory properties, and it reduces colonization of the skin by *Malassezia*. Ketoconazole also affects steroidogenesis locally and it decreases DHT levels at the hair follicle.[46] It should be part of the treatment regimen in women with FPHL who have accompanying inflammatory seborrheic dermatitis or sebopsoriasis. Hyperandrogenic women with FPHL can benefit from the antiandrogenic mechanism of ketoconazole.[47]

Adjunctive Therapies

Hair transplantation

Hair transplant surgery is emerging as an important option for patients with FPHL who do not have success with medical therapies. The hair transplant procedure is an outpatient procedure performed under local anesthesia, in which classically harvested strips from the occipital area are divided into individual hair follicles. The transplanted hair follicles are then placed in recipient sites, where hair grows over the next 3 to 6 months.[48]

A new trend in hair transplants is the adjuvant use of platelet-rich plasma (PRP). The efficacy of adjuvant plasma and platelet growth factors has been well described in wound healing processes.[49] The growth factors and plasma components such as fibrin, fibronectin, and vitronectin can increase hair follicle growth. When used in hair transplant procedures, the hair grafts may be stored in PRP until placed on the scalp, or PRP can be injected directly into the scalp before placement of grafts.[50]

Hair transplantation requires preservation of hair growth over the occipital donor area, which is typically found in men with AGA. In FPHL, there is more diffuse thinning of the scalp, including thinning of the occipital area, which limits the usefulness of hair.[48] The newer techniques of harvesting follicular extraction units, especially the robotic-assisted ones (Restoration Robotics, San Jose, CA), may help increase the usefulness of hair transplants in women.

Camouflage

In recent years, hair extensions and wigs have become widely accepted among women as tools for improving hair appearance. This trend has alleviated some of the stigma associated with their use in FPHL. The medical side effects of hairpieces are limited to irritant dermatitis and traction alopecia. Special attention should be used when choosing attachment methods (eg, glue, pins) to minimize damage to the scalp. The weight of the attached hair needs to be minimized to prevent traction damage.

Camouflage of frontal hair loss in FPHL with hairpieces may create a challenge. In this scenario, the use of camouflaging topical sprays, powders, or keratin fibers may be a better alternative to achieve sufficient density.

Light therapy

A variety of laser and light sources have been tried for treatment of hair loss, with varied success. The idea to use laser light therapy stems from experimental observations that low-powered ruby laser can increase hair growth in mice.[51] Paradoxic increase in hair growth has been observed with the use of 810-nm pulsed laser and intense pulsed light intended for hair removal.[52] The mechanism of low-level lasers on hair growth is not yet known; it is hypothesized that the light enhances mitochondrial respiratory activity and production of adenosine triphosphate.[53]

Several products using low-energy laser light beams are available without a prescription for the treatment of alopecia. They are designed as a hairbrush or comb, which shines red light directly on the scalp. The HairMax LaserComb (Lexington International, LLC, Boca Raton, FL) is a handheld, noninvasive device that was approved by the FDA for treatment of male AGA.[54] It is designed to be used 3 times per week for 15-minute sessions, with noted results in 8 to 16 weeks. In a double-blind study, men treated with the laser comb had a significantly greater increase in hair density and better subjective assessments of hair growth, compared with the control group at 26 weeks. No individual experienced any serious adverse events.[54] The HairMax LaserComb received clearance for use in women with FPHL in 2011.[55]

In addition to low-level lasers, high-energy lasers are being explored for treatment of hair loss. The fractional erbium-glass 1550-nm laser was used successfully to treat FPHL.[56] After 10 treatments with this laser, hair density and fiber thickness markedly increased ($P<.001$). Associated side effects were immediate postprocedural erythema and pruritus in some patients. Although the mechanism of laser treatment in improving hair growth is not clear, the current evidence supports the potential use of lasers for the treatment of alopecia.

Adjuvant therapies

Common topical and nutritional supplements are listed in **Table 2**.

FUTURE DIRECTIONS

Innovative treatments for FPHL are in high demand. The prostaglandin analogues, which are successfully used to treat eyelash hypotrichosis, may present a new option. There are high expectations for the use of topical prostaglandin in patients with alopecia. However, topical applications of prostaglandins have not proved efficacious. A trial of injected bimatoprost solution was ineffective in a patient with FPHL.[68] The efficacy of different prostaglandin analogues and higher concentrations need to be studied in FPHL.

Botulinum toxins have been introduced for treatment of hair loss with some success. In an open-label study, male patients with AGA received 150 units of botulinum toxin into the muscles surrounding the scalp.[69] The botulinum injections reduced hair loss significantly, and in some men, increased hair growth. Botulinum toxin may stop hair loss by improving blood flow to the hair follicle.

Table 2
Adjuvant treatments of FPHL

Product	Mechanism of Action	Treatment Recommendations
Biotin	Regulates mitochondrial carboxylase enzymes in hair roots[57]	No clinical trials showing efficacy treating hair loss[58]
Caffeine	Inhibits phosphodiasterase, stimulates cyclic adenosine monophosphate, counteracts testosterone effects on hair follicles[59]	Caffeine lotion and shampoo, potential increase in hair tensile strength and numbers[60]
Cimetidine	H_2 blocker, a peripheral antiandrogen, blocks binding of DHT to AR[61]	300 g by mouth 5 times per day (1500 mg/d) Not FDA approved for hair loss
Ferritin	Unclear, lack of ferritin causes hair follicles to enter telogen[62,63]	Maintain serum ferritin level >40 ng/mL. Supplement women with anemia and vegetarians
Melatonin	Antiandrogenic effects at the hair follicle[64]	1 mg topical compounded in alcohol and glycerin, no evidence that oral supplementation helps[65]
Zinc	Unclear, deficiency nutritional or iatrogenic causes alopecia[66]	Supplement 8–15 mg by mouth daily (>18 years old)
Zinc pyrithium shampoo	Zinc ions have antiinflammatory and antioxidant effects,[15] and inhibit 5-α reductase in vitro[67]	1% pyrithione zinc shampoo daily use results in significant ($P<.05$) net increase in total visible hair counts[67]

A more oxygenated environment at the hair follicle is believed to favor conversion of testosterone to estrogen, rather than to DHT. The mechanisms are not understood, but botulinum toxin offers a new treatment option for women with FPHL.

SUMMARY

FPHL is the most common cause of hair loss in women, which carries a significant psychosocial burden in affected patients. The currently available treatments offer suboptimal results. Most of the treatments have been developed based on the understanding of AGA mechanisms in men. Clearly, the pathogenesis of FPHL is more complicated, and additional hormonal and growth factors regulators need to be considered. Further studies of FPHL may explain the currently observed variable response to antiandrogen treatments. In the future, FPHL will likely encompass different subtypes based on underlying cause, which can be treated with a better-targeted approach.

REFERENCES

1. Gan DC, Sinclair RD. Prevalence of male and female pattern hair loss in Maryborough. J Investig Dermatol Symp Proc 2005;10(3):184–9.
2. Olsen EA. Female pattern hair loss. J Am Acad Dermatol 2001;45:S70–80.
3. Olsen EA, Messenger AG, Shapiro J, et al. Evaluation and treatment of male and female pattern hair loss. J Am Acad Dermatol 2005;52(2):301–11.
4. Dinh QQ, Sinclair R. Female pattern hair loss: current treatment concepts. Clin Interv Aging 2007; 2(2):189–99.
5. Sellheyer K, Bergfeld WF. Histopathologic evaluation of alopecias. Am J Dermatopathol 2006;28(3): 236–59.
6. Magro CM, Rossi A, Poe J, et al. The role of inflammation and immunity in the pathogenesis of androgenetic alopecia. J Drugs Dermatol 2011;10(12): 1404–11.
7. Futterweit W, Dunaif A, Yeh HC, et al. The prevalence of hyperandrogenism in 109 consecutive female patients with diffuse alopecia. J Am Acad Dermatol 1988;19:831–6.
8. Yip L, Rufaut N, Sinclair R. Role of genetics and sex steroid hormones in male androgenetic alopecia and female pattern hair loss: an update of what we now know. Australas J Dermatol 2011;52(2):81–8.
9. Grino PB, Griffin JE, Wilson JD. Testosterone at high concentrations interacts with the human androgen receptor similarly to dihydrotestosterone. Endocrinology 1990;126(2):1165–72.
10. Hillmer AM, Hanneken S, Ritzmann S, et al. Genetic variation in the human androgen receptor gene is the major determinant of common early-onset androgenetic alopecia. Am J Hum Genet 2005; 77(1):140–8.
11. Cousen P, Messenger A. Female pattern hair loss in complete androgen insensitivity syndrome. Br J Dermatol 2010;162(5):1135–7.
12. El-Samahy MH, Shaheen MA, Saddik DE, et al. Evaluation of androgen receptor gene as a candidate gene in female androgenetic alopecia. Int J Dermatol 2009;48(6):584–7.
13. Niiyama S, Happle R, Hoffmann R. Influence of estrogens on the androgen metabolism in different subunits of human hair follicles. Eur J Dermatol 2001;11:195–8.
14. Muallem MM, Rubeiz NG. Physiological and biological skin changes in pregnancy. Clin Dermatol 2006; 24(2):80–3.
15. Mirmirani P. Hormonal changes in menopause: do they contribute to a 'midlife hair crisis' in women. Br J Dermatol 2011;165(Suppl 3):7–11.
16. Georgala S, Katoulis AC, Georgala C, et al. Topical estrogen therapy for androgenetic alopecia in menopausal females. Dermatology 2004;208(2):178–9.
17. Arias-Santiago S, Gutiérrez-Salmerón MT, Buendía-Eisman A, et al. Sex hormone-binding globulin and risk of hyperglycemia in patients with androgenetic alopecia. J Am Acad Dermatol 2011;65(1):48–53.
18. Arias-Santiago S, Gutiérrez-Salmerón MT, Castellote-Caballero L, et al. Androgenetic alopecia and cardiovascular risk factors in men and women: a comparative study. J Am Acad Dermatol 2010;63(3):420–9.
19. Sato A, et al. Polymorphic CAG repeats in androgen receptor gene and their implication in androgenetic alopecia. Skin Surgery 2006;15(2):67–74.
20. Yamazaki M, Sato A, Toyoshima KE, et al. Polymorphic CAG repeat numbers in the androgen receptor gene of female pattern hair loss patients. J Dermatol 2011;38(7):680–4.
21. Sawaya ME, Shalita AR. Androgen receptor polymorphisms (CAG repeat lengths) in androgenetic alopecia, hirsutism, and acne. J Cutan Med Surg 1998;3(1):9–15.
22. Schweiger ES, Boychenko O, Bernstein RM. Update on the pathogenesis, genetics and medical treatment of patterned hair loss. J Drugs Dermatol 2010;9(11): 1412–9.
23. Sinclair R, Wewerinke M, Jolley D. Treatment of female pattern hair loss with oral antiandrogens. Br J Dermatol 2005;152:466–73.
24. Lowenstein EJ. Diagnosis and management of the dermatologic manifestations of the polycystic ovary syndrome. Dermatol Ther 2006;19(4):210–23.
25. Camacho-Martínez FM. Hair loss in women. Semin Cutan Med Surg 2009;28:19–32.
26. Rogers NE, Avram MR. Medical treatments for male and female pattern hair loss. J Am Acad Dermatol 2008;59(4):547–66.

27. Karrer-Voegeli S, Rey F, Reymond MJ, et al. Androgen dependence of hirsutism, acne, and alopecia in women: retrospective analysis of 228 patients investigated for hyperandrogenism. Medicine (Baltimore) 2009;88(1):32–45.

28. Paradisi R, Porcu E, Fabbri R, et al. Prospective cohort study on the effects and tolerability of flutamide in patients with female pattern hair loss. Ann Pharmacother 2011;45(4):469–75.

29. Yazdabadi A, Sinclair R. Treatment of female pattern hair loss with the androgen receptor antagonist flutamide. Australas J Dermatol 2011;52(2):132–4.

30. Sovak M, Seligson AL, Kucerova R, et al. Fluridil, a rationally designed topical agent for androgenetic alopecia: first clinical experience. Dermatol Surg 2002;28(8):678–85.

31. Kucerova R, Bienova M, Novotny R, et al. Current therapies of female androgenetic alopecia and use of fluridil, a novel topical antiandrogen. Scr Med (Brno) 2006;79(1):35–48.

32. Price VH, Roberts JL, Hordinsky M, et al. Lack of efficacy of finasteride in postmenopausal women with androgenetic alopecia. J Am Acad Dermatol 2000;43:768–76.

33. Shum K, Cullen D, Messenger A. Hair loss in women with hyperandrogenism: four cases responding to finasteride. J Am Acad Dermatol 2002;47:733–9.

34. Iorizzo M, Vincenzi C, Voudouris S, et al. Finasteride treatment of female pattern hair loss. Arch Dermatol 2006;142:298–302.

35. Kohler C, Tschumi K, Bodmer C, et al. Effect of finasteride 5 mg (Proscar) on acne and alopecia in female patients with normal serum levels of free testosterone. Gynecol Endocrinol 2007;23:142–5.

36. Wakisaka N, Taira Y, Ishikawa M, et al. Effectiveness of finasteride on patients with male pattern baldness who have different androgen receptor gene polymorphism. J Investig Dermatol Symp Proc 2005;10(3):293–4.

37. Hajheydari Z, Akbari J, Saeedi M, et al. Comparing the therapeutic effects of finasteride gel and tablet in treatment of the androgenetic alopecia. Indian J Dermatol Venereol Leprol 2009;75(1):47–51.

38. Clark R, Hermann D, Cunningham G, et al. Marked suppression of dihydrotestosterone in men with benign prostatic hyperplasia by dutasteride, a dual 5-alpha-reductase inhibitor. J Clin Endocrinol Metab 2004;89:2179–84.

39. Olszewska M, Rudnicka L. Effective treatment of female androgenic alopecia with dutasteride. J Drugs Dermatol 2005;4:637–40.

40. Ohnemus U, Uenalan M, Handjiski B. Topical estrogen accelerates hair regrowth in mice after chemotherapy-induced alopecia by favoring the dystrophic catagen response pathway to damage. J Invest Dermatol 2004;122:7–8.

41. Gassmueller J, Hoffmann R, Webster A. Topical fulvestrant solution has no effect on male and postmenopausal female androgenetic alopecia: results from two randomized, proof-of-concept studies. Br J Dermatol 2008;158(1):109–15.

42. Olsen E, Whiting D, Bergfeld W, et al. A multicenter, randomized, placebo-controlled, double-blind clinical trial of a novel formulation of 5% minoxidil topical foam versus placebo in the treatment of androgenetic alopecia in men. J Am Acad Dermatol 2007;57:767–74.

43. Tsuboi R, Tanaka T, Nishikawa T, et al. A randomized, placebo-controlled trial of 1% topical minoxidil solution in the treatment of androgenetic alopecia in Japanese women. Eur J Dermatol 2007;17:37–44.

44. Lucky A, Picquadio D, Ditre C, et al. A randomized, placebo-controlled trial of 5% and 2% topical minoxidil solutions in the treatment of female pattern hair loss. J Am Acad Dermatol 2004;50:541–53.

45. Hugo Perez BS. Ketoconazole as an adjunct to finasteride in the treatment of androgenetic alopecia in men. Med Hypotheses 2004;62:112–5.

46. Inui S, Itami S. Reversal of androgenic alopecia by topical ketoconzole: relevance of anti-androgenic activity. J Dermatol Sci 2007;45:66–8.

47. Sonino N, Scaroni C, Biason A, et al. Low-dose ketoconazole treatment in hirsute women. J Endocrinol Invest 1990;13:35–40.

48. Unger WP, Unger RH. Hair transplanting: an important but often forgotten treatment for female pattern hair loss. J Am Acad Dermatol 2003;49(5):853–60.

49. Carter MJ, Fylling CP, Parnell LK. Use of platelet rich plasma gel on wound healing: a systematic review and meta-analysis. Eplasty 2011;11:e38.

50. Rose PT. The latest innovations in hair transplantation. Facial Plast Surg 2011;27:366–77.

51. Avram M, Leonard R Jr, Epstein E, et al. The current role of laser/light sources in the treatment of male and female pattern hair loss. J Cosmet Laser Ther 2007;9:27–8.

52. Desai S, Mahmoud B, Bhatia A, et al. Paradoxical hypertrichosis after laser therapy: a review. Dermatol Surg 2010;36(3):291–8.

53. Oron U, Ilic S, DeTaboada L, et al. Ga-As (808-nm) laser irradiation enhances ATP production in human neuronal cells in culture. Photomed Laser Surg 2007;25:180–2.

54. Leavitt M, Charles G, Heyman E, et al. HairMax LaserComb laser phototherapy device in the treatment of male androgenetic alopecia: a randomized, double-blind, sham device-controlled, multicentre trial. Clin Drug Investig 2009;29(5):283–92.

55. FDA clears HairMax to treat female pattern hair loss and promote hair growth. Available at: http://www.hairmax.com/mediakit/PressReleases/6_04_11_female_clearance_PR.pfd. Accessed February 29, 2012.

56. Lee GY, Lee SJ, Kim WS. The effect of a 1550 nm fractional erbium-glass laser in female pattern hair loss. J Eur Acad Dermatol Venereol 2011;25(12): 1450–4.

57. Zempleni J, Hassan Y, Wijeratne S. Biotin and biotinidase deficiency. Expert Rev Endocrinol Metab 2008;3(6):715–24.

58. Limat A, Suormala T, Hunziker T, et al. Proliferation and differentiation of cultured human follicular keratinocytes are not influenced by biotin. Arch Dermatol Res 1996;288:31–8.

59. Fischer T, Hipler U, Elsner P. Effect of caffeine and testosterone on the proliferation of human hair follicles in vitro. Int J Dermatol 2007;46(1):27–35.

60. Bussoletti C, Mastropietro F, Toluene MV, et al. Use of a cosmetic caffeine lotion in the treatment of male androgenetic alopecia. Journal of Applied Cosmetology 2011;29(4):167–79.

61. Aram H. Treatment of female androgenetic alopecia with cimetidine. Int J Dermatol 1987;26(2): 128–30.

62. Trost LB, Bergfeld WF, Calogeras E. The diagnosis and treatment of iron deficiency and its potential relationship to hair loss. J Am Acad Dermatol 2006;54(5):824–44.

63. Kantor J, Kessler L, Brooks D, et al. Decreased serum ferritin is associated with alopecia in women. J Invest Dermatol 2003;121(5):985–8.

64. Fischer T, Slominski A, Tobin D, et al. Melatonin and the hair follicle. J Pineal Res 2008;44(1):1–15.

65. Fischer TW, Burmeister G, Schmidt HW, et al. Melatonin increases anagen hair rate in women with androgenetic alopecia or diffuse alopecia: results of a pilot randomized controlled trial. Br J Dermatol 2004;150:341–5.

66. Plonka P, Handjiski B, Popik M, et al. Zinc as an ambivalent but potent modulator of murine hair growth in vivo–preliminary observations. Exp Dermatol 2005;14(11):844–53.

67. Berger RS, Fu JL, Smiles K, et al. The effects of minoxidil, 1% pyrithione zinc and a combination of both on hair density: a randomized controlled trial. Br J Dermatol 2003;149(2):354–62.

68. Emer J, Stevenson ML, Markowitz O. Novel treatment of female-pattern androgenetic alopecia with injected bimatoprost 0.03% solution. J Drugs Dermatol 2011;10(7):795–8.

69. Freund B, Schwartz M. Treatment of male pattern baldness with botulinum toxin: a pilot study. Plast Reconstr Surg 2010;126(5):246e–8e.

Pattern Hair Loss in Men
Diagnosis and Medical Treatment

Nusrat Banka, MD[a], M.J. Kristine Bunagan, MD[a],
Jerry Shapiro, MD, FRCPC[a,b,*]

KEYWORDS

- Male pattern hair loss • Androgenetic alopecia • Hair loss • Minoxidil • Finasteride • Dutasteride
- Prostaglandin analogues

KEY POINTS

- Male pattern hair loss is common cause of hair loss in men.
- Androgens and genetic susceptibility predispose to pattern hair loss.
- Diagnosis is mainly by clinical examination.
- The screening test HairDX is available to diagnose susceptible individuals.

INTRODUCTION

Male pattern hair loss (MPHL) is the most common cause of hair loss in men. The incidence of pattern hair loss in men varies from population to population based on genetic background. The highest prevalence is reported in the Caucasian population. In the Asian population the frequency is lower than in Europeans. There is no information on the prevalence in African men.

Hair is an important feature of self-image. Studies have shown men who suffer from MPHL are 75% less confident, especially when interacting with the opposite sex.[1] Young men with hair loss have reported loss of self esteem, introversion, and feeling unattractive to a higher degree than older men with hair loss.[2] Although there is a significant impairment in quality of life in many patients, Alfonso and colleagues[3] revealed that 3 out of 4 men with MPHL had never pursued therapy for hair loss. Men who seek medical help and are successfully treated reported psychological benefits with improvements in self esteem and personal attractiveness. By increasing the level of the patient's knowledge about MPHL, early diagnosis and management can significantly reduce the psychological burden associated with this disease.

PATHOPHYSIOLOGY

MPHL occurs in the presence of androgens in genetically susceptible individuals. The disease onset and progression vary from person to person. Initial signs of MPHL usually develop during teenage years, leading to progressive hair loss with pattern distribution. Bitemporal hair loss starts at the anterior hair line, resulting in a receding hair line followed by hair loss over the vertex and mid-frontal areas, with sparing of the occipital scalp.

Role of Androgen

Locally and systemically derived testosterone either directly binds to the intracellular androgen receptors mainly expressed within the dermal papilla and the hair bulb, or is metabolized into

---

Conflicts of interest: Shapiro is a co-founder and shareholder of Replicel Life Sciences Inc. He is a speaker for Johnson and Johnson and Merck. He is a consultant for Dermagenoma Inc.
[a] Department of Dermatology and Skin Science, University of British Columbia, 835 West, 10th Avenue, Vancouver V5Z 4E8, Canada; [b] Department of Dermatology, New York University, New York City, NY, USA
* Corresponding author. Department of Dermatology and Skin Science, University of British Columbia, 835 West, 10th Avenue, Vancouver V5Z 4E8, Canada.
E-mail address: jerry.shapiro@vch.ca

Dermatol Clin 31 (2013) 129–140
http://dx.doi.org/10.1016/j.det.2012.08.003
0733-8635/13/$ – see front matter © 2013 Elsevier Inc. All rights reserved.

the more potent dihydrotestosterone (DHT) which, in turn, binds to androgen receptors with an approximately 5-fold greater affinity. The conversion of testosterone to DHT in the hair follicle is predominantly mediated by the 5α-reductase (type 1 and 2). It is thought that DHT is the key androgen required for the induction of MPHL.[4] Changes in several factors along the androgen signaling pathway possibly lead to hair-follicle miniaturization, including an increase in the expression of androgen receptors, increased androgen sensitivity to bind more steroid ligand, and higher levels of 5α-reductase.[5] The scalp has a combination of androgen-sensitive and androgen-independent hair follicles. Androgen-sensitive hair follicles are located on the frontal scalp and vertex whereas androgen-independent hair follicles are present on the sides and back of the scalp. This distribution of androgen receptors explains the clinical presentation of pattern hair loss. The success of hair transplantation is based on the fact that hair follicles harvested from the occipital scalp retain their androgen-independent behavior when implanted in the frontal scalp (donor dominance). Dermis of the frontoparietal scalp is derived from the neural crest, whereas dermis of the occipital and temporal scalp is derived from mesoderm. This difference in embryonic origin may explain the differential influence of androgens.[6]

Role of Genetics

A polygenic mode of inheritance has been well established in MPHL. These genes may determine the age of onset, progression, patterning, and severity. Hypermethylation of DNA in gene promoter regions blocks the gene transcription machinery and therefore switches off gene expression, whereas hypomethylated gene promoters engage with gene transcription machinery to switch on gene expression.[7] Partial demethylation of promoters that arises stochastically with age and with the effects of the environment leads to subtle changes in gene expression that are heritable.[8] In balding scalp, differences in androgen receptor gene (AR) sensitivity and expression between vertex and occipital regions may be accounted for by the differential AR methylation patterns, leading to region-specific susceptibility to hair-follicle miniaturization.[9]

The first published genetic link with MPHL was the discovery of a marked association with a particular single-nucleotide polymorphism (SNP) in exon 1 of the AR. This SNP is present in almost 100% of young and older balding men, but is also found in a significant proportion of older men unaffected by baldness, suggesting that this SNP is essential, but not sufficient, for MPHL in men.[10] Genetic testing for MPHL is currently based on genotyping of the nonfunctional SNP in exon 1 of the AR that has been repeatedly associated with MPHL.[10] The AR gene is located on the X chromosome, and men inherit it from their mother. This finding therefore confirms there is a maternal influence on male balding but does not explain the genetic contribution from the father. The identification of new susceptibility genes on chromosomes 3q26 and 20p11 suggest an androgen-independent pathway that is yet to be identified.[11,12]

The difference in clinical presentation in men and women with pattern hair loss may be due to the following observations:

- Females have 3 to 3.5 times less 5α-reductase (types 1 and 2) than men.[13,14]
- The enzyme cytochrome P450 aromatase converts testosterone into estradiol and estrone, which reduces conversion of testosterone into DHT. The aromatase level is significantly higher in the hair follicles of women and also 6 times more in the frontal follicles and 4 times more in the occipital hair follicles, which may explain why women usually retain their frontal hairline in contrast to men with pattern hair loss.[13,15]
- Both men and women have 30% higher AR levels in the frontal hair follicles compared with occipital follicles, but the total receptor level is 40% less in women than in men.[13,15]

Hair-Cycle Dynamics

The key feature in MPHL is follicular miniaturization. The hair cycle has an anagen phase or active growth phase lasting 3 to 5 years, catagen phase or transition phase lasting 1 to 2 weeks, and the telogen or resting phase lasting for 5 to 6 weeks. MPHL results from altered hair-follicle cycling and miniaturization, which leads to the transformation of terminal to vellus hair follicles. A reduction in anagen duration leads to shorter hair length, whereas an increase in telogen duration delays regeneration. This process results in hairs so short and fine that they fail to achieve sufficient length to reach the surface of the scalp, resulting in an increased number of empty pores and a reduction of anagen to telogen ratio. Small hair follicles result in finer hairs. The caliber of the terminal hair shaft is greater than 60 μm, the vellus hair measures less than 30 μm, and the thickness of indeterminate hair is between these two.[16] The exact mechanism of follicular miniaturization remains unknown. The dermal papilla determines the size of the hair bulb and the hair shaft produced; it is likely the target of androgen-mediated events leading to miniaturizations and hair-cycle changes.[17–20]

Histopathology

The characteristic histologic finding is an increase in number of vellus-like hair follicles or miniaturization (**Figs. 1** and **2**).[18]

Vertical section at the level of subcutaneous tissue and reticular dermis shows terminal hairs and follicular stelae. At papillary dermis terminal hairs, vellus hairs and stelae are seen.[21–23] Stelae are the residual fibrous tracts that mark the upward migration of the catagen, telogen, or miniaturizing hair shaft and bulb.

Horizontal section at papillary dermis shows terminal, vellus, and vellus-like hairs. Vellus and vellus-like hairs are less than 30 μm in diameter. Primary vellus hairs are small with a thin outer root sheath, and originate in the upper half of dermis. Vellus-like hairs are miniaturized hairs with thick outer root sheath, and originate from a terminal hair rooted in reticular dermis or subcutaneous fat with underlying stelae. In reticular dermis, no vellus or vellus-like hair follicles are seen.

Follicular counts vary from level to level. In the upper dermis, counts are usually 40 to 50. At reticular dermis this number is reduced to 35, and in the subcutaneous fat it is around 30. The difference in counts between reticular dermis and fat represents the number of telogen hairs. In pattern hair loss, the total number of follicular counts is usually normal in the papillary dermis. The ratios of anagen to telogen and terminal to vellus hairs change in pattern hair loss. The normal terminal

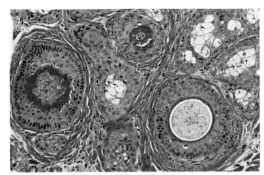

Fig. 2. Androgenetic alopecia: a close-up of a follicular unit showing a normal follicle, a vellus hair, and a telogen hair with normal sebaceous glands (original magnification ×10). (*Courtesy of* M. Martinka.)

to vellus hair ratio is 7:1 and in pattern hair loss it is reduced to 2:1, indicating a marked shift to miniaturization. In late stages variability in follicular sizes is apparent. Sebaceous glands appear enlarged in relation to these miniaturized follicles. Clusters of elastic fibers in the neck of dermal papillae called Arao-Perkins bodies may be seen, which are clumped in catagen and located at the lowest point of origin of follicular stelae. Stacks of Arao-Perkins bodies may be seen, like rungs of ladders, in these stelae of miniaturized hairs. Mild to moderate perifollicular lymphohistiocytic inflammation may be seen. Forty percent of patients with pattern hair loss show moderate lymphocytic inflammation, compared with only 10% of normal controls.[21]

CLINICAL FEATURES

In men hair loss is patterned, involving frontotemporal recession and hair loss over the vertex with sparing of occipital scalp even in the most severe cases. It manifests at an early age and progresses gradually with minimal hair shedding.

Hamilton[24] originally classified MPHL based on frontoparietal/frontotemporal recession and vertex thinning. Norwood[25] later improved this classification, known as Norwood-Hamilton pattern, which divides pattern hair loss in men into 7 stages according to severity. Bitemporal hairline recession is seen in most postpubertal men, but does not necessarily herald the expression of MPHL and is unlikely to reverse with current therapies. A deeper bitemporal recession of greater than 1 inch from the frontal hair line is a part of MPHL, and if treated early may respond to treatment.[26] The onset of hair loss and the rate of progression vary from person to person (**Figs. 3–6**). There is no way to predict what pattern of hair loss a young man with early pattern hair loss will eventually

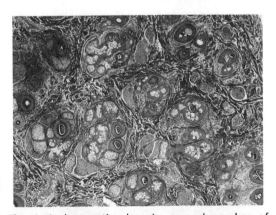

Fig. 1. Androgenetic alopecia: normal number of follicles with variation in follicular size (miniaturization), vellus follicles outnumbering the terminal follicles. Few telogen hairs are present and some follicles show mild perifollicular fibrosis with no significant inflammation. Sebaceous glands are intact and well preserved (original magnification ×4). (*Courtesy of* M. Martinka.)

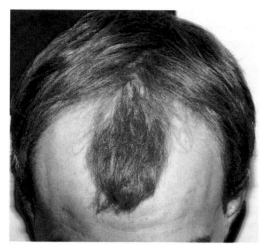

Fig. 3. Male pattern hair loss with frontotemporal recession. Norwood-Hamilton type III.

assume. In general, early onset in the second decade is most progressive compared with delayed onset in late third or fourth decades.

DIAGNOSIS

MPHL is usually diagnosed clinically by examination of hair and scalp showing a pattern distribution of hair loss with no evidence of scarring. The clinical examination should include a pull test, examination of other hair-bearing areas, and nail examination to exclude other differential diagnoses, especially when MPHL is superimposed with diffuse alopecia. In doubtful cases, evaluation of hair roots by scalp biopsy can be helpful. Evaluating hair density and hair caliber using various tools, along with global photography, help in

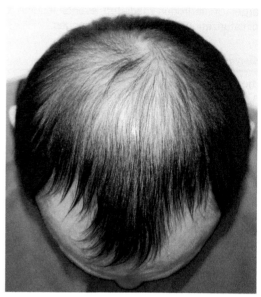

Fig. 5. Male pattern hair loss with diffuse thinning over frontal, mid, and vertex portion of scalp. Norwood-Hamilton type V.

making the correct diagnosis and long-term follow-up of patients with MPHL. In men no laboratory workup is necessary unless there is a superimposed diffuse hair loss.

Pull Test

Approximately 60 hairs are grasped from the proximal portion of the hair shaft at the level of scalp.

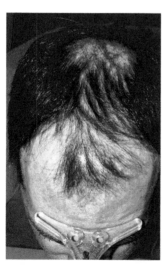

Fig. 4. Male pattern hair loss with frontotemporal recession and hair loss over vertex. Norwood-Hamilton type IV.

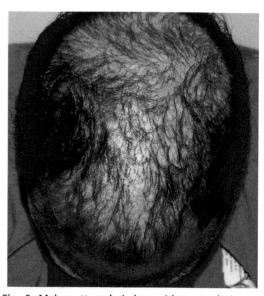

Fig. 6. Male pattern hair loss with sparse hair over frontal, mid, and vertex portion of scalp. Norwood-Hamilton type VI.

The hairs are then tugged from proximal to the distal end. The number of hairs extracted is counted. It is normal to pull 6 of 60 (<10%). More than 6 of 60 hairs is a positive pull test. In pattern hair loss, the pull test is mostly negative. In active disease it may be positive over the top of the scalp and negative over the occipital scalp.

Dermatoscopy

Dermatoscopy demonstrates that scalp hairs exist as compound follicles with 2 or 5 terminal hairs emerging from a single pore. In balding scalp, the terminal hairs within these compound follicles are progressively replaced by finer and shorter vellus hair, such that only 1 or 2 can be seen emerging from a single pore in an affected area. A reduction in the volume of hair can be noticed when the number of terminal hairs per follicular unit decreases; however, balding becomes visible only when the terminal hairs per follicular unit are miniaturized. Dermatoscopy can demonstrate hair-diameter diversity owing to progressive miniaturization before clinical baldness becomes visible, and this is characteristic of MPHL.[27] The reduction in terminal hair in a single pore is a useful feature of early MPHL in patients presenting with increased hair shedding, whereas compound follicles persist on the occipital scalp even in advanced stages of MPHL.

Videodermoscope/Folliscope

This noninvasive technique is used to enhance the images of scalp and hair, and detect the hair shaft in the follicle (if present) and its length, diameter, and possible anomalies (**Fig. 7**). The presence of yellow dots within follicular ostium of both empty and hair-bearing follicles is a characteristic feature

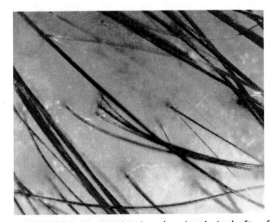

Fig. 7. Folliscope examination showing hair shafts of variable diameters in androgenetic alopecia (original magnification ×100).

of alopecia areata as reported by some investigators. Perifollicular yellow dots may be seen in some advanced cases of MPHL. The yellow dots correspond to degenerated follicular keratinocytes and sebum contained within the dilated ostium of nanogen and miniaturized hair follicles.[28]

Trichogram/Pluck Test

The trichogram is a semi-invasive microscopic method for hair-root and hair-cycle evaluation. The hair should not be washed for 5 days before plucking. A rubber armed forceps is used to pull 60 to 80 hairs. Location depends on the hair disorder. In pattern hair loss, the first site is 2 cm behind the frontal hair line and 2 cm from the midline, with the second site being 2 cm lateral to the occipital protuberance. The hair is grasped at about 0.5 cm above the scalp and rotated to ensure a firm grip. With perpendicular pull the hairs are removed and embedded with roots on a glass slide using medium. The hair roots are evaluated under a magnifying lens or a microscope. This test is painful and time consuming, and in North America is reserved for selected cases.[29]

Phototrichogram

The phototrichogram (PTG) is noninvasive and allows in vivo measurement of the total number of hair, anagen hair, hair density, hair thickness, and hair growth rate. Contrast-enhanced PTG has become a valuable tool in the diagnosis of hair loss. It is used in pattern hair loss to detect early changes of decreased hair density and hair miniaturization before the disorder becomes clinically evident.

In pattern hair loss 2 areas of progression, such as vertex and receding hair line, are chosen, and a control area on the occipital scalp is observed. Photographs are taken. At the first visit all hairs are trimmed 1 mm from the skin surface in all 3 well-defined areas (1 cm²). At both visits the hair sites are covered with transient hair dye for contrast enhancement. At the second visit, a photograph is taken using the scalp immersion proxigraphy method, which involves using close-up photography, whereby the scalp is viewed under a glass slide with a drop of immersion oil (this gives it clarity and improves the resolution of the image).[30] Exactly the same area must be seen on both photographs. The individual hairs on both photographs are located pairwise and compared. Substantial hair growth on the second photograph reflects hair growth and indicates anagen. Moderate elongation reflects catagen, and no elongation reflects resting. A missing hair in the second picture suggests hair shedding.

This method is again time consuming and is used frequently in clinical therapeutic trials.

TrichoScan

TrichoScan is an investigator-independent, automated software program. It is used to monitor and measure hair growth in pattern hair loss. TrichoScan results depend on image quality. A small area between normal and involved scalp is evenly clipped. The dye is then applied to the shaven scalp for 15 minutes. After dying the color area is cleaned and images are obtained with a digital camera equipped with rigid "contact lens," which ensures images are taken at the same distance from the scalp. After taking images the software then analyzes the scalp-hair images for hair density, terminal hair density, vellus hair density, mean and cumulative hair thickness, and rate of hair growth. TrichoScan can be used for patient follow-up during treatment.[31]

Scalp Biopsy

MPHL is essentially a clinical diagnosis. However, in rare cases with diffuse hair loss diagnosis can be confirmed histologically. A 4-mm punch biopsy should be obtained from the involved area and sectioned horizontally.

Screening/Genetic Testing: HairDX

The HairDX test is the first genetic test for predicting the risk of pattern hair loss. This test takes into account both maternal and paternal influences. A personalized analysis of an individual's likelihood of developing pattern hair loss can be estimated. Genetic testing for hair loss is currently based on genotyping of the nonfunctional SNP in exon 1 of AR. A person who tests positive for AR gene variant has a more than 80% chance of developing pattern hair loss despite having a father with a minimal amount of hair loss, whereas a person who tests negative for AR gene variant and has a father with no signs of hair loss has a more than 90% chance of not developing pattern hair loss. The HairDX test collection kit is listed with Japan's Pharmaceuticals and Medical Devices Agency and the US Food and Drug Administration (FDA) as a Class 1 medical device. It is available through doctors only (www.hairdx.com).

Association with Other Diseases

Early-onset MPHL has been associated with an increased risk of coronary heart disease and prostate cancer; however, further studies are needed to find out whether this population of patients will benefit from routine screening or systemic use of 5α-reductase inhibitors as primary prevention.[32,33]

MANAGEMENT

MPHL is a benign medical disorder but can be psychologically disturbing, especially in young men. Body-image satisfaction seems to be globally affected. In some instances, hair loss can be a feature of body dysmorphic disorder.[34] This group of patients may need help from a clinical psychologist or psychiatrist.

Men with pattern hair loss are usually reluctant to see a specialist because of the concern of hair loss being viewed as a trivial problem by their physicians. Many patients end up spending money on unproven hair remedies owing to their lack of knowledge. Patients who seek medical help should be counseled and offered treatment directed toward stabilization, prevention, and induction of hair growth. Treatment options should be cost effective and individualized, as patients often have to bear the full cost of treatment.

MEDICAL TREATMENT

At present, minoxidil and oral finasteride are the only treatments approved by the FDA for MPHL. Both these drugs stimulate hair regrowth in some men and are more effective in preventing progression of hair loss. Because pattern hair loss is an ongoing process, treatments are long term, and both these drugs have a good safety record.

Minoxidil

Minoxidil was discontinued as an antihypertensive drug because of its side effect of developing significant hypertrichosis. In 1988 it was approved by the FDA for treatment of MPHL as 2% scalp lotion, and subsequently 5% lotion was approved in 1997. The recommended dose is 1 mL (25 drops) for both 2% and 5% formulation, or half a cap of foam applied twice daily on the dry scalp and left in place at least for 4 hours. The lotion is spread evenly over the entire dry scalp. Hands should be washed with warm water after application. Both formulations are available over the counter in many countries.

The exact mechanism of action of minoxidil is unclear. Its vasorelaxant action is due to the opening of adenosine triphosphate–sensitive potassium channels in the vascular smooth muscle cells, which renders the intracellular potential more negative, and this negative gradient promotes depletion of intracellular calcium. In the presence of calcium, the epidermal growth factor has been shown to inhibit follicular growth in vitro. The conversion of minoxidil to minoxidil sulfate (active metabolite) is higher in hair follicles than in the surrounding skin and may suppress epidermal growth factor–induced inhibition of growth, prolonging the anagen phase of hair follicles.[35] There is no convincing evidence that minoxidil reverses follicular miniaturization, although it may prevent or delay it. Minoxidil may cause temporary hair shedding during the first month and that lasts for 4 to 6 weeks by inducing anagen from the resting phase. This shedding may be viewed as a clinical indication that the treatment is working, and the patient should be forewarned not to stop treatment. The response to minoxidil in terms of increased hair count and hair weight is rapid and peaks at 16 weeks, although the cosmetic effect may take longer. The mean increase in target area hair count is about 8% with 2% minoxidil lotion and 10% to 12% with 5% formulation. When assessed with global photography, about 60% of men show improvement with 5% formulation and 40% with 2% formulation, compared with 23% with placebo. It is important to stress that treatment is long term, and stopping minoxidil will shed all minoxidil-dependent hair within 4 to 6 months.[36,37]

Adverse effects of minoxidil include skin irritation, hypertrichosis on the face and hands, and tachycardia.[15] Constituents of the vehicle can cause skin irritation, more commonly with the 5% formulation. Allergic reaction to minoxidil or propylene glycol (a component of vehicle) is rare. A propylene glycol–free foam preparation of 5% minoxidil is available, which is potentially less irritating and messy. Contact dermatitis should be excluded by patch test, if it is due to propylene glycol; an alternative vehicle such as butylene glycol can be tried, whereas if irritation and contact dermatitis is due to minoxidil, drug interruption cannot be avoided. To avoid contamination of pillows with subsequent contact with the face, patients should be advised to apply the drug at least 2 hours before going to bed. Facial hypertrichosis mostly affects the forehead, malar areas, and sides of the face. Those women who already have mild hirsutism are more likely to develop this side effect. Hypertrichosis is totally reversible on discontinuation of the drug.[38] Contact with the mucosal surface should be avoided, because it causes burning and irritation.[39] Minoxidil is poorly absorbed after topical application. Only 0.3% to 4.5% reaches systemic circulation and is eliminated within 4 days. Minoxidil should not be used in pregnant or nursing women. There is no evidence of teratogenicity in rats and rabbits, but in humans data are lacking. Minoxidil is secreted in human milk. Studies have not shown any change in blood pressure or any other hemodynamic effect, but minoxidil should be used with caution in patients with cardiovascular disease.[36,39]

Finasteride

Minoxidil monotherapy in MPHL may not halt the process of miniaturization under the influence of androgens. Finasteride is a potent and highly selective inhibitor of 5α-reductase type 2. Taken orally it reduces DHT levels in serum and in scalp by up to 70%.[40] Two types of 5α-reductase inhibitors exist in humans. Type 1 predominates in liver, skin, and scalp, and type II in prostate and genitourinary tract and also in hair follicles. Finasteride is a type II, 5α-reductase inhibitor, and dutasteride inhibits both type 1 and type II 5α-reductase, resulting in a decrease in serum DHT level of 90%. Finasteride was developed for treatment of benign prostate hyperplasia, and in 1993 it was registered in the United States for the treatment of mild to moderate MPHL.[38]

Finasteride is quickly absorbed after oral intake, with peak plasma level occurring 1 to 2 hours after drug intake. The serum half-life is about 6 hours; the biological effect persists much longer. Recommended dosage is 1 mg once daily taken with or without food. If a patient forgets a tablet, talking the double dosage the next day is not recommended. Finasteride is metabolized in liver through the oxidative pathway (cytochrome P450 3A4), although no drug interactions have been noted with drugs metabolized by a similar pathway. Dosage need not be adjusted in the case of renal insufficiency.[39]

Finasteride has been shown to increase both total and anagen hair counts.[41] Finasteride prevents or slows the progression of MPHL, and about two-thirds experience some improvement.[26] The improvement peaks at around 12 months. Finasteride has been shown to produce significant and durable increase in hair growth in men with pattern hair loss. The previously miniaturized hair becomes longer and thicker.[42] Finasteride is more effective over vertex and superior-frontal region of the scalp, compared with a minimal response over the temporal and anterior hairline region.[43] Treatment should be continued because the benefits will not be maintained after ceasing therapy. Baseline photographs of vertex and frontal hair line are helpful and repeated at 6 monthly to yearly intervals to monitor treatment response. Patients are able to observe their regrowth, which serves as a motivating factor in improving long-term compliance to medical treatment.

Patients should be made aware of the pros and cons prior to treatment. Finasteride can cause loss of libido, ejaculatory dysfunction, gynecomastia, and potential depression in a small number of individuals. In a small number of patients adverse sexual effects have been reported to be persistent.[44] Finasteride reduces the level of prostate-specific antigen (PSA). If treatment is started after age 45 years, monitoring of the PSA level should be considered. The PSA level should be doubled to compensate the reduction caused by finasteride, resulting in an interpretation of the test remaining accurate.[38,39]

The level of finasteride in the semen of treated men is very low even with regular intake of finasteride 5 mg/d, and there is no risk in the case of sexual relations with pregnant women. Use of a condom is not necessary for this reason. Finasteride-treated men should avoid donating blood. Women who are or potentially may be pregnant should not handle crushed or broken tablets. Finasteride tablets are coated to prevent contact with the active ingredients during manipulation.[38,39]

Minoxidil Versus Finasteride

Some patients find it more convenient to use a single tablet of finasteride once daily compared with twice-daily minoxidil application. If a patient intends to switch from minoxidil to finasteride, combination therapy is recommended for at least 3, but preferably 6 months before discontinuing minoxidil, to avoid significant hair loss while finasteride can take effect.[38,45]

Dutasteride

Dutasteride has similar characteristics to finasteride but is a more potent, selective inhibitor of the enzyme 5α-reductase types I and II. Dutasteride has been shown to significantly increase hair counts and hair weight, improve the ratio of anagen and telogen hairs, and improve scalp coverage based on assessment of global photography.[26,46–49]

Oral dutasteride 0.5 mg/d can be considered to improve or prevent progression of MPHL in male patients older than 18 years with mild to moderate pattern hair loss. Dutasteride significantly reduces the progression of hair loss in men with pattern hair loss.[50]

Adverse effects of dutasteride are impotence, decreased libido, breast tenderness and enlargement, and ejaculation disorders. These side effects are more common with dutasteride than with finasteride.

One study has compared dutasteride with finasteride.[51] Dutasteride, 2.5 mg was found to be superior to finasteride, 5 mg at 12 and 24 weeks at increasing hair growth in a target area in comparison with placebo in a dose-dependent fashion.

Dutasteride is not FDA approved for MPHL. However, it is approved for men in Korea. More studies are needed comparing the efficacy of dutasteride, 0.5 mg with finasteride, 1 mg.

Miscellaneous Therapies

Often in clinical practice we are confronted with questions concerning the efficacy of a wide range of products available as over-the-counter products. It is therefore important to have some knowledge regarding these products for a better patient-physician relationship. There are insufficient data available regarding the efficacy of these products. Some common over-the-counter hair-growth promoters are saw palmetto, aloe vera, Chinese herbals, Ginseng, millet seeds, and marine extracts, to mention a few. The assumed mechanism of action of miscellaneous therapies has been summarized in an article by Blumeyer and colleagues.[38]

Global Photograph for Monitoring MPHL

Androgenetic alopecia is naturally progressive disease. Treatment is directed toward cessation of hair loss and induction of hair regrowth. A baseline global photograph is helpful in monitoring treatment response and long-term follow-up. Because of the potential impact of subjectivity of clinical investigators, global photographs have been introduced as a more objective record. A global photograph requires a patient with clean, dry hair. Five global views are taken starting from vertex, followed by mid-pattern, frontal, and 2 temporal views.

Surgical Treatment

MPHL is a common cause of hair loss in men. Despite recent advances, medical therapy for this condition remains unsatisfactory in terms of regrowth for many men.

In some patients surgical hair restoration combined with medical treatment can improve cosmetic appearance significantly. Surgical treatment is covered in an article elsewhere in this issue by Bunagan et al.

Combination Therapy

It has been shown in various studies that combination therapy enhances efficacy. Combination of finasteride with topical minoxidil or ketoconazole shampoo showed better results with hair regrowth.[52] Use of topical minoxidil in the preoperative period could prevent the usual shedding that occurs 1 to 2 weeks after hair transplantation and also speed the hair regrowth. Moreover, significantly less grafted hair is lost during shedding periods.[53,54] To achieve good hair density, the use of finasteride and minoxidil in hair transplant patients pre- and postsurgery complement the surgical results by slowing down or stopping further hair loss.[55,56] Minoxidil should be stopped 2 to 3 days before surgery to minimize skin irritation. Therapy should be restarted after 1 to 2 weeks. More randomized, double-blind studies are needed to establish greater efficacy of topical minoxidil, finasteride, and hair transplantation as a combination therapy.

Cosmetic Camouflage

Patients who do not pursue medical treatment or are not ideal candidates for hair transplantation have various camouflage methods available. Spray or scalp dye treatments disguise bald scalp and give the impression of thicker hair. For those with advanced hair loss, good-quality synthetic, acrylic, or natural hairpieces can be offered. Custom-made hair integration systems are available to cover localized areas of hair loss. Hairpieces are discussed in detail in an article elsewhere in this issue by Draelos.

EMERGING TREATMENTS FOR HAIR LOSS
Prostaglandin Analogues

Bimatoprost is a prostaglandin analogue. Lengthening of eyelashes and eyebrows has been observed when prostaglandin analogues are used topically for glaucoma.[57] The precise mechanism of action of prostaglandin analogues is unknown. Bimatoprost 0.03% ophthalmic solution (Latisse) is now approved by the FDA for eyelash hypotrichosis. There is no present evidence to suggest that it can stimulate hair growth over the scalp. Clinical trials are in progress.

Fluridil (Eucapil)

Fluridil is a topical antiandrogen used for the treatment of hyperandrogenic skin syndrome. Topical fluridil, owing to its hydrophobicity, dissolves in the sebum and blocks AR in the hair follicles. Fluridil in the aqueous environment rapidly decomposes into fragments that lack hormonal effects. Fluridil has been widely used in Europe but is still awaiting FDA approval in the United States. A study by Kucerova and colleagues[58] showed 2% fluridil solution in anhydrous isopropanol (Eucapil) to stop progression of pattern hair loss in females after 9 months of use, and anagen hair-stem diameter showed a statistically significant increase at 6 and 9 months. Fluridil has been found to be safe for the treatment of pattern hair loss in men and women.

Laser Therapy

Several lasers have been tried to promote hair regrowth in MPHL, including excimer laser, helium-neon laser, and the HairMax Laser Comb. This technique is discussed in an article elsewhere in this issue by Kalia and Lui.

Cell Therapy/Follicular Cell Implantation

The dermal papilla plays an important role in signaling the epidermis, and thereby influences cell proliferation and differentiation. Cohen and Oliver first demonstrated the inductive role of the dermal papilla, by transplantation of a rat-whisker papilla to the ear skin, which induced formation of a whisker follicle, demonstrating that the dermal papilla specifies the type of hair.[59] The papilla and lower sheath were shown to be essentially equivalent in their hair-inductive capability. The lower portion of the dermal sheath was shown through transplantation to have hair-inductive properties like the papilla,[60] and if the dermal papilla was removed it could be regenerated by cells from the dermal sheath.[61] The idea behind the dermal papilla as a cell therapy to treat hair loss is not new.[62] The dermal papilla was long assumed to play a critical role in follicle morphogenesis,[63] and the first direct evidence was the demonstration in the 1960s that transplanted dermal papillae could induce the formation of new follicles. These experiments first revealed the remarkable hair-inductive power of the adult follicle dermal papilla.

In follicular cell implantation (FCI), dermal papilla cells are taken from a few follicles and expanded in culture and then implanted into the skin to induce the formation of many new follicles. A piece of the patient's nonbalding scalp is removed by a physician in an outpatient clinic. The amount of donor hair required is much smaller than the large donor strips of up to several thousand follicles used for transplantation. The scalp tissue is sent to a laboratory where the follicular cells are isolated from the tissue and expanded in culture. Because the donating scalp contains androgen-insensitive follicles, the dermal papilla cells are "donor dominant" just as in transplanted follicles. After the period of culture expansion, the cells are harvested and then sent back to the clinic for implantation.[64] McElwee and colleagues[65] have shown that intradermally implanted dermal sheath cells have the ability to incorporate into the dermal papillae of preexisting follicles, creating a chimera between preexisting and implanted cells. Thus, implanted cells can potentially hone to and become a part of preexisting dermal papillae in miniaturized follicles. Alternatively, the implanted cells might aggregate to form their own, nascent dermal papilla from which to reactivate the miniaturized follicle.

FCI is an alternative treatment that unlike drugs is permanent, and unlike hair transplantation is not limited by the quantity of donor hair. The ability to expand cells in culture will provide enough cells to induce several new follicles from a small number of donor cells. In the future FCI will offer patients a relatively minimally invasive treatment option for hair loss.

REFERENCES

1. Wells PA, Willmoth T, Russell RJ. Does fortune favour the bald? Psychological correlates of hair loss in males. Br J Psychol 1995;86(Pt 3):337–44.
2. Cash TF. Losing hair, losing points?: the effects of male pattern baldness on social impression formation. J Appl Soc Psychol 1990;20:154–67.
3. Alfonso M, Richter-Appelt H, Tosti A, et al. The psychosocial impact of hair loss among men: a multinational European study. Curr Med Res Opin 2005; 21:1829–36.
4. Kaufman KD. Androgens and alopecia. Mol Cell Endocrinol 2002;198:89–95.
5. Yip L, Rufaut N, Sinclair RD. Role of genetics and sex steroid hormones in male androgenetic alopecia and female pattern hair loss: an update of what we now know. Australas J Dermatol 2011;52:81–8.
6. Ziller C. Pattern formation in neural crest derivatives. In: Van Neste VR, editor. Hair research for the next millennium. Amsterdam: Elsevier Science; 1996. p. 1.
7. Jaenisch R, Bird A. Epigenetic regulation of gene expression: how the genome integrates intrinsic and environmental signals. Nat Genet 2003;33(Suppl): 245–54.
8. Foley DL, Craig JM, Morley R, et al. Prospects for epigenetic epidemiology. Am J Epidemiol 2009; 169:389–400.
9. McGrath J, McLean I. Genetics in relation to the skin: mosaicism. In: Wolff K, Goldsmith L, Katz S, et al, editors. Fitzpatrick's dermatology in general medicine, vol. 1. New York: McGraw Hill Medical; 2008. p. 83–4.
10. Ellis JA, Stebbing M, Harrap SB. Polymorphism of the androgen receptor gene is associated with male pattern baldness. J Invest Dermatol 2001; 116:452–5.
11. Hillmer AM, Flaquer A, Hanneken S, et al. Genome-wide scan and fine-mapping linkage study of androgenetic alopecia reveals a locus on chromosome 3q26. Am J Hum Genet 2008;82:737–43.
12. Hillmer AM, Brockschmidt FF, Hanneken S, et al. Susceptibility variants for male-pattern baldness on chromosome 20p11. Nat Genet 2008;40:1279–81.
13. Sawaya ME, Price VH. Different levels of 5alpha-reductase type I and II, aromatase, and androgen receptor in hair follicles of women and men with androgenetic alopecia. J Invest Dermatol 1997; 109:296–300.
14. Vierhapper H, Maier H, Nowotny P, et al. Production rates of testosterone and of dihydrotestosterone in female pattern hair loss. Metabolism 2003;52:927–9.
15. Shapiro J, Price VH. Hair regrowth. Therapeutic agents. Dermatol Clin 1998;16:341–56.
16. Sinclair RD. Male pattern androgenetic alopecia. BMJ 1998;317:865–9.
17. Jahoda CAB. Cellular and developmental aspects of androgenetic alopecia. Exp Dermatol 1998;7:235–48.
18. Obana NJ, Uno H. Dermal papilla cells in macaque alopecia trigger a testosterone dependent inhibition of follicular cell proliferation. In: Neste DV, Randall VA, editors. Hair research in the next millennium. Amsterdam: Elsevier; 1996. p. 307–10.
19. Oliver RF, Jahoda CA. The dermal papilla and the maintenance of hair growth. In: Roger GA, Reis P, Ward KA, editors. The biology of wool and hair. London: Chapman and Hall; 1989. p. 51–67.
20. Randall VA, Hibberts NA, Hamada K. A comparison of the culture and growth of dermal papilla cells from hair follicles from non-balding and balding (androgenetic alopecia) scalp. Br J Dermatol 1996; 134(3):437–44.
21. Whiting D. Scalp biopsy as a diagnostic and prognostic tool in androgenetic alopecia. Dermatol Ther 1998;8:24–33.
22. Whiting DA. Diagnostic and predictive value of horizontal sectioning of scalp biopsy specimens in male pattern androgenetic alopecia. J Am Acad Dermatol 1993;28:755–63.
23. Headington JT. Transverse microscopic anatomy of the human scalp. A basis for a morphometric approach to disorders of the hair follicle. Arch Dermatol 1984;120(4):449–56.
24. Hamilton J. Patterned loss of hair in man; types and incidence. Ann N Y Acad Sci 1951;53:708–28.
25. Norwood OT. Male pattern baldness: classification and incidence. South Med J 1975;68(11):1359–65.
26. Kaufman KD, Olsen EA, Whiting D, et al. Finasteride in the treatment of men with androgenetic alopecia. Finasteride Male Pattern Hair Loss Study Group. J Am Acad Dermatol 1998;39:578–89.
27. De Lacharriere O, Deloche C, Misciali C, et al. Hair diameter diversity: a clinical sign reflecting the follicle miniaturization. Arch Dermatol 2001;137: 641–6.
28. Tosti A, Whiting D, Iorizzo M, et al. The role of scalp dermoscopy in the diagnosis of alopecia areata incognita. J Am Acad Dermatol 2008;59:64–7.
29. Blume-Peytavi U, Orfanos CE. Microscopy of the hair—the trichogram. In: Serup J, Jemec GB, Grover GL, editors. Handbook of non-invasive methods and the skin. 2nd edition. Boca Raton (FL): CRC Press; 2006. p. 875–81.

30. Van Neste DJ, Dumrotier M, de Brouwer B, et al. Scalp immersion proxigraphy: an improved imaging technique for phototrichogram analysis. J Eur Acad Dermatol Venereol 1992;1:187–91.

31. Hoffmann R, Happle R. Current understanding of androgenetic alopecia. Part II: clinical aspects and treatment. Eur J Dermatol 2000;10:410–7.

32. Arias-Santiago S, Gutierrez-Salmeron MT, Castellote-Caballero L, et al. Androgenetic alopecia and cardiovascular risk factors in men and women: a comparative study. J Am Acad Dermatol 2010; 63:420–9.

33. Yassa M, Saliou M, De Rycke Y, et al. Male pattern baldness and the risk of prostate cancer. Ann Oncol 2011;22:1824–7.

34. Phillips KA. Body dysmorphic disorder: the distress of imagined ugliness. Am J Psychiatry 1991;148: 1138–49.

35. Li M, Marubayashi A, Nakaya Y, et al. Minoxidil-induced hair growth is mediated by adenosine in cultured dermal papilla cells: possible involvement of sulfonylurea receptor 2B as a target of minoxidil. J Invest Dermatol 2001;117:1594–600.

36. Olsen EA, Weiner MS, Amara IA, et al. Five-year follow-up of men with androgenetic alopecia treated with topical minoxidil. J Am Acad Dermatol 1990;22: 643–6.

37. Olsen EA, Dunlap FE, Funicella T, et al. A randomized clinical trial of 5% topical minoxidil versus 2% topical minoxidil and placebo in the treatment of androgenetic alopecia in men. J Am Acad Dermatol 2002; 47:377–85.

38. Blumeyer A, Tosti A, Messenger A, et al. Evidence-based (S3) guideline for the treatment of androgenetic alopecia in women and in men. J Dtsch Dermatol Ges 2011;9:S1–57.

39. Canadian Pharmacists Association monograph, minoxidil and finasteride. In: Compendium of pharmaceuticals and specialities (CPS), 34th edition. Ottawa (Canada): Canadian Pharmacists Association; 1999.

40. Drake L, Hordinsky M, Fiedler V, et al. The effects of finasteride on scalp skin and serum androgen levels in men with androgenetic alopecia. J Am Acad Dermatol 1999;41:550–4.

41. Van Neste D, Fuh V, Sanchez-Pedreno P, et al. Finasteride increases anagen hair in men with androgenetic alopecia. Br J Dermatol 2000;143:804–10.

42. Rossi A, Cantisani C, Scarno M, et al. Finasteride, 1 mg daily administration on male androgenetic alopecia in different age groups: 10-year follow-up. Dermatol Ther 2011;24:455–61.

43. Stough DB, Rao NA, Kaufman KD, et al. Finasteride improves male pattern hair loss in a randomized study in identical twins. Eur J Dermatol 2002;12:32–7.

44. Traish AM, Hassani J, Guay AT, et al. Adverse side effects of 5alpha-reductase inhibitors therapy: persistent diminished libido and erectile dysfunction and depression in a subset of patients. J Sex Med 2011;8:872–84.

45. Price VH. Treatment of hair loss. N Engl J Med 1999; 341:964–73.

46. Roberts JL, Fiedler V, Imperato-McGinley J, et al. Clinical dose ranging studies with finasteride, a type 2 5alpha-reductase inhibitor, in men with male pattern hair loss. J Am Acad Dermatol 1999; 41:555–63.

47. Leyden J, Dunlap F, Miller B, et al. Finasteride in the treatment of men with frontal male pattern hair loss. J Am Acad Dermatol 1999;40:930–7.

48. McClellan KJ, Markham A. Finasteride: a review of its use in male pattern hair loss. Drugs 1999;57: 111–26.

49. Canfield D. Photographic documentation of hair growth in androgenetic alopecia. Dermatol Clin 1996;14:713–21.

50. Stough D. Dutasteride improves male pattern hair loss in a randomized study in identical twins. J Cosmet Dermatol 2007;6:9–13.

51. Olsen EA, Hordinsky M, Whiting D, et al. The importance of dual 5alpha-reductase inhibition in the treatment of male pattern hair loss: results of a randomized placebo-controlled study of dutasteride versus finasteride. J Am Acad Dermatol 2006; 55:1014–23.

52. Khandpur S, Suman M, Reddy BS. Comparative efficacy of various treatment regimens for androgenetic alopecia in men. J Dermatol 2002;29:489–98.

53. Kassimir JJ. Use of topical minoxidil as a possible adjunct to hair transplant surgery. A pilot study. J Am Acad Dermatol 1987;16:685–7.

54. Roenigk HH, Berman MD. Topical 2% minoxidil with hair transplantation. Face 1993;4:213–6.

55. Avram MR, Cole JP, Gandelman M, et al. The potential role of minoxidil in the hair transplantation setting. Dermatol Surg 2002;28:894–900 [discussion: 900].

56. Leavitt M, Perez-Meza D, Rao NA, et al. Effects of finasteride (1 mg) on hair transplant. Dermatol Surg 2005;31:1268–76 [discussion: 1276].

57. Wolf R, Matz H, Zalish M, et al. Prostaglandin analogs for hair growth: great expectations. Dermatol Online J 2003;9:7.

58. Kucerova R, BM, Novotny R, et al. Current therapies of female androgenetic alopecia and use of fluridil, a novel topical antiandrogen. Scripta Med (Brno) 2006;79:35–48.

59. Jahoda CA. Induction of follicle formation and hair growth by vibrissa dermal papillae implanted into rat ear wounds: vibrissa-type fibres are specified. Development 1992;115:1103–9.

60. Horne KA, Jahoda CA. Restoration of hair growth by surgical implantation of follicular dermal sheath. Development 1992;116:563–71.

61. Oliver RF. Whisker growth after removal of the dermal papilla and lengths of follicle in the hooded rat. J Embryol Exp Morphol 1966;15:331–47.

62. Jahoda CA, Horne KA, Oliver RF. Induction of hair growth by implantation of cultured dermal papilla cells. Nature 1984;311:560–2.

63. Chase HB. Growth of the hair. Physiol Rev 1954;34: 113–26.

64. Teumer JC. Follicular cell implantation: an emerging cell therapy for hair loss. Semin Plast Surg 2005;19: 193–200.

65. McElwee KJ, Kissling S, Wenzel E, et al. Cultured peribulbar dermal sheath cells can induce hair follicle development and contribute to the dermal sheath and dermal papilla. J Invest Dermatol 2003; 121:1267–75.

Hair Transplantation Update
Procedural Techniques, Innovations, and Applications

M.J. Kristine Bunagan, MD, Nusrat Banka, MD,
Jerry Shapiro, MD*

KEYWORDS

- Hair transplantation • Update hair transplantation • Follicular unit transplantation
- Follicular unit extraction • Applications hair transplantation • Follicular unit grafts

KEY POINTS

- Follicular unit transplantation yields the most natural looking results and is considered as the current gold standard in hair transplantation.
- Basic steps in hair transplantation consist of donor area harvesting, graft dissection and storage, recipient slit creation and placement of grafts.
- Aside from strip harvesting, follicular unit extraction (FUE) is another newer technique in donor harvesting. Variations in the FUE technique include the use of manual, motorized and automated punches and the utilization of robotic technology.
- Indications for hair transplantation has gone beyond male and female pattern hair loss of the scalp to include transplanting hair over non scalp areas with hair loss such as the eyebrows, eyelashes, moustache, beard and pubic area.
- Scarring alopecias due to secondary causes such as burns, surgery and trauma are mostly amenable to hair transplantation however the utilization of this procedure for primary cicatricial alopecias remains controversial.

INTRODUCTION

Hair transplantation has evolved throughout the years from the larger punch grafts to the smaller mini grafts and finally to the more refined follicular unit graft transplantation performed by most hair restoration surgeons today. This advancement in hair transplantation has its basis in the identification of the follicular unit as the naturally occurring structure of hair follicles on the human scalp. This histologic structure was first described by Headington[1] as a circumscribed unit containing 1 to 4 hair follicles along with its associated sebaceous glands and arrector pili muscle insertion (**Fig. 1**). Because follicular unit transplantation follows the aforementioned natural pattern of hair follicles on the human scalp, the procedure yields the most natural-looking results and is considered the current gold standard in hair transplantation. There are unifying concepts and general steps that characterize this type of surgery; however, there are likewise a lot of variations and innovations in the techniques and applications of this procedure.

PROCEDURAL TECHNIQUES

The basic steps in hair transplantation, including follicular unit transplantation, consist of donor-area harvesting, graft dissection and storage, recipient slit creation, and placement of grafts.

All authors have nothing to disclose.
Department of Dermatology and Skin Science, University of British Columbia, 835 West 10th Avenue, Vancouver, British Columbia, Canada
* Corresponding author.
E-mail address: Jerry.shapiro@vch.ca

Dermatol Clin 31 (2013) 141–153
http://dx.doi.org/10.1016/j.det.2012.08.012
0733-8635/13/$ – see front matter © 2013 Elsevier Inc. All rights reserved.

derm.theclinics.com

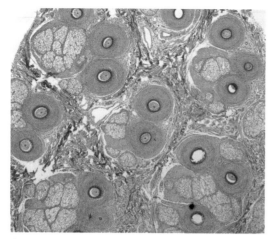

Fig. 1. Horizontal section of a scalp biopsy showing follicular units containing hair follicles, sebaceous glands, and arrector pili muscle. (*Courtesy of* Magdalena Martinka.)

The technique of follicular unit grafting was originated by Limmer[2] and further detailed by Bernstein and Rassman[3,4] in the early 1990s. Since then, the basic procedure remains the same with some variations, modifications, and added applications.

DONOR HARVESTING
Strip Method

Currently, the most common approach in harvesting the donor area is by surgical excision of a strip from the occipital and parietal areas of the scalp, using a single blade or a double-bladed scalpel (**Fig. 2**). To minimize follicular transection, the blade must be held parallel to the angle and the direction of the hair shafts and excision must be made up to the subcutaneous level where the hair bulbs are located. For better visualization of

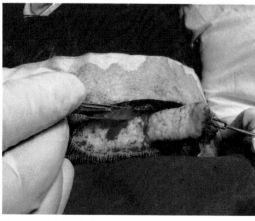

Fig. 2. Single-strip harvesting.

the donor area, some surgeons use magnification devices, such as a loop with 1.5 to 4.0× lens magnification. The ideal donor strip should be taken from the safest and most permanent part of the donor scalp, which is, in most cases, located in between the superior and inferior border of the donor hairs.[5]

To further decrease follicular transection, some surgeons have made some modifications to the basic technique. The Haber spreader is a device with a set of jaws with 4 sharp staggered prongs. The goal is to harvest the strip by separating the skin along the natural tissue dissection plane. A superficial scoring incision is first made to delineate the strip edges, then the instrument is inserted into the incision, and finally the handles are pressed together to separate the wound edges. Although this device may be helpful in some patients, there a certain cases when it may be difficult to separate the skin tissue with the spreader, thus, the surgeon may have to use a scalpel blade to excise the area.[6]

Another modification to the strip harvesting method is through strip excision with the aid of skin hooks. The skin is superficially scored with a scalpel blade and then skin hooks are inserted just below the rim of the wound edges. Once inserted, the skin hooks are then lifted and pulled in opposite directions to allow direct visualization of the follicular units. A scalpel is then used to gently excise the strip without transecting the follicles.[7]

The general guideline for obtaining donor strips that result in very thin linear scars is to obtain strips that are long and narrow. For instance, for regular hair transplantation sessions (1500–2500 grafts), the width may range from 1.0 to 1.5 cm, whereas the length would vary greatly from 20 to 30 cm depending on the patient's follicular unit density and the total graft requirement. Another factor that influences the width size of the strip is the laxity of the donor area. The more lax the skin, the wider the strip that can be excised while still being able to close the donor wound with minimal tension.

For patients who may need more than one hair transplantation session, subsequent procedures may lead to multiple linear scars if the strips are obtained from donor areas separate from the previous scar. To avoid this from occurring, the technique is to incorporate the old scar with the current strip, thus, resulting in a single scar even after multiple surgeries. In general, the subsequent strip has to be narrower than the prior surgeries for lesser tension when closing the wound. In addition, other techniques, such as scalp massage to improve laxity and double-layer closure for wider scars, may help improve the outcome.

Closure Techniques

To close the donor wound, commonly used closure materials include nylon, polypropylene, Vicryl or monocryl sutures, or staples. Techniques include continuous single-layer closure, combined continuous and retention sutures, or the application of staples. Closure with staples may take less time to accomplish; however, patients may complain of more discomfort during the postoperative period. Here at the University of British Columbia (UBC) hair transplant center, for first-session surgeries, a continuous single-layer closure with 3-0 nylon or prolene sutures is typically performed. These nonabsorbable sutures are then removed after 1 week. For subsequent surgeries, when the donor area has less scalp laxity, a double-layer closure with absorbable monocryl or Vicryl may be used.

Trichophytic Closure

The main concern with strip harvesting is the appearance of the resultant donor scar. In most cases when the surgeon has excised a long, thin strip with narrow width (eg, <1 cm) and closure was done without tension, the donor scar would usually be very minimal. However, there are cases when wider strips may have to be excised for larger graft requirements. In addition, for most patients and surgeons, improvement of even a minimal scar has some benefit. Toward this end, Marzola, Rose, and Frechet[8–10] introduced the application of the trichophytic closure in hair transplantation at about the same time period. This technique is performed after the excision of the donor strip and involves the de-epithelialization or removal of the epidermis of either the superior or inferior wound edge (**Fig. 3**A). The two sides would then be approximated together with the de-epithelialized edge underneath the other donor rim. The purpose of removing the epidermis at the wound edge is for the hair follicles, which were superficially cut, to grow within the resultant scar, thus, minimizing the appearance of the scar.[11]

The general guideline is to perform a very superficial excision just below the epidermis not exceeding 1 mm to avoid damaging the permanent portion of the hair follicles at the area of the bulge. This coincides with the results of a study whereby morphometric analysis of the hair follicle and measurement of the depth of the bulge area was done. The mean follicular length was approximately 4.16 mm, whereas that of the bulge area was from 1.0 to 1.8 mm. The depth of the bulge area was determined through immunoreactivity of CK15, a bulge stem cell marker. Thus, to avoid damaging the bulge portion, the trichophytic cut should be less than 1 mm from the surface of the skin.[12]

The instruments used to remove the edge varies, with some surgeons advocating the use of a scalpel[11] to make a right-angle edge, whereas others use scissors.[8,10] Observed effects of the trichophytic closure revealed that there can be problems with resultant hair angles, more so with superior edge de-epithelialization, thus, inferior edge removal is preferred.[11] For surgeons using the trichophytic closure technique, improvement in the appearance of the resultant donor scars is observed in many patients (see **Fig. 3**B).

Follicular Unit Extraction

With the natural looking results of follicular unit transplantation over the recipient area, more attention is being given to improving the scars at the donor area. Although properly done donor strip excision commonly results in minimal linear scars, some surgeons and patients prefer less visible, nonlinear scars. Thus, another technique in donor harvesting, known as follicular unit extraction (FUE), was introduced.[13] The basic procedure involves identifying a follicular unit at the donor area and extracting the individual follicular unit via a punch devise. Variations in the FUE technique are discussed later. Although a linear scar is not produced, this procedure still results in scars that usually appear as dotted hypopigmented macules over the donor area. The proponents of this

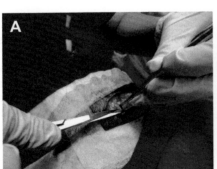
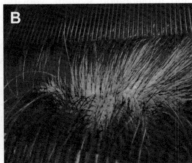

Fig. 3. Trimming of the inferior edge in trichophytic closure (*A*) and minimal donor scar after 1 year (*B*).

procedure have put forth other advantages, such as less postoperative pain over the donor area and the ability to obtain grafts from patients with very tight donor skin caused by multiple surgeries. Critiques of this procedure include potentially high transection rates that may occur with the blind extraction of individual grafts and much longer completion times. And because this procedure is operator driven, a successful outcome would largely depend on the skill of the surgeon.

Manual Punches

The FUE procedure basically uses punches that range from 0.8 to 1.5 mm in diameter. Punches may also have sharp or dull tips, with the choice of tip dependent on the technique preferred by a particular surgeon. One of the main techniques described by Rassman and colleagues[13] is the FOX procedure, which uses a sharp 1-mm punch to make a superficial incision up to level of the mid-dermis followed by the extraction of the individual follicular unit with a forceps. Not all patients are good candidates for this procedure; thus, the proponents of this technique have proposed the FOX test, which is a test session to determine transection rates and, hence, identify which patients would yield positive results.[13]

Another modification of the FUE technique is the Surgically Advanced Follicular Extraction system described by Harris.[14] In this procedure, first a sharp punch creates a superficial scoring incision, which is then followed by a blunt dissecting punch to separate the follicular unit from the surrounding tissue. A variation is the use of a serrated dull tip. A study on patients with male pattern hair loss showed transection rates of 6.14%, with a range of 1.7% to 15.0%. A potential side effect of this procedure is the possible occurrence of buried grafts with the use of dull tips.[15]

Motorized and Automated Punches

Punch devices used for FUE now include motorized and automated punches, such as the automated FUE and implantation system NeoGraft (Medicamat, Malakoff, France). This machine uses pneumatic pressure and automated control to extract individual follicular units. The physician controls the harvesting hand piece, which has a rotating and cutting canula for excision of grafts. After extraction, the grafts are suctioned into a canister. Trimming of the grafts are not necessary. Multiple punch diameter sizes with a depth limiter are provided. Another feature of this machine is the implantation handpiece. A combination of pneumatic pressure automatically loads the graft into the implantation canula then implants

on the recipient site as directed by the physician. The surgeon still has to manually create the recipient slits using regular methods, after which the handpiece can then be used to insert the grafts.[16] A study of 40 FUE cases comparing manual and powered FUE punches showed that the mean harvesting time of the latter group was faster at approximately 100 grafts per 8.9 ± 1.3 minutes. The transection rate reported was 5.5%.[17]

Robotics

Trying to address the disadvantages of FUE, such as long procedural times and high transection rates, a company has come up with a robotic machine (ARTAS System, Restoration Robotics, Mountain View, California) to extract grafts. This machine has recently obtained approval by the Food and Drug Administration. This FUE system has an image-guided set of cameras and computer programming to improve accuracy in extracting follicular units. Physicians control the settings of the machine. The multiple cameras first capture images of the scalp, and then the computer's software analyzes the data through complex algorithms and computations. Through the aforementioned process, the system maps out and monitors the follicular unit location and patient motion. The computer-guided robotic arm with a 1-mm needle and blunt punch then harvests at random based on the follicular unit spacing set by the physician. Their reported transection rate is less than 10% and the extraction rate is 500 to 600 grafts per hour. The surgeon and/or nurses then implant the grafts manually after the recipient slit creation using hypodermic needles or miniblades.[18,19]

Lin X and colleagues[20] reported another hair-harvesting robot with an end-effector arm.[20] This machine has a digital microscope that first localizes and determines follicular units and then guides the punch with a motorized shifting mechanism and rotary guidance design to harvest grafts. The reported end-effector bias and precision was 0.014 mm.

Nonscalp Donor Area

There are patients who are not considered good candidates for hair transplantation because of a poor scalp donor area. Some may have depleted donor supplies from previous hair transplantation procedures. For this subset of patients, there is a need for additional sources of donor supply. Alternative sources from other hair-bearing areas of the body may provide an expanded pool in a select group of hirsute individuals. FUE of nonscalp hairs has been performed by some surgeons with moderately good outcomes. In a case report, this procedure was done because of the extensive scalp scarring with limited donor area. Chest hairs served as donor grafts for the recipient scalp. After more than 1 year, there was acceptable transplanted hair growth. Another observation was the change in length of the chest hairs from 4 cm to and 15 cm (4 times) at about 1.5 years after the hair transplantation.[21]

In another case series whereby some patients had severely depleted donor areas caused by previous surgeries, grafts were sourced from chest, abdomen, beard, arm, and leg areas. There was a reported 80% to 85% survival of the transplanted grafts. In this study, procedural details included the shaving of the donor areas 1 week before surgery to ensure extraction of anagen hairs and the use of hypodermic needles customized at the tip and mounted on a rotary tool as the punch device. The cases had, on average, around 1500 to 1800 grafts per session, with several 2 to 3 consecutive daily sessions done to achieve the total graft requirements. The aforementioned patients were very hirsute individuals, thus, allowing for the extraction of a large number of grafts.[22]

The success of this type of procedure depends heavily on the skill of the surgeon. Other disadvantages include hairs of lesser quality when compared with scalp hairs (eg, caliber and length differences). Although there are some reports of an increase in the length of the transplanted hairs, other surgeons were not able to observe this finding. In certain patients, the body hair supply may be insufficient. In terms of the best source of nonscalp hair, the beard area would most likely yield grafts with the potential to grow longer than the hairs from the other areas of the body.

Hair Regeneration from Bisected Follicles

To further expand the donor supply, various studies have looked into the growth potential of bisected or partial follicular units. A study by Toscani and colleagues[23] bisected hair follicles horizontally resulting in upper and lower portions. The upper part was cut just below the insertion of the arrector pili muscle and was approximately one-third of the length from the dermal papilla. The donor hair follicles were then implanted on the recipient area of a patient with male pattern hair loss. Both the upper and lower portions were stained for epithelial stem cell markers. The hair regrowth evaluation done after 1 year revealed the presence of epithelial markers CD200, beta 1 integrin, and p63 detected over both portions, signifying the possibility of a reservoir of progenitor stem cells capable of regenerating an entire hair follicle. Hair regrowth was $72 \pm 0.4\%$ of the transplanted upper portions and $69.2 \pm 1.1\%$ of the lower portions. The hairs from the bisected follicles had slightly finer caliber hairs compared with intact hairs.

Another study extracted partial longitudinal follicular units. The vertically divided hair follicles (100 and 150 grafts) extracted from the occipital areas of 5 patients were transplanted into their respective recipient areas. After 1 year, there was a mean growth of 95.9% of the partial follicular units transplanted on the recipient area, with the growing hairs possessing the same characteristics as the donor hair.[24]

GRAFT DISSECTION AND HANDLING

After the hair-bearing strip is harvested from the donor area, it is cut into slivers of 1 to 2 rows of follicular units (**Fig. 4**). These slivers are then further dissected into follicular unit grafts with 1, 2, 3, or 4 hairs, depending on the observed natural grouping of the follicular units on a patient's scalp (**Fig. 5**). Proper dissection into follicular unit grafts involve carefully trimming the tissue surrounding

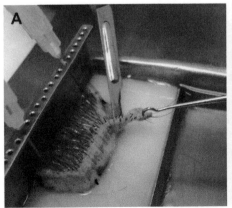 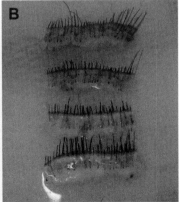

Fig. 4. Slivering technique (*A*) and slivers of single rows of follicular units (*B*).

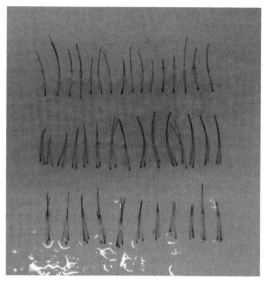

Fig. 5. Follicular unit grafts with 1, 2, and 3 hairs.

ensuring that grafts are properly hydrated throughout the hair transplantation procedure is paramount to graft survival.

Magnification

The binocular stereoscopic microscope provides magnification and proper illumination while dissecting follicular unit grafts (**Fig. 6**). This is especially important in follicular unit transplantation when there can be difficulty in identifying and dissecting tiny follicular unit grafts with the naked eye. This device, with a magnification of ×5 to ×20, enables better visualization of the follicular units to minimize transection of the hair follicles. Surgical technicians commonly use the ×10 magnification setting.[26]

Storage Solutions

Currently, unbuffered normal saline, Plasma-lyte A, and Ringer lactate solution are the most commonly used holding solutions in hair transplantation.[27] Graft survival studies and the surgical experience of hair transplant surgeons with successful outcomes provide a good basis for the use of normal saline solution. At the author's center, chilled normal saline used for surgeries lasting for 6 to 8 hours have consistently yielded a high percentage of graft survival as evidenced by good cosmetic results. The concern of some surgeons is for longer hair transplantation sessions that extend beyond 6 to 8 hours because previous studies have shown a decrease in graft survival with extended duration times.[28,29] More research studies are looking into the use of other holding solutions to improve graft survival.

Intracellular solutions, such as hypothermosol and custodial, have a lower Na+ concentration. For surgical durations within 6 to 8 hours, the survival of grafts in these intracellular solutions

the follicular units, thus, ending up with a pear-shaped graft that is wider at the base where the bulbs of the follicles typically splay and narrower at the top where the hairs converge as they exit the skin. Instruments used for the slivering and dissecting of follicular unit grafts commonly include the number 15 or 10 scalpel blades or double-edged razor blades depending on the training and preference of the surgical assistants.

The possible effect of graft handling injuries on the morphology of the follicular unit graft was analyzed in a study through the use of a light or scanning electron microscope. The grafts were crushed, bent, stretched with forceps, or left drying for 3 minutes. The results showed that there was no change in morphology in the grafts that were stretched, crushed, or bent. Damage was observed only in the grafts left to dry.[25] Therefore,

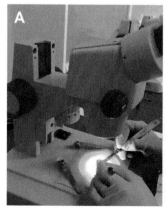
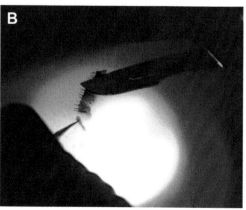

Fig. 6. Stereoscopic microscope (A). Dissecting follicular unit grafts with magnification and illumination (B).

may not vary significantly from grafts in normal saline; however, for much longer sessions, the use of these solutions may have some benefit.[30]

Some studies were focused on the effect of additives to storage solutions primarily in terms of enhancing graft survival. In one study, adding ATP–magnesium chloride and deferoxamine to normal saline solution led to moderate improvement in graft survival. There was 98% graft survival seen with normal saline plus additives compared with 87% with normal saline alone.[31] In another study, DMEM with AMG improved hair shaft elongation after 5 hours. There was also a decrease in cHADF, a measure of apoptotic cell death. DMEM with arachidonic acid inhibitors and AMG (inhibitor of nitric oxide synthase) showed improvement in hair shaft elongation in in vitro and in vivo studies.[32] EET also improved hair shaft elongation.[33]

Uebel[34] conducted a study on the use of platelet-rich plasma (PRP) obtained through the manual centrifuge method. Results revealed that after 1 year of transplanting 20 grafts per centimeter, the hair regrowth was 18.7 grafts per centimeter with PRP compared with 16.4 grafts per centimeter with the control group, signifying an approximately 15% difference in follicular density.[34] Another study by Perez-Meza and colleagues,[35] which obtained PRP via an automated centrifuge machine, had a different finding. After 1 year, hair counts showed similar results for both the PRP and the placebo group.[35]

RECIPIENT GRAFT CREATION AND PLACEMENT

Slit Creation

In creating slits over the recipient area, important considerations include slit size, depth of incision and angle, and direction. In general, over the frontal to midscalp area, the hairs are in an anterior or forward direction with acute angulation. Over the temples and parietal area, the direction is more inferoposterior with very acute angles, especially over the temple points and sideburn areas, which have angles almost flat to the skin. The vertex area can be a complicated area to transplant because hairs may follow a whorl pattern. In terms of the size of the slits, mostly grafts with 1 hair correspond to slits created by 20- to 21-gauge hypodermic needles or 0.7- to 0.9-mm miniblades and 2- to 3-haired grafts to 18- to 19-gauge needles or 1.0- to 1.1-mm miniblades. The depth should depend on the length of the hair follicle, which can be measured along the length of the needle or miniblade to guide the surgeon as to how deep to make the incisions. Follicular lengths range from 4 to 6 mm depending on

ethnicity, with Caucasians usually having shorter follicles and Asians having more on the longer end of the spectrum.

For the frontal hairline, to frame the face well and to create a natural-looking hairline, the slits should be made in an irregular pattern to try to mimic natural hairlines, which are mostly very irregular and slightly asymmetric. Hairlines should only be transplanted with grafts with 1 hair. The 2- to 3-haired grafts should be transplanted behind the 1-hair grafts going more posterior to create more volume or coverage.

Slit orientation can be sagittal or parallel to the direction of hair growth or they can be coronal slits, which are created perpendicular to the hair flow. Traditionally, sagittal slits have been the type of slits created by most surgeons, with good outcomes seen most patients. Surgeons who prefer coronal slits point out that this type of slit orientation causes less tissue damage than sagittal slits, permits closer graft placement, and makes hair strands shingle, creating the illusion of more volume.[36] A microscopic analysis of the natural hair orientation in 100 men showed that multi-hair follicular units were mostly coronal or perpendicular to the radial line from the whorl over the peripheral and midscalp areas.[37]

Density Goals and Size of Sessions

Twenty five to 40 follicular unit grafts per square centimeter are the transplanted densities made by most hair restoration surgeons. This density goal shows a cosmetically acceptable outcome over the recipient area, with most patients being satisfied by the results. Generally, noticeable hair thinning occurs only after a person has greater than 50% hair loss; thus, in most cases, it is not necessary to transplant densities greater than 50%.

In terms of magnitude of sessions, many surgeons are performing hair transplantation surgeries ranging from 1000 to 3000 grafts per session, which is usually adequate to cover small-to moderate-sized areas of hair loss at one time. For patients with larger areas, 2 to 3 sessions may have to be performed, although the possibility of subsequent sessions would depend on the availability of the donor supply.

Implanters

Transplanting over the recipient area is commonly done manually using jeweler's forceps. The graft placer gently grasps the follicular unit graft and, ideally, in one motion should insert the graft inside the recipient slit. This skill requires several months to years to master. This part of the procedure is usually the rate-limiting step, which lengthens the duration of most hair transplantation procedures. Some physicians have come up with instruments to aid in this graft-placement process. Implanters, such as the CHOI and KNU implanters, are used more commonly in Korea and Japan. The original CHOI implanter and the improved KNU version come from Kyungpook National University in Korea. These implanters are shaped liked pencils with a hollow needle at the tip. There are 3 sizes that correspond to 1-, 2-, or 3-haired follicular unit grafts. A single follicular unit is placed inside the hollow end of each device. The device, with its sharp end, can then be injected into the recipient site where it simultaneously creates a slit and inserts the graft inside the slit at the same time. On withdrawal of the implanter, the graft is left inside the incision.[38] A study done to assess the survival rate of 1- and 2-haired follicular unit grafts using the KNU implanter revealed graft growth of 92.0% after 6 months and 90.4% after 1 year.[39] Graft survival at different transplanted densities was also studied, and the results showed that survival rates were higher at 20 to 30 grafts per square centimeter compared with higher transplanted densities of 40 to 50 grafts per square centimeter. The recipient-area density suggested for the KNU implanter is 30 FU/cm^2 per procedure and to perform repeated sessions as necessary.[40] Possible drawbacks to the implanters include potential difficulty in loading finer Caucasian hair; some grafts may be inserted below the skin, resulting in pitting; and blades may not be as sharp, leading to popping of grafts.[41]

POSTOPERATIVE CONSIDERATIONS

It is critical for patients during the postoperative period to ensure that extra care is taken to not cause any trauma to the transplanted grafts when handling the recipient area. Study findings revealed that grafts can still be pulled out 2 days after surgery and that adherent scab removal at 2 to 5 days after the operation resulted in lost grafts. At 9 days, there was no risk of graft removal over the recipient area. Prevention of crusting helps in decreasing the possibility of graft dislodgement during the first 7 days after the hair transplantation procedure.[42]

A common sequela following hair transplantation is the development of forehead edema. The edema may range from mild to severe, with some patients experiencing involvement of both eyelids. A study evaluating the effectivity of several methods to decrease the occurrence of postoperative edema was conducted. The findings showed that incorporating triamcinolone acetonide with the tumescent solution for the recipient area

resulted in the prevention of edema after hair transplantation in 97% of patients (n = 117). Other methods (eg, intramuscular methylprednisolone, triamcinolone with 2% Xylocaine, and oral prednisone) had much lower percentages of patients without edema (47%–70%).[43]

COMPLICATIONS

In general, complications encountered in hair transplantation surgery are uncommon. Exact figures on the incidence rates are not available. In a study of 533 hair transplantation cases, the overall complication rate was low and included enlarged scars, folliculitis, keloid, and necrosis in the donor area.[44] Other complications that may occur over the donor area are neuralgias, donor hair effluvium, and arteriovenous fistulas.[45] Over the recipient area, some complications may include central recipient area necrosis, folliculitis, cyst formation, and an unnatural appearance of transplanted hairs.[45] Although there may be some complications that are unpredictable and may not be avoided because of unforeseen factors, in most cases, complications can be prevented or at least minimized through meticulous planning and utilization of proper surgical techniques.

INDICATIONS
Pattern Hair Loss (Male and Female)

Hair transplantation is most commonly done for male pattern hair loss. According to the 2011 statistics of the International Society of Hair Restoration Surgery, approximately 85% of hair transplantation surgeries performed were for genetic hair loss. The reported success rate and effectivity of this procedure for this hair loss indication is quite high; the benefit to patients is substantial, with excellent growth rates of transplanted grafts (**Fig. 7**).

Although women make up the minority of patients undergoing hair transplantation for pattern hair loss, the advent of the more refined technique of follicular unit transplantation, which yields natural-looking results, opens up this procedure as an effective treatment option for appropriate female patients (**Fig. 8**). The procedural technique for female patients mainly follows the same basic steps as for male patients. For the Ludwig pattern of hair loss, which mainly affects the central aspect of the scalp, transplanting in between the preexisting hairs may lead to the possibility of temporary telogen effluvium or shock loss to these hairs, thus, this has to be discussed with patients. For women who have frontotemporal recession similar to men, the restoration of

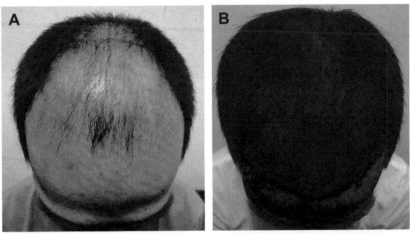

Fig. 7. Before (*A*) and 1 year after (*B*) hair transplantation of a patient with male pattern hair loss.

the hairline follows a different pattern, with hairs transplanted to cover the frontotemporal angles for a feminine look and with hairlines usually brought lower than in men.

Nonscalp Hair Loss

Eyebrow

For various causes of eyebrow loss, such as genetic thinning or hair loss caused by plucking or trauma, hair transplantation over this area has been shown to have successful results (**Fig. 9**). The basic steps of scalp hair transplantation still apply with modifications. In eyebrow transplantation, mostly 1-haired grafts are used in keeping with the natural pattern of human eyebrow hairs occurring as singular follicular units. In Caucasians

with finer hairs, 2-haired follicular units may occur over the central aspect or the body of the eyebrow. Donor hairs are obtained from the sides or the back of the scalp. The follicular unit grafts containing 2 to 3 hairs are further dissected into single-hair grafts and trimmed into skinny grafts before insertion into the recipient area slits over the eyebrows. Smaller slits ranging from 22- to 23-gauge hypodermic needles and 0.6- to 0.7-mm miniblade sizes are used depending on the caliber of the patient's hair. The direction of the grafts would be to follow the natural pattern of the existing hairs if still present. Another technique is the converging method whereby the grafts transplanted over the superior aspect are directed downwards and those over the inferior portion are made to converge upwards creating a more

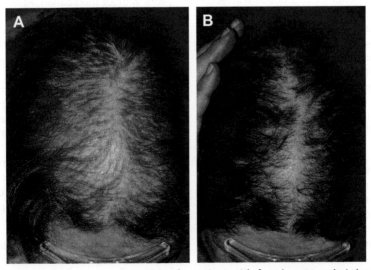

Fig. 8. Before (*A*) and after (*B*) hair transplantation of a patient with female pattern hair loss Ludwig type.

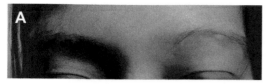 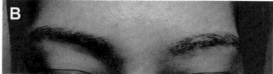

Fig. 9. Enhancement of thin eyebrows (A) through eyebrow transplantation (B).

pleasing shape.[46] In terms of the angulation, the grafts must by inserted as flat as possible to the skin creating a very acute angle.

Moustache and beard

Hair transplantation over the moustache and beard area may be done for men with decreased hair follicles over these areas. Some common causes include congenital absence, surgical or traumatic loss, folliculitis, and so forth. This procedure is more commonly performed for men of Middle Eastern descent because of the cultural and religious significance. The technique is the same as scalp hair transplantation, with some important considerations. In general, coarser hairs occur over the moustache and beard area relative to the scalp; thus, the chosen donor hairs should come from the middle of the occipital area where the thickest hair shafts are most likely to be found. The recommendation is to place 1- to 2-haired grafts at a density of 25 to 30 FU/cm^2 over the beard area and 30 to 45 FU/cm^2 over the moustache area following the common pattern in mature male beards.[47]

Eyelash

There are major concerns with transplanting hairs over the eyelash area, such as the difficulty in transplanting over delicate tissue, postoperative care problems, and lower graft survival rates. Many surgeons prefer to perform this procedure in reconstructive cases rather than cosmetic reasons.

Some surgeons have successfully transplanted grafts over the eyelashes for aesthetic purposes. One technique is through the use of French eye needles to transplant single-hair grafts over the rim of the upper eyelids. In one study, dense packing of 30 to 40 grafts was done over a 4-cm upper lid margin with good resultant growth of more than 95%.[48]

Pubic hair

Hair transplantation over the pubic area is more commonly performed in Korean and Japanese women. In one study, this procedure was performed for pubic atrichosis or hypotrichosis in 507 Korean women of Mongolian origin. The main reason for seeking the procedure was feeling inferior because of their condition. The donor grafts from the scalp were dissected into single-

hair grafts. The mean transplanted hairs was 929 ± 76. The modified horizontal pattern was the pattern created because of its close resemblance to the natural pubic configuration. The reported survival rate was 73.6 ± 6%.[49]

Although rarely done in Caucasians, there are few case reports of this procedure as was the case in a 41-year-old woman with thinning of her pubic hairs causing much psychological distress. The procedure would be the same as mentioned earlier except that, in some Caucasians with finer hairs, 2- to 3-haired follicular unit grafts, aside from the single grafts, may be used. In this particular case, grafts with 1 to 4 hairs per follicular unit were used with a total of 410 grafts transplanted. One- and 2-haired grafts were placed over the periphery and 3 to 4 grafts over the central aspect. The 1-year follow-up showed good growth, with the transplanted hairs developing curl similar to the preexisting hairs.[50]

Cicatricial Alopecia

Primary cicatricial alopecia

Hair transplantation in alopecic areas caused by an active primary scarring disease is contraindicated. There may be some select cases were hair transplantation can be contemplated. This procedure can be considered in primary cicatricial alopecias, which has burnt out or has become inactive for years without medication. At the UBC Hair Transplant Center, a general guideline includes hair transplantation over a small test area with a limited number of grafts (eg, 100–150). The successful take of grafts can then be followed by hair transplantation over the alopecia area. The growth rates are much lower than with hair transplantation for common indications, such as pattern hair loss. Even after acceptable graft survival rates after surgery, there may still be the possibility of disease recurrence, which may lead to the transplanted grafts being affected by the underlying disease process. At this center, there have been moderately successful outcomes in cases of inactive lichen planopilaris and frontal fibrosing alopecia (**Fig. 10**).

Secondary cicatricial alopecia

Scarring alopecias from secondary causes, such as burns, surgery, and trauma, are mostly amenable to hair transplantation. Follicular unit grafts

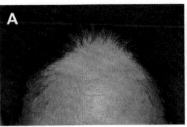
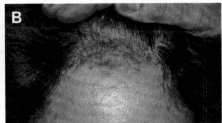

Fig. 10. Before (A) and 5 months after (B) hair transplantation of frontal fibrosing alopecia.

transplanted over scars in hair-bearing areas provide camouflage resulting in an improved cosmetic appearance, especially in highly visible areas, such as the scalp (Fig. 11), eyebrow, and eyelash area. Important considerations include wider spacing of grafts compared with regular hair transplantation of pattern hair loss because of the decreased vascularity over these scarred areas. Staged procedures can be done to increase density and improve coverage.[51] Successful outcomes have been observed with follicular unit transplantation to hide scars and restore hairs lost from rhytidoplasty and other plastic surgeries.[52]

Difficulties arise in cases when there may be larger areas of scarring relative to the scalp donor area. Nonscalp body hair to be harvested via FUE may be potential sources of donor grafts. Another method was undertaken in a study involving facial and scalp burns with a limited donor area. Over the occipital scalp, graft harvest of partial longitudinal grafts was done using hollow wave-tipped needles with an inner diameter of 0.6 mm. The postsurgery evaluation showed that the donor area had reproduced hairs after 2 years. There was a good cosmetic result over the recipient area.[53]

OTHER APPLICATIONS

Hair transplantation may be part of reconstructive procedures performed to improve extensive defects of hair bearing scalp. Successful outcomes have been reported with the use of tissue engineered dermal regeneration templates followed by follicular unit transplantation to reconstruct large scalp defects. A reported case of a traumatized scalp with exposed periosteum/galea underwent a series of procedures consisting of initial coverage with the Integra Dermal Regeneration Template (Integra LifeSciences Corporation, Plainsboro, New Jersey) followed by trial micrografting of 100 grafts into the regeneration template. After there was growth with the test grafts, 2 sessions of 800 grafts per session was performed with a good outcome.[54]

Another study showed the same results with artificial dermis followed by FUT. Their 2-stage procedure first started with the placement over the defect of an artificial dermis (PELNAC, Smith & nephew KK, Japan) that was then allowed to granulate for 1 to 2 months. The follicular unit grafts were subsequently inserted into the granulation tissue. Two cases resulted in a 29% to 43% reduction of the defect, re-epithelialization of the exposed area, and growth of hair grafts with acceptable coverage.[55]

Transplanted follicular unit grafts have been shown to result in repigmentation of depigmented areas of vitiligo. Hair repigmentation may be seen in white donor hairs as was observed in the case of a 57-year-old woman who underwent hair transplantation for frontal scarring alopecia.[56]

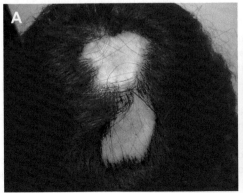
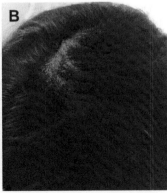

Fig. 11. Before (A) and after (B) transplantation of scarring alopecia caused by hair straightening chemical.

REFERENCES

1. Headington JT. Transverse microscopic anatomy of the human scalp. Arch Dermatol 1984;120:449–56.
2. Limmer BL. Elliptical donor stereoscopically assisted micrografting as an approach to further refinement in hair transplantation. J Dermatol Surg Oncol 1994;20:789–93.
3. Bernstein RM, Rassman WR, Szaniawski W, et al. Follicular transplantation. Intl J Aesthetic Rest Surg 1995;3:119–32.
4. Bernstein RM, Rassman WR. Follicular transplantation: patient evaluation and surgical planning. Dermatol Surg 1997;23:771–84.
5. Unger W, Unger R. Surgical treatment of hair loss. In: Blume Peytavi U, Tosti A, Whiting D, et al, editors. Hair growth and disorders. Springer; 2008. p. 447–65.
6. Haber R. The spreader: technique and indications. In: Unger W, Shapiro R, Unger R, et al, editors. Hair transplantation. 5th edition. Informa Healthcare; 2011. p. 279–81.
7. Pathomvanich D. Skin hook technique. In: Unger W, Shapiro R, Unger R, et al, editors. Hair transplantation. 5th edition. Informa Healthcare; 2011. p. 277–9.
8. Marzola M. Trichophytic closure of donor area. Hair Transplant Forum Intl 2005;15:113–6.
9. Rose P. Ledge closure. Hair Transplant Forum Int 2005;15:113–6.
10. Frechet P. Minimal scars for scalp surgery. J Dermatol Surg 2007;33:45–56.
11. Rose P. Trichophytic closure. In: Unger W, Shapiro R, Unger R, et al, editors. Hair transplantation. 5th edition. Informa Healthcare; 2011. p. 281–4.
12. Jimenez F, Izeta A, Poblet E. Morphometric analysis of the human scalp hair follicle: practical implications for the hair transplant surgeon and hair regeneration studies. Dermatol Surg 2011;37:58–64.
13. Rassman WR, Bernstein RM, Mc Clellan M, et al. Follicular unit extraction: minimally invasive surgery for hair transplantation. Dermatol Surg 2002;28:720–8.
14. Harris JA. Conventional FUE. In: Unger W, Shapiro R, Unger R, et al, editors. Hair transplantation. 5th edition. Informa Healthcare; 2011. p. 291–6.
15. Harris JA. New methodology and instrumentation for follicular unit extraction with lower follicle transection rates and expanded patient candidacy. Dermatol Surg 2006;32:56–61.
16. Vandruff E. Neograft: automated follicular unit extraction and implantation system. In Aesthetic Trends 2010. Available at: http://www.aesthetic-trends.com/news/?p=868.
17. Oada M, Igawa HH, Inone K, et al. Novel technology of follicular unit extraction with a powered punching device. Dermatol Surg 2008;34:1683–8.
18. Bernan D. New computer assisted system may change the hair restoration field. Practical Dermatol 2010;32–5.
19. Vandruff C. Artas system restoration robotics. In: Aesthetic Trends 2011. Available at: http://www.restorationrobotics.com/pdf/Aesthetic_Trends_Tech_10_2011.pdf.
20. Lin X, Nakazawa T, Yasuda R, et al. Robotic hair harvesting system: a new proposal. Med Image Comput Comput Assist Interv 2011;14:113–20.
21. Woods R, Campbell AW. Chest hair micrografts display extended growth in scalp tissue: a case report. Br J Plast Surg 2004;57:789–91.
22. Sanusi U. Hair transplantation in patients with inadequate head donor supply using nonhead hair. Ann Plast Surg 2011;67:332–5.
23. Toscani M, Rotolo S, Seccarella S, et al. Hair regeneration from transected follicles in duplicative surgery: rate of success and cell populations involved. Dermatol Surg 2009;35:1119–25.
24. Gho CG, Martino Neumann HA. Donor hair follicle preservation by partial follicular unit extraction. A method to optimize hair transplantation. J Dermatolog Treat 2010;21:337–49.
25. Gandelman M, Mota AL, Abrahamsohn PA, et al. Light and electron microscopic analysis of controlled injury to follicular unit grafts. Dermatol Surg 2000;26:25–30.
26. Sandoval-Camarena A, Sandoval H. Classic microscope dissection of follicular units. In: Unger W, Shapiro R, Unger R, et al, editors. Hair transplantation. 5th edition. Informa Healthcare; 2011. p. 313–8.
27. Parsley W, Beehner M, Prez-Meza D. Studies on graft hair survival. In: Unger W, Shapiro R, Unger R, et al, editors. Hair transplantation. 5th edition. Informa Healthcare; 2011. p. 328–34.
28. Limmer R. Micrograft survival. In: Stough D, editor. Hair replacement. St. Louis (MO): Mosby Press; 1996. p. 147–9.
29. Kim JC, Hwang S. The effects of dehydration, preservation temperature and time and hydrogen peroxide on hair grafts. In: Unger WP, Shapiro R, editors. Hair transplantation. 4th edition. New York: Marcel Dekker; 2004. p. 285–6.
30. Perez-Meza D, Cooley J, Parsley W. Custodial vs hypothermosol. Hair graft survival at 24 and 48 hours outside the body. San Diego (CA): ISHRS Annual Meeting; 2006.
31. Raposio E, Cella A, Panarese P, et al. Power boosting the grafts in hair transplantation surgery. Evaluation of a new storage medium. Dermatol Surg 1998;24:1342–6.
32. Krugluger W, Moser K, Hugeneck J, et al. New storage buffers for micrografts enhance graft survival and clinical outcome in hair restoration surgery. Hair Transplant Forum Int 2003;13:333–4.

33. Krugluger W, Rohrbacher W, Moser K, et al. Enhancement of in vitro hair shaft elongation in follicles stored in buffers that prevent follicle cell apoptosis. Dermatol Surg 2004;30:1–5.

34. Uebel C. A new advance in baldness surgery using platelet-derived growth factor. Hair Transplant Forum Intl 2005;15:77–84.

35. Perez-Meza D, Leavitt M, Mayer M. The growth factors. Part 1: clinical and histological evaluation of the wound healing and revascularization of the hair graft after the hair transplant surgery. Hair Transplant Forum Intl 2007;17:173–5.

36. Martinick J. Pitfalls of FUT incisions and how to avoid them. In: Unger W, Shapiro R, Unger R, et al, editors. Hair transplantation. 5th edition. Informa Healthcare; 2011. p. 350–6.

37. Yagyu K, Huyashi K, Chang SC. Orientation of multi-hair follicles in non bald men: perpendicular versus parallel. Dermatol Surg 2006;32:651–60.

38. Kim JC. Graft implanters. In: Unger W, Shapiro R, Unger R, et al, editors. Hair transplantation. 5th edition. Informa Healthcare; 2011. p. 404–6.

39. Lee SJ, Lee HJ, Hwang SJ, et al. Evaluation of survival rate after follicular unit transplantation using KNU implanter. Dermatol Surg 2001;27:716–20.

40. Lee W, Lee S, Na G, et al. Survival rate according to grafted density of Korean one hair follicular units with a hair transplant implanter: experience with four patient. Dermatol Surg 2006;32:815–8.

41. Shapiro R, Nagai M. Commentary to graft implanters. In: Unger W, Shapiro R, Unger R, et al, editors. Hair transplantation. 5th edition. Informa Healthcare; 2011. p. 406–7.

42. Bernstein RM, Rassman WR. Graft anchoring in hair transplantation. Dermatol Surg 2006;32:198–204.

43. Abbasi G, Pojhan S, Emami S. Hair transplantation: preventing postoperative oedema. J Cutan Aesthet Surg 2010;3:87–9.

44. Salanitri S, Goncalves AJ, Helene A Jr, et al. Surgical complications in hair transplantation: a series of 533 procedures. Aesthet Surg J 2009;29:72–6.

45. Unger W, Shapiro R, Unger R, et al, editors. Hair transplantation. 5th edition. Informa Healthcare; 2011.

46. Laorwong K, Pathomvanich D. Eyebrow transplant. In: Pathomvanich D, Imagawa K, editors. Hair restoration surgery in Asians. Springer; 2010. p. 215–20.

47. Kulahci M. Moustache and beard hair transplanting. In: Unger W, Shapiro R, Unger R, et al, editors. Hair transplantation. 5th edition. Informa Healthcare; 2011. p. 464–6.

48. Jiang WJ, Jing WM, Wang XP, et al. Aesthetic result of dense packing single hair autologous grafts for eyelashes. Zhonghua Zheng Xing Wai Ke Za Zhi 2011;27:111–3 [in Chinese].

49. Lee YR, Lee SJ, Kin JC, et al. Hair restoration surgery in patients with pubic hair atrichosis or hypotrichosis: review of techniques and clinical considerations of 507 cases. Dermatol Surg 2006; 32:1327–35.

50. Toscani M, Fioramanti O, Ruciani A, et al. Hair transplantation to restore pubic area. Dermatol Surg 2008;34:280–2.

51. Barr L, Barrera A. Use of hair grafting in scar camouflage. Facial Plast Surg Clin North Am 2011;19: 559–68.

52. Radwanski HN, Nuns D, Nazina F. Follicular transplantation for the correction of various stigmas after rhytidoplasty. Aesthetic Plast Surg 2007;31:62–8.

53. Gho CG, Neuman HA. Improved hair restoration method for burns. Burns 2011;37:427–33.

54. Spector CA, Glat PM. Hair bearing scalp reconstruction using a dermal regeneration template and micrograft hair transplantation. Ann Plast Surg 2007; 59:63–6.

55. Narushima M, Mihara M, Yamamoto Y, et al. Hair transplantation for reconstruction of scalp defects using artificial dermis. Dermatol Surg 2011;37: 1348–50.

56. Dinh HV, Sinclair R, Marticnick J. Long term hair repigmentation following a hair transplantation for frontal scarring alopecia. Australas J Dermatol 2007;48:236–8.

Primary Cicatricial Alopecias

Nina Otberg, MD

KEYWORDS

- Primary cicatricial alopecias • Alopecias • Scalp disorders • Hair loss

KEY POINTS

- Primary cicatricial alopecias are defined as idiopathic, inflammatory scalp disorders that result in permanent hair loss.
- Primary cicatricial alopecias can be classified via different approaches, such as clinical presentation, histopathologic findings, or both.
- Primary cicatricial alopecias are rare scalp disorders. Prompt diagnosis and treatment is crucial for a successful management.

INTRODUCTION

Primary cicatricial alopecias refer to a group of rare, idiopathic, inflammatory scalp disorders that result in permanent hair loss. The destructive process is characterized by a folliculocentric inflammatory process that ultimately destroys the hair follicle. Primary cicatricial alopecias are probably the most misdiagnosed scalp disorders and frequently cause major distress for the affected patient. These scalp diseases represent trichologic emergencies because hair follicles are permanently destroyed and therefore the patient might experience disfiguration, psychosocial embarrassment, and a lack of self-esteem. A quick and confident proof of diagnosis and aggressive treatment in the case of active disease are crucial in the management of primary scarring alopecias. Diagnosis and therapy are challenging for the treating dermatologist and the dermatopathologist.

CLASSIFICATION

Primary cicatricial alopecias comprise a diverse group of inflammatory diseases and can be classified via different approaches, such as clinical presentation, histopathologic findings, or both. Each disease shows specific clinical and histopathologic characteristics, although the clinical appearance may show overlapping findings and symptoms.

To classify this diverse group, a consensus meeting on cicatricial alopecia held at Duke University, Durham, North Carolina, in February 2001 came up with a classification based on the predominant inflammatory cells found in and around the follicular epithelium. According to this consensus meeting primary cicatricial alopecias are classified into 3 main groups: 1, lymphocytic; 2, Neutrophilic; and 3, mixed. However, some cases of primary cicatricial alopecia remain unclassifiable and therefore fall in the category "unspecific" (**Table 1**).[1,2]

EPIDEMIOLOGY AND PATHOGENESIS

Primary cicatricial alopecias are rare scalp disorders. Whiting found a prevalence of 7.3% in all patients who sought advice for hair and scalp problems at the Baylor Hair Research and Treatment Center in Dallas between 1989 and 1999.[3] Tan and colleagues[4] found a prevalence of 3.2% of all patients who visited the UBC Hair Clinic in Vancouver between 1997 and 2001.

Pathogenesis is barely understood. The inflammatory process affects mainly the upper portion of the follicle and is followed by a permanent destruction of the hair follicle and continuous deposition of collagen and a loss of sebaceous glands.[5] The follicle loses its capability to regenerate because pluripotent stem cells located in the bulge area are destroyed by inflammation.[3,5–7]

Skin and Laser Center and Hair Transplant Center, Richard-Strauss-Str. 27, Potsdam 14193 Berlin, Germany
E-mail address: otberg@hlcp.de

Dermatol Clin 31 (2013) 155–166
http://dx.doi.org/10.1016/j.det.2012.08.016
0733-8635/13/$ – see front matter © 2013 Published by Elsevier Inc.

derm.theclinics.com

Table 1 Classification of primary cicatricial alopecias		
Lymphocytic	Neutrophilic	Mixed

• Chronic cutaneous lupus erythematosus (DLE)
• LPP
   ○ Classic LPP
   ○ FFA
   ○ Graham-Little syndrome
• Classic PPB
• CCCA
• AM
• KFSD
	• FD
	• Dissecting cellulites/folliculitis (perifolliculitis abscedens et suffodiens)
		Folliculitis (acne) keloidalis
		Folliculitis (acne) necrotica
		Erosive pustular dermatosis

These cells are responsible for the renewal of the upper part of the follicle and the sebaceous gland.[8] Additionally, they restore the lower impermanent part of the follicle and start a new growth (anagen) phase.[9] Damage of sebaceous glands[10] and destruction of the outer root sheath are also believed to be possible pathogenetic factors in the development of cicatricial alopecia.[5,11]

CLINICAL FINDINGS

Primary cicatricial alopecia frequently starts at the central and parietal scalp before progressing to other sites of the scalp. A lack of follicular ostia is the hallmark of scaring alopecia. Isolated alopecic patches showing atrophy and a lack of follicular ostia with inflammatory changes such as diffuse or perifollicular erythema, follicular hyperkeratosis, pigment changes, tufting, and pustules provide hints to the diagnosis.[12,13] However, clinically visible inflammatory changes may be absent in the affected lesions.

DIAGNOSIS

A quick and confident diagnosis is the key to an effective treatment. A thorough examination of the entire scalp, a detailed clinical history, and 1 or 2 biopsy samples of an active lesion are crucial in the diagnosis of cicatricial alopecia. Time of onset and symptoms such as itching or pain can give information on the activity of the disease. Presents of sun sensitivity can lead to diagnose (eg, discoid lupus erythematosus [DLE]). Diffuse or perifollicular erythema, follicular hyperkeratosis, pigment changes, tufting, pustules, and the general pattern (frontal or central location, patchy or reticulated appearance) provide further hints in direction to the diagnosis.[12,13]

A 3-fold magnifying lens or a 10-fold magnifying dermatoscope with and without polarized light can be used as a diagnostic tool. Videodermoscopy has been show to be very helpful in the diagnosis of hair and scalp disorders, especially in cicatricial alopecia.[14–16]

A scalp biopsy is mandatory to confirm the diagnoses and to estimate disease activity. A 4-mm punch biopsy including subcutaneous tissue should be taken from a clinical active area where hair follicles are still present. The punch should be angled according to the growth direction of the hair. The biopsy sample is processed for horizontal sections and stained with hematoxylin and eosin. A second 4-mm punch biopsy sample can be cut vertically into 2 equal pieces. One half provides tissue for direct immunofluorescence studies; the other half can be use for transversal routine histologic sections.[17] Elastin (acid alcoholic orcein), mucin, and periodic acid–Schiff stains may provide additional information.

PATIENT MANAGEMENT

Cicatricial alopecia, especially advanced stages, can cause disfiguration and major distress for the patient. The management and treatment of patients with scarring hair loss require an exceptionally empathetic interaction with the patient. The physician should carefully clarify that hair regrowth is not expected and that the goal of any therapy is the arrest of further loss. Concomitant hair growth problems such as telogen effluvium and androgenetic alopecia should also be addressed and treated. Cicatricial patches can be camouflaged easier when the remaining hair is thick and healthy, even if regrowth is impossible in the lesions. Furthermore, the patient should be advised about different possibilities of camouflage techniques, including hair style, hair pieces, wigs, hair powder, and color. Hair transplantation and scalp reduction surgery are possible once the lesions are burnt out and stable. A scalp biopsy should confirm the absence of inflammatory cells before the surgery. For hair transplantation, the patient needs to have a suitable donor area. Graft survival may not be as good as in androgenetic alopecia and disease reactivation is possible at any time after surgery.

LYMPHOCYTIC PRIMARY CICATRICIAL ALOPECIA
Chronic Cutaneous Lupus Erythematosus (DLE)

DLE and lichen planopilaris represent the most common primary cicatricial alopecia. DLE is a form of chronic lupus erythematosus that can affect the scalp and result in cicatricial alopecia.[12] The typical age of onset is between 20 and 40 years of age. Women are more often affected than men and the disease is more common in adults than in children.[18–20]

Clinical presentation
DLE frequently starts at the occipital and parietal scalp. It presents with 1 or more erythematous patches of alopecia. Early in the process, follicular ostia can still be present in the margin of the lesion. Follicular hyperkeratosis, hyperpigmentation, depigmentation, and teleangiektasia can often be found in or around the lesions.[3,6] The affected patient may report a worsening after ultraviolet exposure, pruritus, or dyesthesia. The clinical features can be very similar those of to lichen planopilaris (**Fig. 1**).

Pathologic examination
Two 4-mm punch biopsies should be taken from a hair-baring margin of an alopecic patch: one for standard histologic horizontal sections and a second for longitudinal sections and direct immunofluorescence.

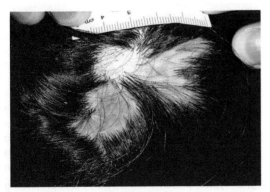

Fig. 1. A 32-year-old female patient with DLE. (*Courtesy of* Dr Jerry Shapiro, UBC Hair Clinic, Vancouver, British Columbia, Canada.)

A lymphocyte-mediated interface dermatitis that shows basilar vacuolar degeneration with necrotic keratinocytes and a thickening of the basement membrane are characteristic for an active DLE lesion. The lymphocytic infiltrate is predominantly found in the upper permanent part of the follicle.[21–24] However, perivascular lymphozytic infiltrate around the periadnexal vessel and the superficial and deep vascular plexus can be found. Plasma cells are seen occasionally. Sebaceous glands can already be destroyed in early lesions.[6,19] The infundibula are filled with laminated keratin, which corresponds to the clinically observed follicular plugging. Older lesions are characterized by a complete loss of follicular units and a perifollicular and interstitial fibrosis.

Direct immunofluorescence shows a linear granular deposition of IgG and C3 at the dermoepidermal junction. IgM, C1q, and, rarely, IgA can also be found.

Additional stains, such as periodic acid–Schiff stain, can be used to identify the characteristic thickening of the basement membrane; elastic stains, such as Verhoeff–van Gieson stain, may help to identify a loss of elastic fibers throughout the reticular dermis.[5,17] Dermal mucin can be increased in older lesions and can be highlighted by Alcian blue and colloidal iron stains.

Risk factors
Patient diagnosed with DLE may develop systemic lupus erythematosus; the risk is higher in children (26%–31% opposed to 5%–10% in adults).[20,25] Therefore, a thorough medical history and physical examination, as well as serum antinuclear antibody titer, complete blood count, and urinalysis should be performed in every patient with DLE.[12,26]

The incidence of alopecia areata is higher in patients with DLE[27]; a close examination of every alopecic area is mandatory to distinguish between different forms of alopecia.

DLE has also been associated with veruciform xanthoma[28] and papulonodular dermal mucinosis. Longstanding DLE lesions are prone to develop squamous cell carcinoma[29] with a high occurrence of metastasis[30]; therefore, every hyperkeratotic or ulcerated lesion in a DLE patch should be biopsied early.[12]

Management and treatment
For rapidly progressive DLE, hydroxychloroqine has been shown to be highly effective. It should be started at a dosage of 200 to 400 mg daily in adults[31,32] or 4 to 6 mg/kg in children.[18,20] A baseline ophthalmologic examination and complete blood count are required before the therapy is started. Bridge therapy with oral prednisone

(1 mg/kg) tapered during the first 8 weeks of treatment might be helpful in patients with very rapid progressive disease.[12,13] For patients with slowly progressive, limited DLE first-line therapy should be intralesional triamcinolone acetonide at a concentration of ideally 10 mg/mL every 4 to 6 weeks[12] with or without topical class I or class II corticosteroids. Topical corticosteroids alone have also been shown to be effective in milder forms of DLE.[13,17,20,22] Oral retinoids have also shown to be effective: acitretin at a dosage of 50 mg daily[32] and isotretinoin at a dosage of 40 mg twice daily.[33]

Oral immunosuppressive therapies such as mycophenolate mofetil, methotrexate, or azathioprine should only be considered when these therapies failed.

Lichen Planopilaris

Lichen planopilaris (LPP) can be subdivided into 3 groups based on clinical presentation: (1) classic LPP, (2) frontal fibrosing alopecia (FFA), and (3) Graham-Little syndrome. The typical age of onset in classic LPP is around 50 years, and women are more often affected than men.[34] Frontal fibrosing alopecia (FFA) predominantly affects postmenopausal women.[5]

Clinical presentation

LPP most commonly starts at the parietal scalp. Patients may report itching, burning, and sensitivity of the scalp. The clinical features of classic LPP overlap with those of DLE. The alopecic plaques are often smaller and interconnected, which can lead to a reticulated pattern. The typical LPP lesion presents with follicular hyperkeratosis and perifollicular erythema (**Figs. 2** and **3**).[22]

FFA is characterized by a frontal or, in some cases, a circumferential recession of the hair line.[5] The cicatricial hair loss appears as a bandlike area of variable width of 1 to 8 cm[12,35] and typically spares a few hairs. Clinical features of classic LPP, such as follicular hyperkeratosis and perifollicular erythema, can often be found in the first rows of hairs in the hair line. Alopecia of the eyebrows is an additional typical finding in FFA (**Fig. 4**).

Graham-Little syndrome presents with lesions of classic LPP on the scalp, nonscarring alopecia of axillary and pubic hair, and keratosis pilaris on the trunk and extremities; in some cases, alopecia of the eyebrows can be found.[36]

Pathologic examination

All 3 subgroups show more or less the same histopathologic features. Similar to DLE lymphocyte-mediated interface, dermatitis can be found especially in the permanent part of the follicle. The

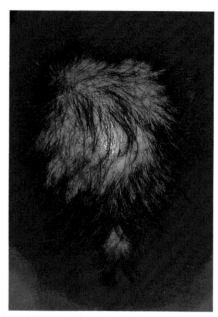

Fig. 2. A 36-year-old male patient with LPP. (*Courtesy of Dr Jerry Shapiro, UBC Hair Clinic, Vancouver, British Columbia, Canada.*)

interfollicular epidermis is often spared, and often nonaffected hair follicles can be found next to affected follicles in the biopsy sample. Unlike DLE, the vascular plexus is not affected by inflammation and mucin deposits are absent.[5] The lymphocytic infiltrate is predominantly found in the upper permanent part of the follicle, mostly at the bottom of the dilated, keratin-filled, infundibulum.[37,38] Sebaceous glands are already destroyed in early lesions.

Direct immunofluorescence may show globular cytoid depositions of IgM, and rarely IgA, IgG, or C3, in the dermis around the infundibulum.[39]

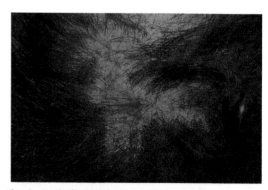

Fig. 3. Typical presentation of classic LPP presenting with erythema and follicular hyperkeratosis. (*Courtesy of Dr Jerry Shapiro, UBC Hair Clinic, Vancouver, British Columbia, Canada.*)

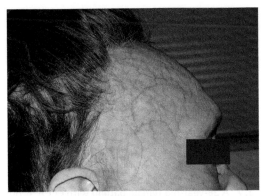

Fig. 4. A 69-year-old female patient with FFA. (*Courtesy of* Dr Jerry Shapiro, UBC Hair Clinic, Vancouver, British Columbia, Canada.)

Whereas in DLE the lack of elastic fibers can be found throughout the entire reticular dermis, in LPP a wedge-shaped scar in the area of the infundibulum can be found with a loss of elastic fibers only in that area.[40] Elastic stains can be useful to distinguish between DLE and LPP.

Risk factors
Extracranial lichen planus can be found in 17% to 28% of patients with LPP.[4,41] A higher incidence of hepatitis C in patients with lichen planus had been described.[42] Patients with extensive lesions should undergo hepatitis C virus testing.

Management and treatment
A thorough review of the patient's medications is necessary to identify possible triggering drugs.

Literature on the treatment of LPP is limited. Oral cyclosporine of 300 mg daily for 3 to 5 months and low-dose tretinoin at a dosage of 10 mg daily have been reported to be effective in a small number of patients with LPP.[43,44] Oral acitretin at a dosage of 30 mg daily has been shown to be most effective in lichen planus.[45] Antimalarias[3,6] and griseofulvine[46] showed also a positive outcome. Oral corticosteroids in the first weeks of treatment as bridge therapy should be considered in very active, rapidly progressive cases.

First-line treatment of moderately active LPP lesions is intralesional triamcinolone acetonide at a concentration of ideally 10 mg/mL every 4 to 6 weeks optional in combination with topical class I or class II corticosteroids.[12,33] In frontal fibrosing alopecia, a lower dose of intralesional triamcinolone acetonide (2.5–5 mg/mL) and topical application of corticosteroids and minoxidil can be considered. The treatment of Graham-Little syndrome equals the management of classic LPP. Alopecia of the eyebrows may be treated with intralesional triamcinolone acetonide (2.5 mg/mL) and topical minoxidil,

although an effective treatment has not yet been reported in literature.

Classic Pseudopelade of Brocq

Pseudopelade of Brocq (PPB) is the second most common cause of primary cicatricial alopecia.[4] Women between 30 and 50 years of age are most frequently affected.

Clinical presentation
PPB frequently starts on the parietal scalp and presents with small flesh-toned alopecic patches with irregular margins. This particular pattern has been described as "foot prints in the snow."[47] Follicular hyperkeratosis and perifollicular or diffuse erythema are mostly absent.[6] However, clinical overlap with DLE and LPP is possible (**Figs. 5** and **6**).

Pathologic examination
A sparse or moderate lymphocytic infiltrate around the infundibulum and the absence of sebaceous glands are pathologic hallmarks for an early PPB lesion.[48] In later lesions, the follicular epithelium becomes more and more atrophic and follicles are often surrounded by concentric lamellar fibroplasias[3,23,24] until finally the follicle is replaced by fibrous tracts. Unlike in DLE and LPP, the elastic fiber network is preserved and elastin stain might

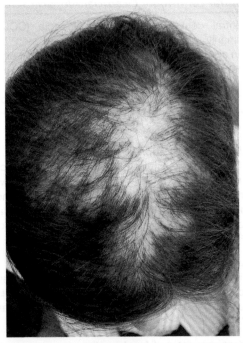

Fig. 5. A 46-year-old female patient with PPB. (*Courtesy of* Dr Jerry Shapiro, UBC Hair Clinic, Vancouver, British Columbia, Canada.)

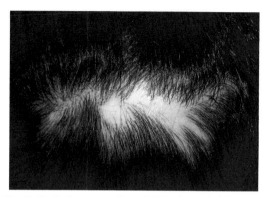

Fig. 6. Typical presentation of PPB, cicatricial alopecia with lack of follicular ostia, and very few clinical signs of inflammation. (*Courtesy of* Dr Jerry Shapiro, UBC Hair Clinic, Vancouver, British Columbia, Canada.)

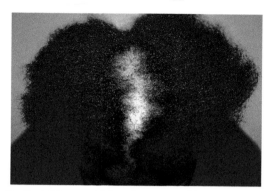

Fig. 7. A 28-year-old female patient with CCCA. (*Courtesy of* Dr Jerry Shapiro, UBC Hair Clinic, Vancouver, British Columbia, Canada.)

show markedly thickened elastic fibers.[40] Occasionally, granular deposits of IgM can be found on direct immunofluorescence.[48]

Management and treatment
Disease activity in patients with no clinical signs and symptoms of inflammation can be difficult to track. Measurements and photographs of the lesion may help to document progression.

Topical and intralesional triamcinolone acetonide at a concentration of ideally 10 mg/mL every 4 to 6 weeks, hydroxychloroquine, oral prednisone, and isotretinoin have shown some effectiveness.[4,6,49]

Central Centrifugal Cicatricial Alopecia

Central centrifugal cicatricial alopecia (CCCA) primarily affects African American women but can also rarely been seen in whites ("central elliptical pseudopelade") and African American men. It remains unclear exactly which role hair care practices such as chemical processing, heat, traction, or other traumas play in the pathogenesis of this cicatricial alopecia.

Clinical presentation
CCCA presents with a patch of scarring alopecia similar to PPB on the central scalp that slowly progresses centrifugally. It remains unclear if chemical processing, heat, traction, or other traumas contribute to the development of this condition (**Fig. 7**).[2,22,50]

Pathologic examination
Histopathologic features of CCCA seem to be identical to those of PPB. Therefore, it has been discussed that CCCA might be considered a variant of PPB.[3,22]

Management and treatment
Topical corticosteroids and tetracycline have shown to be effective in active progressive cases.[22]

Because a multifactoral cause is discussed for CCCA, some authors recommend a switch to more natural, less traumatizing hair care practices.[6,17,51] Hair restoration surgery can give satisfying results but is reserved for burnt-out stages. Wigs and hairpieces are frequently used by women with CCCA to camouflage the alopecia.

Alopecia Mucinosa

Clinical presentation
Alopecia mucinosa (AM) presents with erythematosus or skin colored, sometimes indurated, well-demarcated patches of scarring or nonscarring alopecia. The condition can be accompanied by diffuse hair loss[52] and alopecia of the eyebrows.[53] AM can clinically be mistaken for other cicatricial hair loss conditions or alopecia areata. Grouped follicular papules, follicular cysts, and follicular hyperkeratosis can be found in some cases. Lesions on the neck, the trunk, and the extremities have been described.[53]

Risk factors
AM can occur idiopathically or in the setting of cutaneous T-cell lymphoma or mycosis fungoides.[54] Cell atypia and monoclonal populations of T-lymphocytes can be present in the idiopathic form of AM in addition to in the latter form.[54]

Pathologic examination
Histologic findings in AM is characterized by mucin deposition in the outer root sheath and later by a replacement of the entire follicle including the sebaceous gland by pools of mucin.[5,53] AM, strictly speaking, is not a primary cicatricial alopecia because the hair follicle is not replaced by a true scar.[5] A lymphocytic infiltrate can be found in the follicular epithelium, and with varying expression around the superficial and/or deep vascular plexus and diffusely in the dermis. Cell atypia and monoclonal populations of

T-lymphocytes can be present in the idiopathic form and in the mycoides fugoides related form.[54] A mucin staining is mandatory to confirm the diagnosis.

Management and treatment
No effective standard therapy for AM is available. Oral corticosteroids,[55] minocycline,[56] and isotretoin[57] have been shown to be effective. Topical and intralesional corticosteroids,[58] dapsone,[59] indomethacin,[60] and light therapy[61] have also been used with variable outcome. Most important is a complete workup to rule out an underlying malignancy such as mycosis fungoides and Sézary syndrome.

Keratosis Follicularis Spinulosa Decalvans

Keratosis follicularis spinulosa decalvans (KFSD) is a rare inherited keratinizing disorder. Family studies suggest an X-linked dominant inheritance pattern. Men are more severely affected than women. A mutation in the gene encoding spermidine/spermine N-(1)-acetyltransferase (SSAT) located in the Xp22.13-p22.2 region has been identified in patients with KFSD.[62] It is closely related to keratosis atrophicans faciei (or ulerythema ophrygenes) and atrophodermis vermiculata, which mostly affects the face. KFSD usually develops during adolescence.

Clinical features
The condition presents with noninflammatory, flesh-colored, scarring alopecic patches lesions, mostly on the scalp. However, the eyelashes, eyebrows, hands, and trunk can be affected. KFSD can present with tufted folliculitis and may show similar clinical findings to folliculitis decalvans.[5]

Risk factors
Photophobia is seen in many patients with KFSD. Punctuate corneal defects can be found in some patients.[63]

Pathologic examination
KFSD is characterized by follicular plugging and hypergranulosis.[63] An inflammatory infiltrate consisting of lymphocytes and neutrophils can be seen in the infundibular epithelium in early stages, similar to late-stage folliculitis decalvans. Later, the infiltrate is predominantly lymphocytic and the follicle is replaced by fibrous tissue.

Management and treatment
Because KFSD is a disease of adolescence, careful calculation of risks and benefits of any treatment is important. Topical and intralesional corticosteroids[63] and oral retionids[64] have shown some effectiveness.

NEUTROPHILIC CICATRICIAL ALOPECIAS
Folliculitis Decalvans

Approximately 10.7% to 11.2% of all patients with primary cicatricial alopecias are diagnosed with folliculitis decalvans (FD). FD predominantly occurs in young and middle-aged adults with a slight preference of the male gender.[3,4] The cause of FD remains unclear. It may be a complex combination of a bacterial infection, particularly Staphylococcus aureus hypersensitivity reaction to the "superantigens" and defect in host cell–mediated immunity.[3,65,66]

Clinical presentation
FD frequently starts at the vertex area of the scalp with erythematous patches, follicular pustules or papules, and follicular hyperkeratosis.[65] The inflammatory process is followed by the formation of alopecic, sometimes slightly hypertrophic, ivory-like patches.[17,67] Patients frequently complain about pain, itching, and/or burning sensations. Tufted folliculitis is typically found in FD but can also occur in other cicatricial inflammatory alopecias. Tufted folliculitis is characterized by multiple hairs (5–15) emerging from 1 dilated follicular orifice.[68] In older lesions, pustules may be absent but progressive scarring may continue. An overlap with acne keloidalis is possible because some patients with acne keloidalis not only develop cicatricial lesion on the nape of the neck but also develop progressive cicatricial alopecia that resembles FD in other areas of the scalp (**Fig. 8**).

Pathologic examination
Keratin aggregation in the infundibulum with numerous intraluminal neutrophils, as well as an intrafollicular and perifollicular neutrophilic infiltrate, is found in early lesoins.[3,5,6] Sebaceous glands are destroyed early in the process. In advanced lesions, the infiltrate may consist of neutrophils, lymphocytes, and plasma cells and extend into the dermis.[6,12] Hair shaft granulomas with foreign-body giant cells can frequently be found.[3,6] In end-stage lesions, follicular and interstitial dermal fibrosis and hypertrophic scarring can be observed.[6]

Management and treatment
FD can be very aggressive and resistant to therapy.[65,69] Attempts to eradicate S aureus infection is the first goal of therapy. Bacterial cultures with antibiotic sensitivities should be obtained from every patient.

Antistaphyloccocal and broad-spectrum antibiotics such as minocycline erythromycin, cephalosporins, and sulfamethoxazoletrimethoprim showed

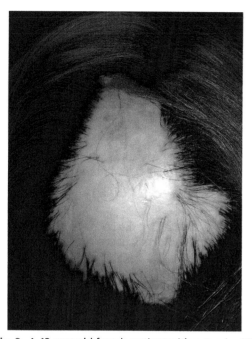

Fig. 8. A 43-year-old female patient with extensive FD and hypertrophic scarring. (*Courtesy of* Dr Jerry Shapiro, UBC Hair Clinic, Vancouver, British Columbia, Canada.)

variable effectiveness. Relapse can often be observed after the antibiotics are discontinued.[13,65,69] Other antibiotics that might induce longer remissions are rifampin, clindamycin, and fucidic acid. Rifampin 600 mg in combination with or without clindamycin 600 mg daily has shown good response and no relapse for 1 year.[65,70] Oral fucidic acid can be used alone or in combination with other agents. A triple therapy with oral fusidic acid 1500 mg daily for 3 weeks, zinc sulfate 400 mg daily for 6 months, and topical 1.5% fusidic acid cream for 2 weeks has shown some good response. The treatment was sustained with zinc sulfate 200 mg daily for longer than 1 year.[71] Intralesional corticosteroids can be added to control the acute inflammation. Intralesional triamcinolone acetonide (10 mg/mL) injected into the surrounding hair areas every 4 to 6 weeks can slow down further progression and reduce symptoms such as itching and burning.[4,13] Topical antibiotics such as mupirocin, 1.5% fusidic acid, and 2% erythromycin[70,71] are usually used in combination with oral antibiotics. Intranasal eradication of S aureus with topical antibacterial agents have been described to be useful.[6] Only limited data are available on the effectiveness of oral isotretinoin or oral L-tyrosine administration.[70,72]

Dissecting Folliculitis

Dissecting folliculitis (DF) (or dissecting cellulites or perifolliculitis capitis abscedens et suffodiens of Hoffman) is related to acne conglobata and hidradenitis suppurativa. These 3 diseases have been described as the follicular occlusion triad. DF predominantly occurs in young men between 18 and 40 years of age.[12] African American men seem to be more commonly affected compared with white men. DF can also occur in men of other ethnicity; women and children are rarely affected.[73,74] The pathogenesis of DF may include follicular occlusion, seborrhea, androgens, and secondary bacterial overpopulation, as well as an abnormal host response to bacterial antigens.[75]

Clinical presentation
DF frequently starts at the vertex region. Follicular pustules and papules expand into patches of perifollicular pustules, firm or fluctuant nodules, and eventually abscesses and sinuses.[17,76] Multifocal lesions can coalesce to form cerebriform ridges. Seropurulent exudates can be discharged when pressure is applied to one region of the scalp and an adjacent intercommunicating ridge.[77] Chronic and relapsing courses result in cicatricial alopecia, which can occur as hypertrophic or keloidal scars.[76]

Risk factors
DF can coexist with acne conglobata, hidradenitis suppurative, and pilonidal cysts, together composing the follicular occlusion tetrad.[78] It has been reported to occur with spondyloarthropathy, sternoclavicular hyperostosis, SAPHO syndrome (synovitis, acne, palmoplantar pustulosis, hyperos osis, osteitis), marginal keratitis, secondary squamous cell carcinoma, S aureus osteomyelitis, pyoderma vegetans, and pityriasis rubra pilaris.[76,79–85]

Pathologic examination
In the early stage, dissecting cellulitis displays follicular occlusion by keratin plugs with intrafollicular and perifollicular neutrophilic infiltration.[5] In later stages, follicular perforation, perifollicular and deep dermal abscesses with infiltrative neutrophils, lymphocytes, and plasma cells are present. Interconnecting sinus tracts lined by squamous epithelium are the hallmark of the disease.[5,6,24] In later stages, hair follicles are destroyed; the inflammatory areas around sinus tracts are replaced by extensive fibrosis and scar tissue.[86]

Management and treatment
Prolonged remission of the disease was achieved with isotretinoin 1 mg/kg daily for a minimum of 4 months, maintained by 0.75 to 1 mg/kg daily

for an additional 5 to 7 months or 0.75 mg/kg daily for 6 months, followed by 0.5 mg/kg daily for 3 additional months.[87,88] Oral and topical antibiotics include tetracyclines, minocycline, cloxacillin, erythromycin, cephalosporin, and clindamycin.[73,77,89] Other options include intralesional triamcinolone acetonide, zinc sulfate, dapsone, antibacterial soaps, and colchicine daily.[4,13,73,90–93] Multimodality treatment has been reported with successful results, such as systemic antibiotics (minocycline), intralesional corticosteroids, and oral prednisolone.[94,95]

Surgical therapy should only be considered if medical treatment fails to work and the lesion are very symptomatic. Laser epilation with long-pulse, non–Q-switched ruby and 800-nm pulsed diode has been reported with good results.[92,95,96] Modern external beam radiation therapy has also been reported.[97] Incision and drainage of painful nodules and complete scalp extirpation with skin grafting have been reported but should be an exception for extreme and therapy refractory cases.[73,88]

MIXED PRIMARY CICATRICIAL ALOPECIA
Acne Keloidalis

Acne keloidalis (also named acne keloidalis nuchae, dermatitis papillaris capillitii, or folliculitis keloidalis) occurs predominantly in African American men between 14 and 25 years of age.[50] Acne keloidalis is a chronic idiopathic, inflammatory process leading to hair loss and hypertrophic scarring in papules and plaques.[77] The exact cause of acne keloidalis is unknown. Probable participating factors include constant irritation from shirt collars, excoriation, and seborrhea; infection; shaving of the neck, coarse hair; and autoimmunity.[12,98] In isolated case reports, acne keloidalis can be induced by drugs, such as cyclosporine, diphenyl-hydantoin, and carbamazepine.[99,100]

Clinical presentation
The initial lesions are dome-shaped, firm, skin-colored follicular papules and pustules, which are mostly located in the occipital scalp and the nape of the neck, although they may also be found in the vertex and parietal area.[50,101] In the course of the disease, papules and pustules may enlarge and coalesce into keloid-like plaques, with with the formation of a cicatricial alopecia. Abscesses and sinuses can be presented in rare advanced cases.[50,101] The patients sometimes complain about itching and burning sensations of the lesions. If the lesions become very extensive, the disease will have a significant impact on quality of life (**Fig. 9**).[98]

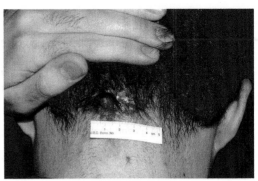

Fig. 9. A 24-year-old male patient with acne keloidalis nuchae presenting a hypertrophic nodule, pustules, crust, and follicular tufting. (*Courtesy of* Dr Jerry Shapiro, UBC Hair Clinic, Vancouver, British Columbia, Canada.)

Pathologic examination
The earliest event in acne keloidalis is characterized by an acute inflammation with neutrophilic or lymphocytic infiltration in the isthmus and the lower infundibulum. The infundibulum is dilated, which is similar to early folliculitis decalvans and dissecting cellulites.[5] Chronic granulomatous inflammatory can be found around the lower isthmus, ensued by hypertrophic scarring.[50,102] Sebaceous glands are destroyed early. True keloids do not occur and keloidal collagen bundles are uncommon.[5]

Management and treatment
Acne keloidalis often presents a therapeutic challenge. First-line therapy is prevention.[98] Avoiding any trauma and infection is very important. For mild cases, there are some reports of success with class I or II topical steroids alone or in combination with topical antibiotics and monthly intralesional triamcinolone acetonide (10–40 mg/mL) alone or combined with topical 2% clindamycin or oral (tetracyclines) antibiotics.[3,17,50,103,104]; Cryotherapy and laser therapy (carbon dioxide, 1064-nm Nd:YAG, 810-nm diode) have been noted to treat this condition with some success.[98,105] For the extensive keloidal plaques or recalcitrant disease, surgical excision may be necessary. Most approaches include excision with primary closure or secondary intention healing.[98,106] Good results could be obtained when patients underwent cold-steel excision and the excision includes the posterior hairline area and extends to muscle fascia or deep subcutaneous tissue.[98,106] Any surgical intervention should be reserved for therapy-refractory, extensive, and symptomatic cases.

REFERENCES

1. Olsen EA, Bergfeld WF, Cotsarelis G, et al. Summary of North American Hair Research Society

(NAHRS)-Sponsored Workshop on Cicatricial Alopecia, Duke University Medical Center, February 10 and 11, 2001. J Am Acad Dermatol 2003;48: 103–10.

2. Olsen EA, Stenn K, Bergfeld W, et al. Update on cicatricial alopecia. J Investig Dermatol Symp Proc 2003;8:18–9.

3. Whiting DA. Cicatricial alopecia: clinico-pathological findings and treatment. Clin Dermatol 2001;19:211–5.

4. Tan E, Martinka M, Ball N, et al. Primary cicatricial alopecias: clinicopathology of 112 cases. J Am Acad Dermatol 2004;50:25–32.

5. Sellheyer K, Bergfeld WF. Histopathologic evaluation of alopecias. Am J Dermatopathol 2006;28: 236–59.

6. Headington JT. Cicatricial alopecia. Dermatol Clin 1996;14:773–82.

7. Kossard S. Diffuse alopecia with stem cell folliculitis: chronic diffuse alopecia areata or a distinct entity? Am J Dermatopathol 1999;21:46–50.

8. Cotsarelis G, Sun TT, Lavker RM. Label-retaining cells reside in the bulge area of pilosebaceous unit: implications for follicular stem cells, hair cycle, and skin carcinogenesis. Cell 1990;61:1329–37.

9. Taylor G, Lehrer MS, Jensen PJ, et al. Involvement of follicular stem cells in forming not only the follicle but also the epidermis. Cell 2000;102:451–61.

10. Stenn KS, Sundberg JP, Sperling LC. Hair follicle biology, the sebaceous gland, and scarring alopecias. Arch Dermatol 1999;135:973–4.

11. Maroon M, Tyler WB, Marks VJ. Keratosis pilaris and scarring alopecia. Keratosis follicularis spinulosa decalvans. Arch Dermatol 1992;128:397–400.

12. Ross EK, Tan E, Shapiro J. Update on primary cicatricial alopecias. J Am Acad Dermatol 2005;53: 1–37.

13. Shapiro J. Hair loss: principles of diagnosis and management of alopecia. 1 edition. London: Martin Dunitz; 2002.

14. Rakowska A, Slowinska M, Kowalska-Oledzka E, et al. Trichoscopy of cicatricial alopecia. J Drugs Dermatol 2012;11:753–8.

15. Duque-Estrada B, Tamler C, Sodré CT, et al. Dermoscopy patterns of cicatricial alopecia resulting from discoid lupus erythematosus and lichen planopilaris. An Bras Dermatol 2010;85:179–83.

16. Ross EK, Vincenzi C, Tosti A. Videodermoscopy in the evaluation of hair and scalp disorders. J Am Acad Dermatol 2006;55:799–806.

17. Olsen EA. Disorders of hair growth: diagrosis and treatment. 2 edition. New York: McGraw-Hill Companies; 2003.

18. Callen JP. Chronic cutaneous lupus erythematosus. clinical, laboratory, therapeutic, and prognostic examination of 62 patients. Arch Dermatol 1982; 118:412–6.

19. Wilson CL, Burge SM, Dean D, et al. Scarring alopecia in discoid lupus erythematosus. Br J Dermatol 1992;126:307–14.

20. George PM, Tunnessen WW Jr. Childhood discoid lupus erythematosus. Arch Dermatol 1993;129:613–7.

21. Kossard S. Lymphocytic mediated alopecia: histological classification by pattern analysis. Clin Dermatol 2001;19:201–10.

22. Sperling LC, Solomon AR, Whiting DA. A new look at scarring alopecia. Arch Dermatol 2000;136:235–42.

23. Solomon AR. The transversely sectioned scalp biopsy specimen: the technique and an algorithm for its use in the diagnosis of alopecia. Adv Dermatol 1994;9:127–57.

24. Templeton SF, Solomon AR. Scarring alopecia: a classification based on microscopic criteria. J Cutan Pathol 1994;21:97–109.

25. Moises-Alfaro C, Berrón-Pérez R, Carrasco-Daza D, et al. Discoid lupus erythematosus in children: clinical, histopathologic, and follow-up features in 27 cases. Pediatr Dermatol 2003;20:103–7.

26. Tebbe B, Mansmann U, Wollina U, et al. Markers in cutaneous lupus erythematosus indicating systemic involvement. A multicenter study on 296 patients. Acta Derm Venereol 1997;77:305–8.

27. Werth VP, White WL, Sanchez MR, et al. Incidence of alopecia areata in lupus erythematosus. Arch Dermatol 1992;128:368–71.

28. Meyers DC, Woosley JT, Reddick RL. Verruciform xanthoma in association with discoid lupus erythematosus. J Cutan Pathol 1992;19:156–8.

29. Garrett AB. Multiple squamous cell carcinomas in lesions of discoid lupus erythematosus. Cutis 1985;36:313–4.

30. Sulica VI, Kao GF. Squamous-cell carcinoma of the scalp arising in lesions of discoid lupus erythematosus. Am J Dermatopathol 1988;10:137–41.

31. Lo JS, Berg BR, Tomecki KJ. Treatment of discoid lupus erythematosus. Int J Dermatol 1989;28:497–507.

32. Ruzicka T, Sommerburg C, Goerz G, et al. Treatment of cutaneous lupus erythematosus with acitretin and hydroxychloroquine. Br J Dermatol 1992;127:513–8.

33. Newton RC, JJ, Solomon AR Jr, et al. Mechanism-oriented assessment of isotretinoin in chronic or subacute cutaneous lupus erythematosus. Arch Dermatol 1986;122:170–6.

34. Chieregato C, ZA, Barba A, et al. Lichen planopilaris: report of 30 cases and review of the literature. Int J Dermatol 2003;74:784–6.

35. Kossard S, LM, Wilkinson B. Postmenopausal frontal fibrosing alopecia: a frontal variant of lichen planopilaris. J Am Acad Dermatol 1997;37:215–7.

36. Bianchi L, PVA, Piemonte P, et al. Graham little-piccardi-lassueur syndrome: effective treatment with cyclosporin A. Clin Exp Dermatol 2001;26: 518–20.

37. Mehregan AH. Histopathology of alopecias. Cutis 1978;21:249–53.

38. Alopecia Pinkus H. Clinicopathologic correlations. Int J Dermatol 1980;19:245–53.

39. Mehregan DA, VHH, Muller SA. Lichen planopilaris: clinical and pathologic study of forty-five patients. J Am Acad Dermatol 1992;27:935–42.

40. Elston DM, MM, Warschaw KE, et al. Elastic tissue in scars and alopecia. J Cutan Pathol 2000;27:147–52.

41. Eisen D. The evaluation of cutaneous, genital, scalp, nail, esophageal, and ocular involvement in patients with oral lichen planus. Oral Surg Oral Med Oral Pathol Oral Radiol Endod 1999;88:431–6.

42. Gimenez-Garcia R, P-CJ. Lichen planus and hepatitis C virus infection. J Eur Acad Dermatol Venereol 2003;17:291–5.

43. Ott F, BW, Geiger JM. Efficacy of oral low-dose tretinoin (all-trans-retinoic acid) in lichen planus. Dermatology 1997;192:334–6.

44. Mirmirani P, WA, Price VH. Short course of oral cyclosporine in lichen planopilaris. J Am Acad Dermatol 2003;49:667–71.

45. Cribier B, FC, Chosidow O. Treatment of lichen planus. An evidence-based medicine analysis of efficacy. Arch Dermatol 1998;134:1521–30.

46. Massa MC, RRr. Griseofulvin therapy of lichen planus. Acta Derm Venereol 1981;61:547–50.

47. Ronchese F. Pseudopelade. Arch Dermatol 1960;82:336–43.

48. Braun-Falco O, IS, Schmoeckel C, et al. Pseudopelade of Brocq. Dermatologica 1986;172:18–23.

49. Bulengo-Ransby SM, HJ. Pseudopelade of Brocq in a child. J Am Acad Dermatol 1990;23:944–5.

50. Sperling LC, HC, Pratt L, et al. Acne keloidalis is a form of primary scarring alopecia. Arch Dermatol 2000;136:479–84.

51. Callender VD, MA, Cohen GF. Medical and surgical therapies for alopecias in black women. Dermatol Ther 2004;17:164–76.

52. Gibson LE, MS, Peters MS. Follicular mucinosis of childhood and adolescence. Pediatr Dermatol 1988;5:231–5.

53. van Doorn R, SE, Willemze R. Follicular mycosis fungoides, a distinct disease entity with or without associated follicular mucinosis: a clinicopathologic and follow-up study of 51 patients. Arch Dermatol 2002;138:191–8.

54. Boer A, GY, Ackerman AB. Alopecia mucinosa is mycosis fungoides. Am J Dermatopathol 2004;26:33–52.

55. Passaro EM, SM, Valente NY. Acneiform follicular mucinosis. Clin Exp Dermatol 2004;29:396–8.

56. Anderson BE, MC, Helm KF. Alopecia mucinosa: report of a case and review. J Cutan Med Surg 2003;7:124–8.

57. Arca E, KO, Tastan HB, et al. Follicular mucinosis responding to isotretinoin treatment. J Dermatolog Treat 2004;15:391–5.

58. Emmerson RW. Follicular mucinosis. A study of 47 patients. Br J Dermatol 1969;81:395.

59. Harthi FA, KA, Ajlan A, et al. Urticaria-like follicular mucinosis responding to dapsone. Acta Derm Venereol 2003;83:389–90.

60. Kodama H, US, Nohara N. Follicular mucinosis: response to indomethacin. J Dermatol 1988;15:72–5.

61. von Kobyletzki G, KJ, Nordmeier R, et al. Treatment of idiopathic mucinosis follicularis with UVA1 cold light phototherapy. Dermatology 2000;201:76–7.

62. Van de Vosse E, VdBP, Heus JJ, et al. High-resolution mapping by YAC fragmentation of a 2.5-Mb Xp22 region containing the human RS, KFSD and CLS disease genes. Mamm Genome 1997;8:497–501.

63. Baden HP, BH. Clinical findings, cutaneous pathology, and response to therapy in 21 patients with keratosis pilaris atrophicans. Arch Dermatol 1994;130:469–75.

64. Richard G, HW. Keratosis follicularis spinulosa decalvans. Therapy with isotretinoin and etretinate in the inflammatory stage. Hautarzt 1993;44:529–34 [in German].

65. Powell JJ, Dawber RP, GK. Folliculitis decalvans including tufted folliculitis: clinical, histological and therapeutic findings. Br J Dermatol 1999;140:328–33.

66. Powell J, DR. Successful treatment regime for folliculitis decalvans despite uncertainty of all aetiological factors. Br J Dermatol 2001;144:428–9.

67. Sullivan JR, KS. Acquired scalp alopecia. Part 2: a review. Australas J Dermatol 1999;40:61–70.

68. Dalziel KL, TN, Wilson CL, et al. Tufted folliculitis. A specific bacterial disease? Am J Dermatopathol 1990;12:37–41.

69. Brooke RC, GC. Folliculitis decalvans. Clin Exp Dermatol 2001;26:20–2.

70. Brozena SJ, CL, Fenske NA. Folliculitis decalvans: response to rifampin. Cutis 1988;42:512–5.

71. Abeck D, KH, Braun-Falco O. Folliculitis decalvans. Long-lasting response to combined therapy with fusidic acid and zinc. Acta Derm Venereol 1992;72:143–5.

72. Salinger D. Treatment of folliculitis decalvans with tyrosine. Exp Dermatol 1999;8:363–4.

73. Stites PC, BA. Dissecting cellulitis in a white male: a case report and review of the literature. Cutis 2001;67:37–40.

74. Ramesh V. Dissecting cellulitis of the scalp in 2 girls. Dermatologica 1990;180:48–50.

75. Salim A, DJ, Holder J. Dissecting cellulitis of the scalp with associated spondylarthropathy: case report and review. J Eur Acad Dermatol Venereol 2003;17:689–91.

76. Scheinfeld NS. A case of dissecting cellulitis and a review of the literature. Dermatol Online J 2003; 9:8.

77. Hay RJ, AB. Rook's textbook of dermatology. 7 edition. London: Blackwell Scientific; 2004.

78. Chicarilli ZN. Follicular occlusion triad: hidradenitis suppurativa, acne conglobata, and dissecting cellulitis of the scalp. Ann Plast Surg 1987;18: 230–7.

79. Sivakumaran S, MP, Burrows NP. Dissecting folliculitis of the scalp with marginal keratitis. Clin Exp Dermatol 2001;26:490–2.

80. Ramasastry SS, GM, Boyd JB, et al. Severe perifolliculitis capitis with osteomyelitis. Ann Plast Surg 1987;18:241–4.

81. Ongchi DR, FM, Harris CA. Sternocostoclavicular hyperostosis: two cases with differing dermatologic syndromes. J Rheumatol 1990;17: 1415–8.

82. Libow L, FD. Arthropathy associated with cystic acne, hidradenitis suppurativa, and perifolliculitis capitis abscedens et suffodiens: treatment with isotretinoin. Cutis 1999;64:87–90.

83. Curry SS, GD, King LE Jr. Squamous cell carcinoma arising in dissecting perifolliculitis of the scalp. A case report and review of secondary squamous cell carcinomas. J Am Acad Dermatol 1981;4:673–8.

84. Boyd AS, ZA. A case of pyoderma vegetans and the follicular occlusion triad. J Dermatol 1992;19: 61–3.

85. Bergeron JR, SO. Follicular occlusion triad in a follicular blocking disease (pityriasis rubra pilaris). Dermatologica 1968;136:362–7.

86. Sperling LC. Dissecting cellulitis of the scalp (perifolliculitis capitis abscedens et suffodiens). New York: Parthenon Publishing Group; 2003.

87. Scerri L, WH, Allen BR. Dissecting cellulitis of the scalp: response to isotretinoin. Br J Dermatol 1996; 134:1105–8.

88. Koca R, AH, Ozen OI, et al. Dissecting cellulitis in a white male: response to isotretinoin. Int J Dermatol 2002;41:509–13.

89. Brook I. Recovery of anaerobic bacteria from a case of dissecting cellulitis. Int J Dermatol 2006;45: 168–9.

90. Kobayashi H, AS, Tagami H. Successful treatment of dissecting cellulitis and acne conglobata with oral zinc. Br J Dermatol 1999;141:1137–8.

91. Halder RM. Hair and scalp disorders in blacks. Cutis 1983;32:378–80.

92. Boyd AS, BJ. Use of an 800-nm pulsed-diode laser in the treatment of recalcitrant dissecting cellulitis of the scalp. Arch Dermatol 2002;138:1291–3.

93. Berne B, VP, Ohman S. Perifolliculitis capitis abscedens et suffodiens (Hoffman). Complete healing associated with oral zinc therapy. Arch Dermatol 1985;121:1028–30.

94. Goldsmith PC, DP. Successful therapy of the follicular occlusion triad in a young woman with high dose oral antiandrogens and minocycline. J R Soc Med 1993;86:729–30.

95. Adrian RM, AK. Perifolliculitis capitis: successful control with alternate-day corticosteroids. Ann Plast Surg 1980;4:166–9.

96. Chui CT, BT, Price VH, et al. Recalcitrant scarring follicular disorders treated by laser-assisted hair removal: a preliminary report. Dermatol Surg 1999; 25:34–7.

97. Chinnaiyan P, TL, Brenner MJ, et al. Modern external beam radiation therapy for refractory dissecting cellulitis of the scalp. Br J Dermatol 2005; 152:777–9.

98. Kelly AP. Pseudofolliculitis barbae and acne keloidalis nuchae. Dermatol Clin 2003;21:645–53.

99. Grunwald MH, B-DD, Livni E, et al. Acne keloidalis like lesions on the scalp associated with antiepileptic drugs. Int J Dermatol 1990;29:559–61.

100. Carnero L, SJ, Guijarro J, et al. Nuchal acne keloidalis associated with cyclosporin. Br J Dermatol 2001;144:429–30.

101. Goette DK, BT. Acne keloidalis nuchae. A transepithelial elimination disorder. Int J Dermatol 1987;26:442–4.

102. Herzberg AJ, DS, Kerns BJ, et al. Acne keloidalis. Transverse microscopy, immunohistochemistry, and electron microscopy. Am J Dermatopathol 1990;12:109–21.

103. Halder RM. Pseudofolliculitis barbae and related disorders. Dermatol Clin 1988;6:407–12.

104. Dinehart SM, HA, Kerns BJ, et al. Acne keloidalis: a review. J Dermatol Surg Oncol 1989;15:642–7.

105. Kantor GR, RJ, Wheeland RG. Treatment of acne keloidalis nuchae with carbon dioxide laser. J Am Acad Dermatol 1986;14:263–7.

106. Gloster HM Jr. The surgical management of extensive cases of acne keloidalis nuchae. Arch Dermatol 2000;136:1376–9.

Nutrition and Hair
Deficiencies and Supplements

Andreas M. Finner, MD

KEYWORDS

- Nutrition • Hair • Hair loss • Alopecia • Malnutrition • Deficiency • Diet • Supplements

KEY POINTS

- A caloric deprivation or deficiency of several components, such as proteins, minerals, essential fatty acids, and vitamins, caused by inborn errors or reduced uptake, can lead to structural abnormalities, pigmentation changes, or hair loss, although exact data are often lacking.
- Acquired reasons for nutrition-related hair growth disorders are combined or specific deficiencies due to malnutrition, inadequate diets, or insufficient parenteral alimentation or malabsorption in gastrointestinal disease.
- The evidence on dietary supplements in hair disorders is limited, combinations containing l-cystine are studied best.

INTRODUCTION

Hair follicle cells have a high turnover. Their active metabolism requires a good supply of nutrients and energy. A caloric deprivation or deficiency of several components, such as proteins, minerals, essential fatty acids, and vitamins, caused by inborn errors or reduced uptake can lead to structural abnormalities, pigmentation changes, or hair loss, although exact data are often lacking.[1] Combined deficiencies are not uncommon, especially in malnutrition.

In developed countries, hair growth disorders caused by nutritional deficiencies in healthy individuals are rare and tend to be overestimated by patients and physicians, especially concerning vitamins. National and International Institutions have established recommended daily allowances of many nutritional components. In the United States, the National Institutes of Health has published recommendations for the daily reference intake of micronutrients and macronutrients and the maximum daily intake that will likely not cause adverse effects.

Dietary supplements have traditionally been used unspecifically to improve hair growth, a few of which have been studied systematically in animals and humans.

CLINICAL DIAGNOSIS

The diagnosis is based on a careful history of nutritional habits including 3 to 4 months before the hair problem. Clinical signs include a diffusely positive pull test, hair diameter, color, and quality changes or fragility as well as skin and nail changes. The latter changes are easier to recognize by holding a contrasting white or black paper (hair card) behind the tips of the hairs and by using trichoscopy and videotrichoscopy. A trichogram or digital phototrichogram may reveal increased rates of telogen. Laboratory blood tests should be targeted based on the suspected deficiency.

Hair analysis is often marketed as a tool to diagnose deficiencies and intoxications as causes of hair loss and structural hair changes. However, the use of hair analysis in a hair clinic is very limited, because there are no laboratory standards and no clear correlation between hair components and the nutritional status has been established. The hair content can be influenced by polluted air and other external factors. Concentrations can also be influenced by changes in hair growth speed because of variations in nutritional status.

Trichomed Clinic for Hair Medicine and Hair Transplantation, Berlin, Germany
E-mail address: info@trichomed.com

Dermatol Clin 31 (2013) 167–172
http://dx.doi.org/10.1016/j.det.2012.08.015
0733-8635/13/$ – see front matter © 2013 Elsevier Inc. All rights reserved.

SPECIFIC DEFICIENCIES
Malnutrition and Weight Loss Diets

Marasmus is a diet low in calories, whereby amino acids are used to provide energy and are not available for tissue and plasma protein synthesis and other functions. The glycogen content of the follicular sheath is reduced, providing less energy for cell mitosis. The hair is thin, sparse, fragile, and even more easily shed than in kwashiorkor (see later discussion), whereas lanugo body hair may be increased.[2] Organs show atrophy. Hair morphology in children and their mothers has been used to detect malnutrition in developing countries.

Diets for weight loss can also lead to hair loss, especially if the daily calorie intake is less than 1000 kcal and if protein intake is inadequate. This cause should be suspected especially in young obese women.[3] The hair loss may be more profound in diets with a negative nitrogen balance (loss of lean body mass) and be partly due to reduced thyroid activity.

Proteins

Protein is the major constituent of hair fibers. Therefore, a reduced protein uptake can impair hair growth, even before serum albumin levels are decreased.[4]

Kwashiorkor is a result of a low protein intake in a calorically normal diet. It is characterized by reddish, short, dull hair and a telogen and dystrophic effluvium. Hairs can be plucked easily.[5]

In early stages, anagen bulbs are atrophic,[6] and hairs are already reduced in diameter, often intermittently. Hair elasticity is reduced, and hairs feel weaker and softer. Hair color changes may also vary along the hair shaft depending on the nutritional situation,[7] leading to red or light bands in dark hair. Brown hair may become blonde. The skin is hypopigmented and partly dry. Edema and anemia are typical.

Other situations of low protein uptake are infants on special diets, such as in urea-cycle disorders, milk-free diets, gastrointestinal disease, blood loss and blood donations, anorexia nervosa,[8] depression, drug addiction, or malignancy.

Vitamin C

Ascorbic acid is essential for collagen synthesis and cross-linkage of keratin fibers. The reference daily intake for men is 90 mg and for women is 75 mg. A deficiency is called scurvy and often occurs in elderly patients, alcoholics, and patients with chronic disease. Hair changes are corkscrew hairs, perifollicular hyperkeratosis and hemorrhage, follicular plugging, and curling caused by changes in the perifollicular fibrous tissue. Other symptoms include ecchymoses, bleeding gums, chronic wounds, and infections.

Biotin

Vitamin H is a crucial cofactor of carboxylases in the mitochondria.[9] Biotin deficiency is rare because it is also produced by intestinal bacteria. It has been seen in congenital or acquired biotinidase or carboxylase deficiency,[10] parenteral alimentation, impaired gastrointestinal flora caused by antibiotics, and after excessive ingestion of raw white eggs due to binding by avidin. Symptoms include structural changes of the hair and nails, perioral dermatitis, conjunctivitis, and infections. Alopecia is not a typical symptom of biotin deficiency but trichorrhexis nodosa and other structural anomalies can occur. The reference daily intake for adults is 30 μg. Antiepileptic drugs can reduce biotin levels; a prophylactic supplementation can therefore be recommended.

It has not been sufficiently shown that additional supplementation of biotin in patients with normal blood levels can improve hair loss, although an effect on hair and nail structure is possible.

Vitamin B12

A deficiency of cyanocobalamin is seen in vegetarians, fish bandworm infestation, and various gastrointestinal disorders, including atrophic gastritis with antibodies to intrinsic factors leading to pernicious anemia. It can cause gray hair, megaloblastic anemia, peripheral neuropathy, Hunter glossitis, and angular cheilitis. The reference daily intake for adults is 2.4 μg.

Zinc

Zinc is an essential cofactor of several metaloenzymes and transcription factors. The required daily zinc uptake of 8 to 10 mg per day is usually supplied through a normal diet, but deficiencies are still common in developing countries.[11]

Zinc deficiency can lead to telogen effluvium, thin white and brittle hair, as well as nail dystrophy, a seborrhoic and later psoriasiform acral and perioral dermatitis, cheilitis, blepharoconjunctivitis, infection, and skin superinfection with *Candida albicans* and *Staphylococcus aureus*.[12] Other symptoms are diarrhea, neurologic disturbances, and growth retardation. Histology shows pale superficial epidermal cells and single-cell necrosis.

The deficiency can be genetic, presenting after weaning because of an autosomal-recessive absorption disorder called acrodermatitis enteropathica, with an additional reduced uptake of desaturated fatty acids and inadequate desaturation of linoleic acid and alpha-linoleic acid to their long-chain metabolites.[13] The hair shows diameter narrowing,[14] and polarized microscopy may show irregular bands, such as in trichothiodystophy.[15] Occasionally, serum zinc levels are normal. A clinical response to zinc supplementation confirms the diagnosis.

Acquired zinc deficiency occurs in elderly persons, in persons with alcoholism, anorexia nervosa, nephropathy, pancreatitis, after prolonged breast feeding without supplementation, following gastrointestinal bypass surgery, from cereals containing phytate, because of excessive intake of iron, and because of drugs that chelate zinc, such asangiotensin-converting enzyme inhibitors.

During treatment, zinc levels should be monitored because overdose can lead to copper or calcium deficiency, drowsiness, and headache. The daily reference intake for men and pregnant women is 11 mg and for women is 8 mg. In deficiency, the recommended dose for adults is 25 to 50 mg of elemental zinc and 0.5 to 1 mg/kg for children.

Although traditionally used in unspecific hair treatments, an effect of zinc supplementation on hair growth in patients with normal serum zinc levels has not been sufficiently proved.[16]

Niacin

Vitamin B3 is an essential component of amide adenine dinucleotide connecting the citric acid cycle to the oxidative phosphorylation required for adenosine triphosphate production and thus cell energy supply. The recommended daily intake is at least 13 mg. A deficiency is called pellagra, meaning "rough skin." The major symptoms are a photosensitive dermatitis with hyperpigmentation, diarrhea, dementia, and finally, death (the 4 Ds). Early signs are diffuse hair loss, weakness, irritability, glossitis, and stomatitis.

Pellagra occurs in areas where maize and millet are the main food, such as parts of Asia, Africa, and India. Other reasons are impaired food intake, Crohn disease, tumors that impair niacin metabolism such as carcinoid, and drugs such as isonicotine hydrazide. The reference daily intake for male adults is 16 mg and for women is 14 mg.

Essential Fatty Acids

Linoleic acid and alpha-linoleic acid are required for normal human metabolism. They are an important component of cell membranes and lamellar bodies of the stratum corneum. A deficiency was seen in inappropriate parenteral nutrition and in children with impaired uptake, such as in children with biliar atresia, who were put on a diet rich in triglycerides, and in cystic fibrosis patients. Hair loss of the scalp and eyebrows and depigmentation are symptoms, among other complaints.[17]

Iron

Iron deficiency is ranked as the world's most common deficiency by the World Health Organization, affecting up to 80% of humankind.

Iron works as a catalyst in oxidation and reduction reactions, and it may control DNA synthesis through the enzyme ribonuclease in dividing cells. Its deficiency causes microcytic and hypochromic anemia. Even in the absence of anemia, diffuse hair loss and other skin symptoms, such as glossitis, cheilitis, and kolonychia, can occur. The impaired keratin production can lead to thinner anagen hairs. In African hair, band-like color changes have been reported.

Severe deficiency can cause fatigue, weakness, pale conjunctivae, and tachycardia because of anemia.

Iron is functional in hemoglobin within erythrocytes and in myoglobin and enzymes, stored in ferritin and transported in transferrin. For laboratory tests, sufficient ferritin levels are essential, reflecting the iron reserve.

In premenopausal women, iron deficiency is often due to menorrhagia or pregnancy, whereas, especially in older patients, gastrointestinal bleeding should be excluded. Other reasons may include a vegetarian or vegan diet, hookworms, nephropathy and dialysis, frequent blood donations, surgery, or chronic inflammatory bowel disease.

In at-risk groups, sufficient intake of red meat is important; other heme iron sources include clams and fish. Non-heme iron sources, such as beans, peas, and cereals, should be eaten together with sources of vitamin C. Excessive consumption of coffee and tea should be avoided.

The daily reference intake is 8 mg for men and 18 mg for women between 19 and 50 years of age; different values apply for children, seniors, and pregnant or lactating women.

The required iron levels and their significance for hair loss are still an object of scientific discussion, with several studies coming to different conclusions.[18–22]

Most authors consider a ferritin level of at least 40 mg/L as adequate in their female patients; others only require 10 mg/L, and some require 70 mg/L. To correct iron deficiency, ferrous fumarate, ferrous lactate, ferrous gluconate, or ferrous sulfate should be taken for several weeks in 2 to

3 daily doses, because absorption is lower in high doses. The latter 2 doses may be better tolerated. For the treatment of low iron deficiency anemia, the Centers for Disease Control and Prevention recommends 50 to 60 mg of oral elemental iron twice daily for 3 months, which corresponds to 325 mg ferrous sulfate twice a day. Gradually increasing the dose or intake with food may minimize gastrointestinal side effects. Iron overload is more common in adult men and postmenopausal women. It should be avoided, because it can cause tissue damage and fibrosis and exacerbate hemochromatosis.

Copper

Copper is crucial for aminoxydases required for oxidation of thiol groups to dithio- crosslinks, which are essential for keratin fiber strength. Some enzymes also depend on copper, such as ascorbic acid oxidase and tyrosinase.

In children, a rare autosomal-recessive malabsorption disorder may be present. Hypopigmented hair and pili torti are typical in Menkes kinky hair syndrome,[23] as well as a degeneration of brain, bones, and connective tissue. including arterial occlusion, and pale and lax skin. The treatment consists of infusions with copper salts.

An acquired deficiency is also seen in premature babies, inadequate cow milk, or parental alimentation and after a longer zinc therapy.[24] It presents with hypopigmented hair, microcytic anemia, leukopenia, and myelopathy. The reference daily intake for adults is 900 μg.

Selenium

Selenium is an important component of glutathione peroxidase, an antioxidant system. A deficiency has been reported in areas of soil with low selenium content and in parenteral nutrition. Although symptoms are mostly muscular and cardiac, hypopigmentation of the hair and skin can occur. The reference daily intake for adults is 55 μg. Selenium intoxicants from overdosed supplements have been reported.

Vitamin A

Although vitamin A deficiency is not an established cause of hair loss, an excessive intake can lead to general hair loss and dry skin. The recommended maximum daily intake is 10,000 IU.

Vitamin D

The role of vitamin D for hair growth is still under investigation.[25] Several studies in animals in vitro and in vitamin D–resistant rickets suggest a role for vitamin D in hair growth,[26,27] although no relation to male baldness or alopecia areata could be shown.[28,29] Therefore, obtaining a Vitamin D3 level in patients with telogen effluvium can be helpful. The reference daily intake for adults is 5 to 10 μg (1 μg calciferol = 40 IU vitamin D).

TOXINS

The ingestion of toxins such as thallium, arsen, and mimosin in a plant called *Leucenia glauca* and others can cause hair loss and/or hair breakage. Acrodynia after mercurium intoxication has become rare. It is characterized by scalp hair alopecia and hypertrichosis on the arms, legs, and sometimes the trunk.

NUTRITIONAL SUPPLEMENTS

Although many nutritional supplements have been used traditionally to treat hair disorders, there is limited evidence of their use in non deficient patients.

Long-term effects of antioxidants on hair aging may be possible, but are difficult to assess. The amino acid taurin has been shown to promote follicle cell survival in vitro[30]; it is combined with the polyphenol katechin and other ingredients. L-carnitine has been shown to stimulate hair follicle cells in vitro.[31] Components derived from soybeans may also have an effect on hair growth through anti-inflammatory and estrogen-dependent mechanisms,[32,33] but studies in vivo are lacking and an increase of angioma rubi has been reported.[34]

Orthosilicic acid increased hair tensile strength and thickness in a controlled study after 6 months[35] and decreased hair brittleness in a study after 20 weeks.[36]

From studies with sheep, it has been snown that additional intake of L-cysteine can improve wool production.[37] An antioxidant effect of L-cysteine is also suspected. Later, studies in humans have shown a significant effect in the treatment of diffuse telogen effluvium. In a randomized, placebo-controlled study in 30 women, a supplement of L-cysteine in combination with medicinal yeast and pantothenic acid led to a normalization of the rate of anagen after 6 months, whereas a placebo did not.[38] Clinically, this supplement of L-cysteine would correspond to avoiding a temporary loss of several thousands of long hairs. Further studies are needed to increase the evidence on nutritional supplements on hair.

SUMMARY

Various genetic or acquired malabsorption deficiencies or insufficient uptake of nutrients can influence hair growth. The diagnosis is established through a careful history and clinical examination. Typical clues are a diffusely positive pull test confirmed by a trichogram or digital phototrichogram, changes in hair diameter, structure and strength including broken or brittle hairs, and pigment changes seen in trichoscopy.

Laboratory blood tests confirm the specific deficiency. Relevant iron deficiency can be assumed at ferritin levels less than 40 mg/L. Specific treatment of the deficiency will lead to improved hair parameters within 3 to 6 months. Unspecific treatment of hair loss without confirmed deficiencies has only been effective in telogen effluvium with a supplement containing L-cysteine, but otherwise can not generally be recommended.

REFERENCES

1. Rushton DH. Nutritional factors and hair loss. Clin Exp Dermatol 2002;27(5):396–404.
2. Castellani A. Hypertrichosis of the lanugo hair in malnutrition. Br Med J 1947;2(4517):188.
3. Rooth G, Carlström S. Therapeutic fasting. Acta Med Scand 1970;187(6):455–63.
4. Jordan VE. Protein status of the elderly as measured by dietary intake, hair tissue, and serum albumin. Am J Clin Nutr 1976;29(5):522–8.
5. Sims RT. Hair growth in kwashiorkor. Arch Dis Child 1967;42(224):397–400.
6. Bradfield RB. Protein deprivation: comparative response of hair roots, serum protein, and urinary nitrogen. Am J Clin Nutr 1971;24(4):405–10.
7. McKenzie CA, Wakamatsu K, Hanchard NA, et al. Childhood malnutrition is associated with a reduction in the total melanin content of scalp hair. Br J Nutr 2007;98(1):159–64.
8. Strumia R. Dermatologic signs in patients with eating disorders. Am J Clin Dermatol 2005;6(3):165–73.
9. Zempleni J, Hassan YI, Wijeratne SS. Biotin and biotinidase deficiency. Expet Rev Endocrinol Metabol 2008;3(6):715–24.
10. Williams ML, Packman S, Cowan MJ. Alopecia and periorificial dermatitis in biotin-responsive multiple carboxylase deficiency. J Am Acad Dermatol 1983; 9(1):97–103.
11. Prasad AS. Discovery of human zinc deficiency: 50 years later. J Trace Elem Med Biol 2012;26(2–3):66–9.
12. Weismann K, Høyer H. Zinc deficiency dermatoses. Etiology, clinical aspects and treatment. Hautarzt 1982;33(8):405–10 [in German].
13. Moynahan EJ. Letter: acrodermatitis enteropathica: a lethal inherited human zinc-deficiency disorder. Lancet 1974;2(7877):399–400.
14. Dupré A, Bonafé JL, Carriere JP. The hair in acrodermatitis enteropathica—a disease indicator? Acta Derm Venereol 1979;59(2):177–8.
15. Traupe H, Happle R, Gröbe H, et al. Polarization microscopy of hair in acrodermatitis enteropathica. Pediatr Dermatol 1986;3(4):300–3.
16. Garcia-Machado R. Letter: zinc and hair. Lancet 1975;2(7929):322.
17. Skolnik P, Eaglstein WH, Ziboh VA. Human essential fatty acid deficiency: treatment by topical application of linoleic acid. Arch Dermatol 1977;113(7): 939–41.
18. Olsen EA. Iron deficiency and hair loss: the jury is still out. J Am Acad Dermatol 2006;54(5):903–6.
19. Trost LB, Bergfeld WF, Calogeras E. The diagnosis and treatment of iron deficiency and its potential relationship to hair loss. J Am Acad Dermatol 2006;54(5):824–44.
20. Bregy A, Trueb RM. No association between serum ferritin levels >10 microg/l and hair loss activity in women. Dermatology 2008;217(1):1–6.
21. Kantor J, Kessler LJ, Brooks DG, et al. Decreased serum ferritin is associated with alopecia in women. J Invest Dermatol 2003;121(5):985–8.
22. Rushton DH, Ramsay ID. The importance of adequate serum ferritin levels during oral cyproterone acetate and ethinyl oestradiol treatment of diffuse androgen-dependent alopecia in women. Clin Endocrinol (Oxf) 1992;36(4):421–7.
23. Aguilar MJ, Chadwick DL, Okuyama K, et al. Kinky hair disease. I. Clinical and pathological features. J Neuropathol Exp Neurol 1966;25(4): 507–22.
24. Olivares M, Uauy R. Copper as an essential nutrient. Am J Clin Nutr 1996;63(5):791S–6S.
25. Amor KT, Rashid RM, Mirmirani P. Does D matter? The role of vitamin D in hair disorders and hair follicle cycling. Dermatol Online J 2010;16(2):3.
26. Demay MB, MacDonald PN, Skorija K, et al. Role of the vitamin D receptor in hair follicle biology. J Steroid Biochem Mol Biol 2007;103(3–5):344–6.
27. Marx SJ, Bliziotes MM, Nanes M. Analysis of the relation between alopecia and resistance to 1,25-dihydroxyvitamin D. Clin Endocrinol (Oxf) 1986;25(4):373–81.
28. Bolland MJ, Ames RW, Grey AB, et al. Does degree of baldness influence vitamin D status? Med J Aust 2008;189:674–5.
29. Akar A, Orkunoglu FE, Tunca M, et al. Vitamin D receptor gene polymorphisms are not associated with alopecia areata. Int J Dermatol 2007;46: 927–9.
30. Collin C, Gautier B, Gaillard O, et al. Protective effects of taurine on human hair follicle grown in vitro. Int J Cosmet Sci 2006;28(4):289–98.
31. Foitzik K, Hoting E, Förster T, et al. L-carnitine-L-tartrate promotes human hair growth in vitro. Exp Dermatol 2007;16(11):936–45.
32. Tsuruki T, Takahata K, Yoshikawa M. Anti-alopecia mechanisms of soymetide-4, an immunostimulating

peptide derived from soy beta-conglycinin. Peptides 2005;26(5):707–11.

33. McElwee KJ, Niiyama S, Freyschmidt-Paul P, et al. Dietary soy oil content and soy-derived phytoestrogen genistein increase resistance to alopecia areata onset in C3H/HeJ mice. Exp Dermatol 2003;12(1):30–6.

34. Ramalho R, Correia O, Delgado L. Adverse effect of a nutritional supplement for hair loss. Eur J Dermatol 2011;21(2):283–4.

35. Wickett RR, Kossmann E, Barel A, et al. Effect of oral intake of choline-stabilized orthosilicic acid on hair tensile strength and morphology in women with fine hair. Arch Dermatol Res 2007;299(10):499–505.

36. Barel A, Calomme M, Timchenko A, et al. Effect of oral intake of choline-stabilized orthosilicic acid on skin, nails and hair in women with photodamaged skin. Arch Dermatol Res 2005;297(4):147–53.

37. Downes AM, Reis PJ, Sharry LF, et al. Metabolic fate of parenterally administered sulphur-containing amino acids in sheep and effects on growth and composition of wool. Aust J Biol Sci 1970;23(5): 1077–88.

38. Lengg N, Heidecker B, Seifert B, et al. Dietary supplement increases anagen rate in women with telogen effluvium: results of a randomized, placebo-controlled study. Therapy 2007;(7).

Shampoos, Conditioners, and Camouflage Techniques

Zoe Diana Draelos, MD

KEYWORDS

- Scalp hair • Scalp-hair cleansers • Dimethicone • Hair loss

KEY POINTS

- Shampoos are used to cleanse the scalp and beautify the hair. These activities must occur simultaneously.
- Conditioning shampoos are valuable for patients with hair loss in maintaining adequate hygiene while smoothing the cuticle to maintain hair shine and manageability.
- Dimethicone is a valuable conditioner in the hair-loss patient because it does not make thinning hair limp, while providing decreased static electricity and improved hair styling.

INTRODUCTION

Scalp-hair appearance assumes great importance in both men and women. Hair can be cut, shaved, styled, combed, brushed, braided, twisted, glued, shampooed, conditioned, dyed, curled, straightened, and teased. Why are there so many techniques to modify human scalp hair? The answer lies in human behavior patterns whereby such services and products are purchased to support the hair-care industry. The amount of money spent on beautifying scalp hair signifies the preoccupation humans have with their hair. This preoccupation is even more challenging in persons who are experiencing hair loss. This article examines hair care in persons with hair loss. The use of shampoos, conditioners, and hair styling products to camouflage hair loss is discussed.

SHAMPOOS

Shampoos are designed to primarily clean the scalp and secondarily clean the hair, even though most consumers believe otherwise.[1] In fact, shampoo is a relatively modern invention. Until the mid-1930s bar soap was used to cleanse the

hair. This method was somewhat unsatisfactory because hard water in combination with bar soap left behind a scum that dulled the hair appearance. Early shampoo formulations were liquid coconut-oil soaps that lathered and rinsed better than bar soap. Surfactant shampoos were introduced in the late 1930s and represented a significant advance because they performed well even with the hardest water.[2] These new surfactants have allowed the hair-care formulator to develop shampoos that meet a variety of hair and scalp needs, including those of the patient with hair loss.

The act of shampooing involves the following steps: (1) hair and scalp are wetted and the liquid shampoo distributed; (2) shampoo is foamed and massaged into the scalp; (3) shampoo foam is distributed throughout the hair; (4) water is used to thoroughly rinse the hair and scalp; (5) hair is towel dried to absorb excess water; (6) wet hair is combed. Shampooing is actually a very complex procedure because the average woman has 4 to 8 m of hair surface area to clean.[3] It is easy to formulate a shampoo that will remove all of the sebum from the hair and scalp, but this will leave the hair frizzy, dry, and unattractive. The challenge

No conflicts of interest pertain to this article.
Department of Dermatology, Duke University School of Medicine, Durham, 2444 North Main Street, High Point, NC 27262, USA
E-mail address: zdraelos@northstate.net

Dermatol Clin 31 (2013) 173–178
http://dx.doi.org/10.1016/j.det.2012.08.004

is to remove just enough sebum to allow the hair to appear clean and leave behind enough conditioning agents, actually representing synthetic sebum, to beautify the clean hair. The basic formulation for shampoo is listed in **Box 1**.[4]

The cleansing ingredient found in shampoos is known as a detergent or surfactant. These agents are soap-free synthetic substances that possess both lipophilic and hydrophilic structures. The lipophilic end binds to the sebum and the hydrophilic end allows the sebum to rinse away with water down the drain. Chemical moieties that possess this chemical structure are amphiphilic.[5] The most commonly used detergents in shampoos are listed in **Box 2**.[6]

The art of shampoo formulation is mixing together detergents to achieve the desired balance between cleansing and hair beautification. Typically several detergents are combined together to achieve the desired end result. For example, if the shampoo is intended for oily hair, detergents with strong sebum removal qualities are selected; conversely, if the shampoo is intended for permanently waved or dyed hair, mild detergents are selected to reduce sebum removal. Persons with hair loss typically want to maximize hair cleansing, because sebum makes the hair appear flat, and then beautify the hair to make it shiny, smooth, and easy to untangle. This action is best accomplished with a product known as a 2-in-1 shampoo. Two-in-1 shampoos are so named because they clean and condition, performing 2 functions, in 1 product. The detergents that can be combined to achieve these results and their attributes are listed in **Table 1**.[7]

Shampoos for Hair Loss

A shampoo for hair loss should remove adequate sebum, but not overdry the hair to make it harsh, rough, subject to static electricity, dull, and difficult to untangle. Sodium lauryl sulfate is a strong surfactant while sodium laureth sulfate is slightly milder. Most shampoos for hair loss use sodium laureth sulfate as the primary surfactant and then combine a secondary surfactant that is milder.

Box 1
Basic shampoo ingredient formulation and function

1. Detergents

   Function to remove environment dirt, styling products, sebum, and skin scale from the hair and scalp

2. Foaming agents

   Allow the shampoo to form suds, because consumers equate cleansing with foaming even though the two are unrelated

3. Conditioners

   Leave the hair soft and smooth after sebum removal by the detergent

4. Thickeners

   Thicken the shampoo, because consumers believe that a thick shampoo works better than a thin shampoo

5. Opacifiers

   Added to make a shampoo opaque as opposed to translucent for aesthetic purposes unrelated to cleansing

6. Sequestering agents

   Function to prevent soap scum from forming on the hair and scalp in the presence of hard water: the basic difference between a liquid shampoo and a bar cleanser

7. Fragrances

   Added to give the shampoo a consumer acceptable smell

8. Preservatives

   Prevent microbial and fungal contamination of the shampoo before and after opening

9. Specialty additives

   Treatment ingredients or marketing aids added to impart other benefits to the shampoo besides hair and scalp cleansing

The detergent listed first is the primary cleanser in highest concentration and the detergent listed second is the secondary cleanser designed to complement the shortcomings of the primary detergent.

Sodium laureth sulfate is an anionic detergent representing only one category of surfactants. Anionic detergents are named for their negatively charged polar group. A second detergent group, known as cationic detergents, possesses a positively charged polar group. Cationic detergents have limited ability to remove sebum and do not produce much lather, but are excellent at imparting softness and manageability to damaged hair.[3] A third detergent category is the nonionics, which have no polar group. Nonionic detergents are the mildest of all surfactants and are used in combination with ionic surfactants as a secondary cleanser.[8] Examples of commonly used nonionic detergents include polyoxyethylene fatty alcohols, polyoxyethylene sorbitol esters, and alkanolamides. The final and fourth group of detergents is the amphoterics, named for the fact that they possess both a negatively charged and a positively charged polar group. Amphoteric detergents are unique in that they contain both an anionic and a cationic group, which allows them to behave as cationic detergents at lower pH values and as anionic detergents at higher pH values. The amphoteric detergent category includes the betaines, sultaines, and imidazolinium derivatives. Amphoteric detergents, such as cocamidopropyl betaine and sodium lauraminopropionate, are used in shampoos for hair loss because they foam moderately well, leaving the hair manageable and soft.

Conditioning Shampoos

The best shampoos for hair loss combine the cleansers previously discussed with a conditioning agent. The conditioner in the shampoo functions to impart manageability, gloss, and antistatic properties to the hair.[9,10] Substances that perform this function are usually fatty alcohols, fatty esters, vegetable oils, mineral oils, or humectants. Commonly used conditioning substances in shampoos include hydrolyzed animal protein, glycerin, dimethicone, simethicone, polyvinylpyrrolidone, propylene glycol, and stearalkonium chloride.[11,12]

Protein-derived substances are popular in conditioning shampoos because they can temporarily mend split ends, medically known as trichoptilosis. Split ends arise when the protective cuticle has been lost from the distal hair shaft and the exposed cortex splits. Protein is attracted to the keratin, a property known as substantivity, and the protein adheres the cortex fragments together until the next shampooing occurs.[13] However, the effectiveness of proteins in shampoos is not great because the contact time between the shampoo protein and the hair is minimal. Conditioners that remain on the hair for a longer period have a more profound effect on beautifying hair in the hair-loss patient.

Table 1
Shampoo detergent characteristics

Surfactant Type	Chemical Class	Characteristics
Anionics	Lauryl sulfates, laureth sulfates, sarcosines, sulfosuccinates	Deep cleansing, may leave hair harsh
Cationics	Long-chain amino esters, ammonioesters	Poor cleansing, poor lather, impart softness and manageability
Nonionics	Polyoxyethylene fatty alcohols, polyoxyethylene sorbitol esters, alkanolamides	Mildest cleansing, impart manageability
Amphoterics	Betaines, sultaines, imidazolinium derivatives	Nonirritating to eyes, mild cleansing, impart manageability
Natural surfactants	Sarsaparilla, soapwort, soap bark, ivy, agave	Poor cleansing, excellent lather

pH and Shampoos

Another key shampoo consideration in hair-loss patients is shampoo pH. Hair shampoos contain pH adjusters to minimize hair damage from alkalinization. Most shampoo detergents have an alkaline pH, which causes hair-shaft swelling. This swelling loosens the protective cuticle predisposing the hair shaft to damage. Hair-shaft swelling can be prevented by "pH-balanced" shampoos formulated with the addition of an acidic substance, such as glycolic acid. Shampoos formulated at a neutral pH are most important for chemically treated hair from either permanent dyeing or permanent waving.

CONDITIONERS FOR HAIR LOSS

Additional beautification of the hair can be achieved by using a separate conditioner following shampooing. The role of a conditioner is to mimic sebum in making the hair manageable, glossy, and soft. Conditioners also attempt to recondition hair that has been damaged by chemical or mechanical trauma.[14] Common sources of trauma include excessive brushing, hot blow-drying, detergent shampoos, alkaline permanent waves, and bleaching. Because hair is nonliving tissue, obviously any reconditioning that occurs is minimal and temporary until the next shampooing. Because hair-loss patients frequently possess hair damage, the use of additional conditioning is important.

Additional conditioning is imparted to the thinning hair by applying a separate conditioner after shampooing. These conditioners are applied in the shower to wet hair and then rinsed immediately before exiting; they are known as instant conditioners, because they are left on the hair a very short time.[15] All formulations of instant conditioners are good at detangling hair by smoothing the cuticle and reducing friction. However, if the hair has been severely damaged and the cuticular scales are sparse, only a protein-containing conditioner can penetrate the hair shaft and temporarily increase hair strength. Because hair breakage is an important cause of accelerated hair loss in the alopecia patient, strengthening the hair to resist breakage is important. Protein-containing conditioners can increase hair strength by up to 5%, but the protein that penetrates the hair shaft during conditioning will exit the hair shaft during the next shampoo, requiring reapplication. Proteins can also coat the hair shaft, temporarily increasing its thickness; this is the basis of many of the "hair-thickening" conditioners. These conditioners do not increase hair thickness by promoting growth, but temporarily increase hair-shaft thickness until the subsequent shampoo. Although the concept of hair thickening may be misleading, these conditioners do lead to hair with a better cosmetic appearance in the hair-loss patient, thus accounting for their continued marketing success.

Occasionally it is necessary to impart more conditioning benefits to thinning hair than an instant conditioner can deliver; this is especially the case in hair that has underdone chemical processing, such as permanent dyeing, bleaching, permanent waving, or chemical straightening. These procedures all intentionally disrupt the cuticular scale to reach the cortex and medulla of the hair shaft to induce a change in color or configuration. Once the cuticle has been disrupted with chemical processing, it can never be fully restored. Thus, there is a trade-off for the hair-loss patient between the cosmetic value of chemically treating the hair shaft and its reduced ability to function optimally. Some of the damage can be minimized with a deep conditioner.

Deep conditioners are creams, rather than the liquid instant conditioners, which remain on the hair for 20 to 30 minutes and may include the application of heat from a hair dryer or warm towel.[3] The extended application time allows more conditioner to coat the hair shaft, while heat causes hair-shaft swelling and allows increased conditioner penetration. These products are intended for damaged hair and work very well in the hair-loss patient.

Hair Conditioner Formulation

As discussed previously for shampoos, a variety of ingredients are used in combination to create a hair conditioner that beautifies thinning hair. Although some conditioners are labeled for thinning hair, individuals with thinning hair usually can use products developed for damaged hair, as the formulations are usually identical even though the packaging contains different wording.

Some instant hair conditioners applied immediately following shampooing and rinsed are based on ingredients previously discussed for hair shampoos.[16] Cationic detergents, also known as quaternaries or quaternary ammonium compounds or quats, are excellent at increasing adherence of the cuticular scales to the hair shaft, which increases the light-reflective abilities of the hair, adding shine and luster. In addition, they are able to electrically neutralize static electricity based on the negative (anionic) charge of processed or damaged hair, which attracts the positively (cationic) charged quaternary compound to adhere to the hair shaft, thus improving manageability.[17] These qualities make them an excellent conditioner choice in patients with permanently dyed or permanently waved hair, in addition to hair loss.

Another category of conditioners, known as leave-in conditioners, are designed to stay on the hair shaft until removal by the next shampooing. These film-forming conditioners apply a thin layer of polymer, such as polyvinylpyrrolidone (PVP), over the hair shaft.[18] The polymer fills hair-shaft defects, creating a smooth surface to increase shine and luster while eliminating static electricity owing to its cationic nature. The polymer also coats each individual hair shaft, thus "thickening" the hair shaft. This type of conditioner is excellent for hair-loss patients because the hair feels thicker and retains a style better.

HAIR GROOMING FOR THE HAIR-LOSS PATIENT

The dermatologist should also provide some hair-grooming tips to hair-loss patients, focused on using the patient's remaining natural hair to camouflage thinning where possible. Because hair is nonliving, any hair damage that results from grooming should be minimized. The first rule of hair care is to avoid manipulating wet hair. Hair shafts are most subject to fracture when wet, because of increased elasticity. Thus, it is much easier to stretch wet hair to breaking point than dry hair. Wet hair should be initially detangled with the fingers and slightly dried, before detangling with a wide-toothed comb. Brushes should not be used for detangling wet hair. Further, all combing and brushing should be kept to a minimum to avoid hair damage. In short, the less done to thinning hair, the better.

HAIR-STYLING PRODUCT CAMOUFLAGE TECHNIQUES

Hair-styling products are the easiest way to decrease the appearance of thinning hair besides wearing a hairpiece. Most patients are highly motivated to take measures to prevent the purchase of a wig, making the understanding of hair-styling products very important. Styling products can keep the hair in place and add volume by allowing the hair to stand away from the scalp, defying gravity and creating the illusion of fullness. Available styling product categories include styling gels, sculpturing gels, mousses, and hair sprays. Styling gels, sculpturing gels, and mousses are generally applied to towel-dried hair whereas hair sprays are used to improve the hold of a finished hairstyle. Sculpturing gels provide a stiffer hold than styling gels, which provide a better hold than mousses.

One quick way to increase the appearance of hair volume is to massage a small amount of styling gel or mousse into the base of the hair shafts followed by drying the hair with a blow dryer, while combing the hair away from the scalp or bending over with the hair falling away from the scalp because of gravity. This maneuver stiffens and fixes the hair in place away from the scalp, creating the illusion of fullness. The styling products create temporary bonds between adjacent hair strands and allow the hair to defy gravity. These styling products contain polymers, such as vinyl acetate and polyvinyl pyrrolidone, which coat the hair shaft with a clear stiff layer, allowing the hair to stand away from the scalp. The products are easily removed with shampooing, and must be reapplied after water contact or if the bonds are broken with pulling, combing, or brushing. The products can be reapplied daily or as needed, to restore the hair style or create a new hair style with fresh shampooing or between shampoos.

A variant of hair gel is hair spray, the most important styling product for hair-loss patients. Hair spray is dispensed from an aerosol can or nonaerosol bottle to create a thin polymer film that can be used to keep the final hairstyle in place. For example, hair can be rearranged to cover thinning areas and then kept in place with a high-hold hair spray. This camouflage technique is the easiest to master and can be used in men, women, and children. The pump aerosol hair sprays are preferred because of their safety, and can be easily removed with shampooing.

SUMMARY

Hair loss is a traumatic condition for any patient. Providing shampoo, conditioner, and hair-styling product advice is important because it lets patients know that the dermatologist understands their concerns and wants to move forward with treatment. Most hair-loss treatments do not produce immediate results; however, proper hair-care measures can increase the cosmetic value of the hair following one application. Because hair is nonliving, medical treatments are limited to only inducing change in the follicles within the scalp skin and do not improve the hair loss actually witnessed by the patient. This aspect explains the need to accompany the medical treatment of hair loss with cosmetic hair treatment to optimize patient satisfaction.

REFERENCES

1. Robbins CR. Interaction of shampoo and creme rinse ingredients with human hair. In: Chemical and

physical behavior of human hair. 2nd edition. New York: Springer-Verlag; 1988. p. 122–67.

2. Markland WR. Shampoos. In: deNavarre MG, editor. The chemistry and manufacture of cosmetics, vol. IV, 2nd edition. Wheaton (IL): Allured Publishing Corporation; 1988. p. 1283–312.

3. Bouillon C. Shampoos and hair conditioners. Clin Dermatol 1988;6:83–92.

4. Fox C. An introduction to the formulation of shampoos. Cosmet Toilet 1988;103:25–58.

5. Zviak C, Vanlerberghe G. Scalp and hair hygiene. In: Zviak C, editor. The science of hair care. New York: Marcel Dekker; 1986. p. 49–86.

6. Shipp JJ. Hair-care products. In: Williams DF, Schmitt WH, editors. Chemistry and technology of the cosmetics and toiletries industry. London: Blackie Academic & Professional; 1992. p. 32–54.

7. Tokiwa F, Hayashi S, Okumura T. Hair and surfactants. In: Kobori T, Montagna W, editors. Biology and disease of the hair. Baltimore (MD): University Park Press; 1975. p. 631–40.

8. Powers DH. Shampoos. In: Balsam MS, Gershon SD, Reiger MM, et al, editors. Cosmetics science and technology. 2nd edition. New York: Wiley-Interscience; 1972. p. 73–116.

9. Hunting ALL. Can there be cleaning and conditioning in the same product? Cosmet Toilet 1988;103:73–8.

10. Gruber J, Lamoureux B, Joshi N, et al. The use of x-ray fluorescent spectroscopy to study the influence of cationic polymers on silicone oil deposition from shampoo. J Cosmet Sci 2001;52:131–6.

11. Harusawa F, Nakama Y, Tanaka M. Anionic-cationic ion-pairs as conditioning agents in shampoos. Cosmet Toilet 1991;106:35–9.

12. Sun J, Parr J, Travagline D. Stable conditioning shampoos containing high molecular weight dimethicone. Cosmet Toilet 2002;117:41–50.

13. Karjala SA, Williamson JE, Karler A. Studies on the substantivity of collagen-derived peptides to human hair. J Soc Cosmet Chem 1966;17:513–24.

14. Swift JA, Brown AC. The critical determination of fine change in the surface architecture of human hair due to cosmetic treatment. J Soc Cosmet Chem 1972;23:675–702.

15. Menkart J. Damaged hair. Cutis 1979;23:276–8.

16. Allardice A, Gummo G. Hair conditioning. Cosmet Toilet 1993;108:107–9.

17. Idson B, Lee W. Update on hair conditioner ingredients. Cosmet Toilet 1983;98:41–6.

18. Finkelstein P. Hair conditioners. Cutis 1970;6:543–4.

Long-Term Removal of Unwanted Hair Using Light

Soodabeh Zandi, MD[a,b], Harvey Lui, MD, FRCPC[a,*]

KEYWORDS

- Hair removal • Photoepilation • Laser • Intense pulsed light

KEY POINTS

- Photoepilation is based on the extended theory of selective photothermolysis, which aims to destroy follicular cells via heat. Follicular melanin is the target chromophore that locally converts the treatment light into heat.
- Different types of laser or light systems are available for photoepilation. Commonly used options include the alexandrite, diode, or long-pulsed Nd:YAG lasers and intense pulsed light (IPL) devices.
- For best results and least side effects, appropriate selection of parameters and patients is essential. The four most important treatment parameters to consider are fluence, pulse duration, wavelength, and spot size.

INTRODUCTION

Cultural and sociologic norms dictate that hair growth not only should be luxuriant and healthy but also must appear only in certain specific body sites according to gender roles. Removal of hair that is not supposed to be visible at certain sites has been performed by peoples of different cultural backgrounds all over the world for centuries. Like clothing fashions, preferences for displaying or removing hair can change dramatically over time. With occasional exceptions, such as pseudofolliculitis barbae, acne keloidalis, pilonidal sinus, trichiasis, and hidradenitis suppurative, hair removal is driven almost exclusively by personal preferences and societal pressures rather than being medically necessary. Social customs also influence whether a given hair removal process should preferably be long-term (ie, permanent) as opposed to temporary. For example, the daily ritual of removing facial hair temporarily becomes a rite of passage among maturing adolescent men, and for the rest of their lives men are more

or less conditioned to dutifully attend to this practice to varying degrees without ever wishing that their facial hair be permanently gone. In contrast, body hair among men is no longer the preferred esthete, with a corresponding demand by both sexes for smooth bodies. A range of physical, chemical, and pharmacologic approaches exist for dealing with unwanted hair, and most deliver excellent short-term results. The development of lasers and other high-intensity light sources for removing hair, also known as *photoepilation*, has raised the realistic specter of effective and efficient long-term hair removal and is the focus of this review. The extent to which light-based hair removal remains a medical procedure will depend largely on the development of devices that can be used safely by consumers without the need for physician supervision. In this article, unless otherwise specified, the term *light* when used alone without qualification refers collectively to lasers and other (ie, nonlaser) high-intensity sources.

Once the principle of selective photothermolysis for highly targeted therapy was proven via the

[a] Photomedicine Institute, Department of Dermatology and Skin Science, University of British Columbia, 835 West 10th Avenue, Vancouver, BC, Canada V5Z 4E8; [b] Department of Dermatology, Kerman University of Medical Sciences, Kerman, Iran
* Corresponding author.
E-mail address: harvey.lui@ubc.ca

Dermatol Clin 31 (2013) 179–191
http://dx.doi.org/10.1016/j.det.2012.08.017
0733-8635/13/$ – see front matter © 2013 Elsevier Inc. All rights reserved.

effective destruction of port wine stain blood vessels[1] using pulsed lasers, it was only a matter of time until the hair follicle could be similarly targeted. The initial systematic approach to laser hair removal used millisecond ruby laser pulses with the goal of achieving permanent effects.[2,3] Prior studies on laser hair removal had focused on medically abnormal hair growth, such as pilonidal sinuses. In 1996, the U.S. Food and Drug Administration (FDA) approved the use of lasers for removing hair, and since then hair removal has grown to become the most common medical application of high-intensity photonic devices.[4] The transformation of the hair removal industry since the mid-1990s is paralleled by an extensive literature documenting the exploration of dosimetry, novel devices, and clinical methods for using this technology (**Fig. 1**).

The FDA permits device companies to claim permanent *reduction*, but not permanent *removal* of hair for their lasers or intense light sources. Permanent hair reduction is defined as the long-term, stable reduction in the number of hairs regrowing after a treatment regime, which may include several sessions, but does not necessarily imply that all hairs within the treatment area are eliminated.[5]

More specifically, the number of regrowing hairs must be stable over a period greater than the duration of the complete growth cycle of hair follicles, which varies from 4 to 12 months according to body location. Mechanistically, the energy required to induce thermal follicular destruction is mediated through the photobiologic targeting of melanin within the hair follicle complex.

EXCESSIVE OR UNWANTED HAIR GROWTH

Excessive hair growth can perhaps be distinguished from unwanted hair largely by the notion that "unwanted hair" refers specifically to a subjective patient expectation, whereas "excessive hair" growth implies either a significant deviation from normal physiology or a pathologic process. Excessive hair growth is usually also unwanted by patients, but no question exists that a large

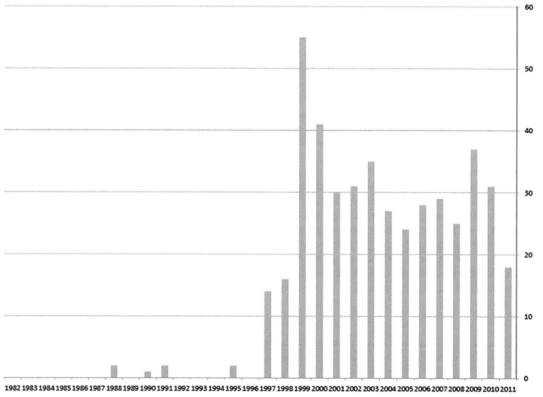

MEDLINE articles on removing hair with light

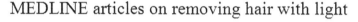

Fig. 1. The development of lasers and high-intensity light sources can be tracked indirectly through the MEDLINE database. Note the abrupt and sustained rate of publications beginning in 1997, 1 year after the FDA approved the first laser for hair removal.

proportion of patients who have unwanted hair have absolutely no physiologic or pathologic hair excess. In these cases, the unwanted hair is fundamentally a cosmetic concern. Racial variations in normal hair pigmentation and growth can be the source of unwanted hair, particularly for women.

Pathologically excessive hair growth can be classified to 2 groups: hypertrichosis and hirsutism.

Hypertrichosis

Hypertrichosis generally refers to diffuse or localized hair growth in androgen-independent areas of the body. Hypertrichosis develops when vellus hairs convert to terminal hairs. Diffuse hypertrichosis may be caused by medications, anorexia nervosa, or genetic, developmental, and metabolic disorders.

Hirsutism

Hirsutism is defined as excessive terminal hair growth in androgen-dependent areas of face or body of women, including the lip, sideburn area, chin, and chest. Hirsutism affects 5% to 15% of women,[6] and is usually related to qualitative changes in hair fiber, such as diameter, pigmentation, and length, rather than the number of hair follicles. The hair count is genetically determined and the number of hair follicles depends on factors such as race and ethnicity. Hirsutism affects quality of life and can induce anxiety, depression, embarrassment, low self-confidence, and body dissatisfaction.[7,8] In hirsutism treatment, the goals are destruction of the hair follicle and/or reduction in the hair shaft caliber.[9]

Polycystic ovary syndrome is the most common cause of androgen overproduction. Adrenal hyperplasia, hyperandrogenic insulin-resistant acanthosis nigricans syndrome, androgen-secreting tumors and androgenic drug intake are less frequent causes.[6] Idiopathic hirsutism is caused by increased sensitivity of hair follicles to normal levels of circulating androgen and/or increased peripheral conversion of testosterone to dihydrotestosterone by 5α-reductase.

LASER AND LIGHT BIOPHYSICS AND HAIR REMOVAL

The extended theory of selective photothermolysis is the principal mechanism of laser hair removal.[10] Melanin in the hair shaft, outer root sheath of infundibulum, and matrix is the main chromophore for laser hair removal. Melanin as a chromophore absorbs certain wavelengths in the red and infrared parts of the electromagnetic spectrum. After laser beam energy is absorbed, it transforms

to heat in the tissue and causes damage to the hair follicle. For permanent hair removal, follicular stem cells in the bulge region and/or dermal papilla should be destroyed by heat diffusion from the melanin to the stem cells. Because the actual chromophore and target are not identical, the pulse duration should be longer than the chromophore thermal relaxation time to conduct heat diffusion to hair follicle stem cells.[11] Because of the relative or absolute absence of melanin within light-colored, red, gray, white, or vellus hair, photon absorption is insufficient to cause photothermal follicular alteration. Dark hair on a background of light skin represents the best target for treatment.

Optimizing Hair Removal Via Skin Cooling

To remove unwanted hairs from any given area, light must pass through the epidermis and then be absorbed by target hair follicles in the dermis. During laser hair removal, the delivered fluence at the skin surface must be high enough so that sufficient photons are delivered to and absorbed at the depth of the follicle to cause irreversible damage to the hair-producing apparatus. Melanin within the interfollicular epidermis competes with hair follicle melanin for laser energy absorption. When the epidermal temperature is 45°C or greater, epidermal thermal damage can occur. If the heat produced within the epidermis can be dissipated or prevented from exceeding the 45°C threshold, the risk of damage will be decreased. Therefore, cooling the skin surface, especially in darker skin types, can decrease epidermal thermal damage and minimize laser-induced side effects.[12] Cooling also permits treatment with higher fluences, thereby increasing the overall effectiveness of laser hair removal.[13]

PHOTOEPILATION DEVICES FOR HAIR REMOVAL (TABLE 1)
Ruby

Long-pulsed ruby lasers were the first laser used for hair removal. A xenon flash lamp excites a ruby crystal that emits a laser beam of 694 nm. Ruby lasers are indicated in Fitzpatrick skin types I through III with dark hair. Primarily because of their relative inefficiency and high cost, ruby lasers are no longer commercially available in North America.

Neodymium:Yttrium-Aluminum-Garnet

Initially, the Q-switched neodymium:yttrium-aluminum-garnet (Nd:YAG) laser was used in combination with a carbon particle suspension that was applied topically to the skin before laser treatment. Subsequently, the carbon suspension was shown to be not necessary and that long-pulsed rather than ultrashort Q-switched pulsed lasers were more effective for hair removal.[14] The long-pulsed Nd:YAG laser is best indicated for patients with Fitzpatrick skin phototype VI. The Nd:YAG laser system operates at a longer wavelength (1064 nm) than the alexandrite laser, allowing deeper penetration into the dermis.[15] The Nd:YAG laser is less absorbed by epidermal melanin, and therefore is possibly more suitable for darker skin types because of lesser side effects in these patients. Clinical studies have shown less hair removal with the Nd:YAG laser than with the ruby or alexandrite lasers.[15]

Alexandrite

The long-pulsed alexandrite (755 nm) laser has been shown to be effective for hair removal. Patients with Fitzpatrick skin phototypes I through IV can be treated with long-pulse alexandrite lasers.[11]

Diode

The long-pulsed diode laser has been used for laser hair removal, and is recommended for patients with Fitzpatrick skin phototypes I through V. Multiple arrays of semiconductor diodes provide a laser light of 800 to 810 nm.[15] Diode lasers are generally considered reliable devices.

Nonlaser Devices

Intense pulsed light (IPL) devices emit polychromatic noncoherent light with wavelengths ranging from 400 to 1400 nm. With these light sources, different filters are used to target different chromophores. The light delivery systems for IPLs consist of broad rectangular crystal probes that are held in contact with the skin. Good alignment of each adjacent rectangular exposure pulse and maintenance of skin contact over the entire crystal surface are important for uniform treatment.

Radiofrequency Combined with IPL

Dual-energy technology is based on the delivery of synchronous pulses of bipolar radiofrequency current and pulsed visible light within the same pulse to reduce the light intensity and side effects.

PHOTOEPILATION TECHNIQUES
Patient Preparation and Selection

Before treatment, patient evaluation should focus on identifying treatable causes of hirsutism or hypertrichosis, reviewing previously used methods for hair removal and checking for a history of herpes labialis or genitalis if perioral or pubic areas are to be treated. The informed consent process should include a review of potential complications, such as blistering and crusting, and side effects such as hypopigmentation, hyperpigmentation, scarring, keloid formation, paradoxical hypertrichosis, and infection. In addition, patients must have realistic expectations of what is possible with light-based hair removal, particularly the fact that these procedures lead to long-term reduction of hair but not necessarily complete and permanent removal. Patients should be informed that lasers are less effective for treating vellus hair or hair that is light-colored, red, gray, or white.

For up to 6 weeks before and after treatment, patients should use a broad-spectrum sunscreen and avoid tanning or applying sunless tanners. They should also avoid plucking, waxing, or electrolysis 2 weeks before treatment, because this can make it difficult to visualize and delineate the target sites during treatment. Relative contraindications to using light to remove hair include gold therapy, isotretinoin therapy in the previous 6 months, photosensitizing drugs, pregnancy, and photosensitive disorders. In darker skin patients, test spot treatments are often appropriate for determining the appropriate laser parameters and also predicting the degree to which postinflammatory dyspigmentation may occur. Other situations that warrant caution include patients

Table 1				
Devices used to remove hair with light				
	Wavelength	Pulse Duration (ms)	Fluence (J/cm^2)	Spot Size (mm)
Ruby	694	No longer commercially available in North America		
Nd:YAG	1064	0.1–10000	Up to 900	1.5–30 x 30
Diode	800–810	5–500	Up to 100	5–22 x 35
Alexandrite	755	0.1–300	Up to 600	1.5–18
IPL	400–1400	0.3–500	Up to 500	Up to 50 x 25

who have disorders that may koebnerize (eg, vitiligo, psoriasis) or who have a tendency to form keloids.

Anesthesia and Pain Control

Topical anesthetics reduce pain for laser hair removal. There is no difference between lidocaine and EMLA cream for pain control in laser hair removal. Therefore, cost and potential side effects are important factors in selecting the appropriate anesthetic.[16] One to 2 hours before the laser treatment, a topical anesthetic cream may be applied and covered to reduce pain. Moistened gauze can be used to cover the skin after applying topical anesthetic to maximize its effects and ensure its adherence to the target sites. Topical piroxicam and EMLA provided similar pain relief in female patients after 1064-nm Nd:YAG laser-assisted hair removal. Topical piroxicam has fewer inflammatory side effects.[17] Various skin-cooling systems also reduce pain and discomfort. Pneumatic skin flattening (PSF) technology is believed to reduce pain by invoking the "gate theory" of pain transmission (see later section on "vacuum-assisted treatment").

Primary Laser and Light Treatment Parameters

There are 4 main parameters to consider when using lasers and light: wavelength, fluence, spot size, and pulse duration. The wavelength is usually fixed according to the specific device type, whereas the operator selects the fluence, spot size, and pulse duration.

Wavelength

Melanin within the hair shaft is the chromophore for laser hair removal. Although melanin is absorbed by all wavelengths throughout the ultraviolet, visible, and near-infrared (NIR) regions, only the longer-wavelength photons (ie, red to NIR) are capable of penetrating the skin to the level of the growing hair follicle. NIR lasers may be associated with a lower risk of skin dyspigmentation after treatment because of their lower absorption by epidermal melanin compared with red photons.

Spot size

The spot size is the diameter of the laser beam or the overall linear dimensions of the IPL skin contact probe. Because of the phenomenon of lateral scattering of light once it penetrates the skin, the spot size has an effect on the effective depth of light penetration. If all other parameters are held constant, a larger spot size will result in an overall greater depth of effect, which is desirable for targeting hair follicles.

Pulse duration

Pulse duration refers to the subsecond duration of each light exposure, and is inversely proportional to the peak power density of the laser or light pulses. According to the theory of selective photothermolysis, thermal effects within tissue can be confined to a specific structure through heating that structure faster than it cools. The rate at which any tissue component cools is largely dependent on the square of its physical diameter and is usually specified by its thermal relaxation time, which in turn is the time it takes for the target to dissipate half of its heat to the surrounding tissue. To achieve selective photothermolysis, the optimal pulse duration is roughly equal to or shorter than the thermal relaxation time.

Hair-bearing skin contains melanin as a chromophore both within the hair shaft and the interfollicular surface epidermis. During laser hair removal, epidermal melanin represents an unintended bystander target. Clinical effects on the epidermis can be minimized through selecting pulse durations that are longer but do not exceed the follicular thermal relaxation time. Longer pulse durations allow for more gentle heating of the epidermis by slowing the deposition of the light energy into the skin; the more gradually the pigmented epidermis absorbs light, the slower its conversion to heat, making cooling more efficient and limiting any deleterious thermal effects on the interfollicular epidermis.[12] This mechanism is essentially an extension of the concept of selective photothermolysis, and has been referred to as *thermokinetic selectivity*, which states that smaller structures (eg, epidermal melanin) will lose heat more quickly than larger structures (eg, dermal hair follicles). The pulse durations in laser and light devices have a range from 1 to 600 ms; usually pulse durations longer than 100 ms are preferred in darker skin types.

Fluence

The amount of energy delivered to a unit area in a single pulse is defined as fluence. Higher fluences deliver more photons to the hair follicle, and therefore higher energy results in more hair reduction. However, the risk of inducing side effects will be increased with higher fluences. Some authors recommend test treatment spots to determine suitable energy and pulse duration settings, particularly in dark-skinned patients. The test spot should be selected to match with the treatment area in terms of skin color and hair density.[12] From a practical point of view, the fluence should be gradually titrated upward until the clinical threshold of immediate perifollicular erythema and edema is reached; this determines the appropriate optimal fluence setting.[11] Another useful immediate treatment end point is whether hairs within the treatment site can be easily pulled and released from the skin using epilating forceps. The fluence should be gradually increased until this is observed.

Secondary Parameters and Techniques for Photoepilation

Skin cooling

A variety of techniques for skin cooling have been devised to lower the epidermal temperature through direct contact (ie, aqueous gel or chilled transparent optical handpiece tips) or the delivery of cold air or cryogen sprays to the skin surface. Aggressive cooling with cryogen spray and cold air has been associated with blistering and discoloration of the skin.[12]

Scanners

Many laser hair removal systems are equipped with automated scanners that will direct a series of laser pulses uniformly over defined treatment areas. This feature is important for increasing treatment efficiency, especially when treating broader areas such as the back, chest, or extremities.

Vacuum-assisted treatment

Vacuum-assisted hand pieces are currently featured in diode lasers and work by stretching the skin through suction, which essentially positions the hair follicle closer to the skin surface. The stretched epidermis also means that the laser energy is distributed over a larger area, such that the density of epidermal melanin and heating within that layer are reduced. This handpiece design is promoted as being capable of removing hair at lower fluences and greater coverage rates.[18]

PSF technology decreases pain based on Melzack and Wall's[19] "gate theory" of pain transmission, in which activation of nerves that do not transmit pain signals interferes with signal transmission from pain fibers. The PSF suction device stimulates the tactile and pressure receptors on skin before the laser pulse and blocks the transmission of pain. PSF also decreases blood flow in dermal vessels, removing a competing chromophore from the treatment area. PSF has reduced pain associated with hair removal by laser or IPL.[20]

Frequency and Number of Treatments

Multiple laser treatments are necessary to achieve long-term reduction of hair, typically in the range of 5 to 7 sessions spaced approximately 4 to 8 weeks apart. With each session, an estimated 15% to 30% of hairs are removed.[11] Treated hairs usually shed 2 weeks after the laser treatment. Treated sites will manifest a decrease in the total hair density with treatment and/or miniaturization of hairs.

TREATMENT EFFICACY OF LIGHT-BASED HAIR REMOVAL

Multiple studies have shown efficacy of different lasers in reducing unwanted hairs. Relevant controlled studies were selected from the MEDLINE database up to 2012 based on the following key criteria: randomized controlled trials with more than 1 treatment applied to the same individual, with or without observer blinding; randomized controlled trials with 1 treatment were excluded. The results are presented in **Table 2**. In long-term clinical trials, photoepilation devices have been shown to reduce hair counts by approximately 50% after a series of multiple treatments.[37]

Comparing Photoepilation with Other Methods of Hair Removal

Physical methods for removing excess hair include waxing (including sugar forms), shaving, threading, plucking, chemical depilation, electrolysis, and bleaching. Waxing removes hair down to the root, diminishing the required frequency of physical hair removal. Shaving is a frequently used method of reducing hair, but it only has a short-term effect. Depilatory creams decrease hair by dissolving the disulfide bonds and peptides of hair keratin.[9] Electrolysis is the only form of physical epilation that produces a permanent hair reduction through destroying the hair follicle via electric current or heat delivered through a needle that is manually inserted into the hair follicle. Electrolysis can reduce nonpigmented and pigmented hair. This method is completely dependent on operator technique and results are variable.[38] In 2000, Görgü and colleagues[39] compared the effectiveness of long-pulse alexandrite laser hair removal with electrolysis in 12 patients. The average clearance rate of the hairs was 74% by laser and 35% by electrolysis 6 months after the initial treatment.

Eflornithine hydrochloride 13.9% cream or difluoromethylornithine is an irreversible inhibitor of ornithine decarboxylase that slows the growth phase of hair and is effective for excessive facial hair caused by medical or hereditary conditions.[40]

Combination Approaches to Hair Removal

Pharmacologic treatments are often used in combination with laser hair removal. In a randomized, double-blind, placebo-controlled, right–left

Table 2
Randomized controlled trials of laser and light-based hair removal

Author, Year	Number of Patients	Blinding	Primary Outcome	Laser or IPL	Follow-Up	Side Effects	Number of Treatments	Results
Allison et al,[21] 2003	68	None	Hair count	Ruby laser, 2 treatments vs 3 treatments	5 mo after treatment	Superficial burn, hypopigmentation, herpes	2 or 3	2 treatments = 3 treatments
Nouri et al,[22] 2004	17	Blind photo	Hair count	Alexandrite, 8-mm and 12-mm spot size vs control	6 mo after treatment	None	3	12-mm alexandrite <18-mm alexandrite
Fiskerstrand et al,[23] 2003	41	Blind photo	Hair count	Diode laser, 800 vs 810 nm	6 mo after treatment	Redness	3	810-nm diode = 800-nm diode
Handrick & Alster,[24] 2001	20	Blind photo	Hair count	Alexandrite/diode, 35 J/cm² vs 40 J/cm²	6 mo after treatment	Hyperpigmentation	3	Alexandrite = diode
Clayton et al,[25] 2005	88/PCOS	None	(1) Self-reported severity of facial hair (2) Depression score	Alexandrite laser, low-fluence vs high-fluence	6 mo during treatment	None	5	High fluence > low fluence
Toosi et al,[26] 2006	232	None	(1) Hair reduction (2) Side effects	Alexandrite vs diode vs IPL	6 mo after treatment	Diode > IPL and alexandrite	3-6	Alexandrite = diode = IPL
Smith et al,[27] 2006	44	Yes	(1) Physician's global assessment (2) Physician comparison (3) Subject's self-assessment	Nd:YAG or alexandrite plus eflornithine vs Nd:YAG or alexandrite	34 wk during treatment	Equal in both groups	2	Eflornithine plus laser > laser
Hamzavi et al,[28] 2007	31	Double-blind	(1) Investigator global scoring (2) Patient self-assessment (3) Hair count analysis	Alexandrite plus eflornithine or placebo	2 wk after last treatments	None	Up to 6	Eflornithine plus laser > laser

(continued on next page)

Table 2
(continued)

Author, Year	Number of Patients	Blinding	Primary Outcome	Laser or IPL	Follow-Up	Side Effects	Number of Treatments	Results
Sand et al,[29] 2007	32 Blonde, white and gray hair	Double-blind	(1) Hair count (2) Patient satisfaction	Liposomal melanin spray (Lipoxome) plus diode laser vs physiologic saline spray plus diode laser	6 mo after treatments	Perifollicular urticaria Erythema Folliculitis	3	Disappointing results in both groups
Davoudi et al,[30] 2008	20	Single-blind	Hair count	Nd:YAG laser vs alexandrite laser (12-mm spot size) vs alexandrite laser (18-mm spot size) vs combination of Nd:YAG and alexandrite	18 mo	Hyperpigmentation Side effects more common in combination group	4	No significance difference among 4 groups
Rezvanian et al,[31] 2009	70/PCOS	None	(1) Hair diameter (2) Hair count (3) Free androgen index (4) Hirsutism score (5) Homeostasis model assessment for insulin resistance	IPL plus metformin vs IPL	6 mo	Nausea, diarrhea, and abdominal pain from metformin	5	IPL plus metformin > IPL
Braun,[32] 2009	25	Single-blind	(1) Hair count (2) Pain score	Low-fluence, high-repetition diode laser vs high-fluence, low-repetition diode	6 mo	Superficial burn	5	No statistically difference between groups Pain less in low-fluence group

Study	N	Blinding	Outcomes	Comparison	Follow-up	Side effects	Score	Results
Haak et al,[33] 2010	31	Single-blind	(1) Hair count (2) Patient evaluation in hairiness and (3) Patient satisfaction (4) Pain (5) Side effects	IPL vs long-pulse diode	6 mo after treatments	Transient hypopigmentation and hyperpigmentation Pain	6	No difference between IPL and long-pulse diode
Bakus et al,[34] 2010	11 Fine hair	Single-blind	(1) Hair count (2) Patient satisfaction	Single-pulse vs double-pulse Nd:YAG	6 mo and 24 mo after treatment	Erythema and edema were less in double-pulse mode	4	No difference
Braun,[35] 2011	22	Single-blind	Hair count	High-fluence, single-pass diode vs low-fluence, multiple-pass diode	18 mo	Less pain in low-fluence, multiple-pass group	5	No difference
Pai,[36] 2011	42/PCOS	None	(1) Hair count (2) Pain assessment	Low-fluence, high-repetition rate vs high-fluence, low-repetition-rate 810-nm diode laser	End of 6 treatments	Less pain in low-fluence, multiple-pass group	6	No significant difference in hair reduction between groups Significant reduction in hair thickness

Abbreviation: PCOS, polycystic ovary syndrome.

The search strategy used was as follows: 1. hirsutism/; 2. hypertrichosis/; 3. hyperandrogenism/; 4. hair.ti. or hair.ab.; 5. hair-removal.mp. or Hair Removal/; 6. hair-follicle.mp. or Hair Follicle/; 7. hirsutism.ti. or hirsutism.ab.; 8. hypertrichosis.ti. or hypertrichosis.ab.; 9. hyperandrogenism.ti. or hyperandrogenism.ab.; 10. 1 or 2 or 3 or 4 or 5 or 6 or 7 or 8 or 9; 11. exp light/; 12. exp laser-surgery/; 13. exp light coagulation/; 14. laser*.ti. or laser*.ab.; 15. light*.ti. or light*.ab.; 16. 11 or 12 or 13 or 14 or 15; 17. 10 and 16; 18. randomized controlled trial.pt.; 19. controlled clinical trial.pt.; 20. randomized.ab.; 21. placebo.ab.; 22. drug therapy.fs.; 23. randomly.ab.; 24. trial.ab.; 25. groups.ab.; 26. 18 or 19 or 20 or 21 or 22 or 23 or 24 or 25; 27. exp animals/not humans.sh.

comparison study, Hamzavi and colleagues[28] showed significantly better results in favor of eflornithine cream plus alexandrite laser versus laser treatment alone for treating unwanted hair on the upper lip. The combination approach resulted in more rapid hair reduction and was associated with greater patient satisfaction. In a randomized controlled trial, 70 women with polycystic ovary syndrome received metformin with IPL therapy or IPL therapy alone; 52 patients finished the study. Hair reduction and patient satisfaction was significantly better in the metformin plus IPL group at the end of the 6 months' follow-up.[31]

Treating Other Localized Hair-Bearing Sites

Laser hair removal has been used to treat pseudofolliculitis barbae. In 2009, Schulze and colleagues[41] reported that low-fluence 1064-nm laser treatment can improve pseudofolliculitis barbae. Acne keloidalis is another skin disease that can be improved by laser hair removal through the destruction of tufted hairs that act as foreign bodies. The treatment results for acne keloidalis will be more satisfactory if laser hair removal is combined with other treatments, such as antibiotics.[12] For pilonidal sinus, laser hair removal after surgery can decrease the risk of recurrence of disease.[42] The long-pulse Nd:YAG laser is also effective for treating of hidradenitis suppurativa, although the end point of this laser indication is the reduction of inflammatory nodules and scarring rather than hair removal per se.[43]

WHERE IS PHOTOEPILATION PERFORMED?

In 2011, laser hair removal was the third most common minimally invasive cosmetic procedure after botulinum toxin and hyaluronic acid injections.[4] Laser hair removal was originally performed in medical clinics and offices under the direct supervision of physicians, because class IV laser devices were used. Over time, laser hair removal has come to be performed in a variety of medical and nonmedical settings (eg, spas, beauty salons, hair salons), all governed by a multiplicity of differing regulations and standards, depending on the specific legal jurisdiction. In reality, laser operators can range from minimally trained lay individuals to cosmeticians, laser technicians, nurses, and physicians. One study has compared the outcome of 100 patients who underwent laser hair removal performed by a trained supervised nurse versus a trained physician and found no differences in overall efficacy, adverse effects, or patient satisfaction.[44]

Home Photoepilation

In 2008, the FDA approved laser hair removal devices for home use. The first home-use lasers required a prescription, but consumers can now buy these devices without a prescription.

No trials have compared the relative efficacies of home-use lasers with office-based devices.

Tria

The Tria laser (Tria Beauty, Inc, Dublin, CA) is an 810-nm hand-held device that has 3 energy fluence settings (high: 22.0 J/cm^2; medium: 17.5 J/cm^2; and low: 13.0 J/cm^2) with 3 respective pulse widths (600, 450, and 300 ms). The spot size is 1.0 cm^2. Different studies using this laser have shown varying degrees of hair reduction, from 10% to 72%. In one clinical trial, the mean hair reduction at 1, 6, and 12 months after 3 treatments was found to be 60%, 41%, and 33%, respectively.[45]

E-One

The E-One is a compact IPL-type flash device that is filtered to 580 nm (E-Swin, Paris, France). Its pulse duration is 34 ms and it operates at lower fluences than office IPLs. E-One has been compared with hot wax for axillary depilation and found to be more efficient.[46]

No! No!

The No! No! is a hand-held self-treatment device (Thermicon, Radiancy Inc, Orangeburg, NY) that consists of an AC/DC power converter and a handpiece that houses a replaceable thermal filament. The filament delivers heat to the hair shaft, which is then transferred to the follicle. In 2009, Spencer[47] showed that the No! No! device cleared approximately 43% of hair from the legs and 15% from the umbilicus/bikini line areas at 12 weeks after stopping treatment.

Silk'n

Silk'n (Home Skinovations Ltd, Israel) is an IPL device with wavelengths of 475 to 1200 nm, a spot size of 6 cm^2, and 2 energy settings. Silk'n is suitable for light-skin phenotypes (types I–IV) and the FDA has approved it for nonfacial skin hair removal. SensEpil, a newer model of the Silk'n, has a sensor for increasing safety; it will not fire on skin types V and VI. The built-in skin sensor will determine skin types and fire only on lighter skin types. It also does not allow the device to flash when not in contact with skin. In 2009, Alster and Tanzi[48] studied the Silk'n device on 20 women with skin types I through IV. The response was better in the legs, which showed between 37% and 53% hair reduction at 6 months.

LASER SAFETY AND COMPLICATIONS

Eye protection is essential for any type of laser or light-based hair removal device, and both the patient and operator must use goggles. Each goggle protects against specific wavelengths, so goggles cannot be exchanged between lasers. Because of the potential risk of eye damage, laser hair removal devices should not be used within the bony orbit.[49] When working around the lips, the enamel of the teeth should also be covered by gauze.[12]

Skin color, body location, and sun exposure are the major factors that influence laser hair removal complications. The extremities show the highest rate of side effects, whereas sun-protected areas, such as the axillary and inguinal areas, are associated with lower risk. Complications usually occur more in individuals with tanned or darker skin phototypes.[50]

Discoloration (Hyperpigmentation and Hypopigmentation)

Pigmentary changes are the most common side effects of photoepilation and can manifest as either hypopigmentation or hyperpigmentation. Hyperpigmentation occurs in 14% to 25% of individuals, and hypopigmentation in 10% to 17%.[15] The selection of the proper wavelength, pulse duration, and fluence will decrease the risk of side effects. Optimal cooling of epidermis also reduces the risk of pigmentary changes, which are usually transient and improve over a weeks to months, although hypopigmentation can be permanent, particularly in individuals at risk for vitiligo.

Paradoxical Hypertrichosis

Paradoxical hypertrichosis is an increase in hair density, color, or coarseness at laser hair removal sites or adjacent areas occurring in the absence of any known cause of hypertrichosis. All types of laser and light sources can induce paradoxical hypertrichosis.[51] Paradoxical hypertrichosis can occur in 0.01% to 1.9%[52] and up to 10%[53] of treated patients. The pathogenesis for this effect is poorly understood. Subtherapeutic thermal injury to hair follicles may cause induction of active hair cycling,[51] or the overall effect may be related to hair cycle synchronization within the treated sites. Paradoxical hypertrichosis mostly occurs on the face and neck of female patients. Individuals with darker skin and black hair may be at higher risk.[40] Other factors that may contribute to developing paradoxical hypertrichosis are the presence of posttreatment side effects (crusting, erythema, and hyperpigmentation), superficial

depth of treatment, suboptimal treatment fluences, and presence of hormonal conditions, such as polycystic ovary syndrome.[51] Laser-induced paradoxical hair growth can be treated with subsequent laser therapies at moderate to high fluences.[50] Patients should be informed about paradoxical hypertrichosis during the consent form process.[40]

Scarring

Fortunately scarring is a less common complication that usually only occurs at high laser fluences or with inexperienced operators.

Urticaria

Urticaria can occur 24 to 72 hours after laser photoepilation. It may be caused by rupture of hair follicles by laser and induction of delayed hypersensitivity reactions.[54,55]

Other Side Effects

Fox-Fordyce disease[56] has been reported after laser hair removal. Local anesthetic toxicity can be induced through applying topical agents to large surface areas with or without occlusion for prolonged periods.[57]

SUMMARY

Laser and light-based hair removal has become one of the most ubiquitous procedures performed on the skin. Dermatologists should be familiar with the principles of photoepilation and the expected outcomes, limitations, and complications. No single device is considered to be superior to the others, and optimal treatment outcomes require individual customization of specific treatment parameters.

REFERENCES

1. Anderson RR, Parrish JA. Selective photothermolysis: precise microsurgery by selective absorption of pulsed radiation. Science 1983;220:524–7.
2. Grossman MC, Dierickx C, Farinelli W, et al. Damage to hair follicles by normal-mode ruby laser pulses. J Am Acad Dermatol 1996;35:889–94.
3. Dierickx CC, Grossman MC, Farinelli WA, et al. Permanent hair removal by normal-mode ruby laser. Arch Dermatol 1998;134:837–42.
4. Celebrating 15 years of trustworthy plastic surgery statistics. Available at: http://www.surgery.org/media/news-releases/celebrating-15-years-of-trustworthy-plastic-surgery-statistics. Accessed August 20, 2012.
5. Radiation-emitting products. Available at: http://www.fda.gov/Radiation-EmittingProducts/ResourcesforYou

RadiationEmittingProducts/ucm252761.htm. Accessed August 20, 2012.

6. Azziz R. The evaluation and management of hirsutism. Obstet Gynecol 2003;101:995–1007.

7. Jackson J, Caro JJ, Caro G, et al. The effect of eflornithine 13.9% cream on the bother and discomfort due to hirsutism. Int J Dermatol 2007;46:976–81.

8. Keegan A, Liao LM, Boyle M. 'Hirsutism': a psychological analysis. J Health Psychol 2003;8:327–45.

9. Brodell LA, Mercurio MG. Hirsutism: diagnosis and management. Gend Med 2010;7:79–87.

10. Altshuler GB, Anderson RR, Manstein D, et al. Extended theory of selective photothermolysis. Lasers Surg Med 2001;29:416–32.

11. Ibrahimi OA, Avram MM, Hanke CW, et al. Laser hair removal. Dermatol Ther 2011;24:94–107.

12. Battle EF Jr. Advances in laser hair removal in skin of color. J Drugs Dermatol 2011;10:1235–9.

13. Zenzie HH, Altshuler GB, Smirnov MZ, et al. Evaluation of cooling methods for laser dermatology. Lasers Surg Med 2000;26:130–44.

14. Nanni CA, Alster TS. Optimizing treatment parameters for hair removal using a topical carbon-based solution and 1064-nm q-switched neodymium: YAG laser energy. Arch Dermatol 1997;133:1546–9.

15. Sanchez LA, Perez M, Azziz R. Laser hair reduction in the hirsute patient: a critical assessment. Hum Reprod Update 2002;8:169–81.

16. Guardiano RA, Norwood CW. Direct comparison of EMLA versus lidocaine for pain control in Nd: YAG 1,064 nm laser hair removal. Dermatol Surg 2005;31:396–8.

17. Akinturk S, Eroglu A. A clinical comparison of topical piroxicam and EMLA cream for pain relief and inflammation in laser hair removal. Lasers Med Sci 2009;24:535–8.

18. Xia Y, Moore R, Cho S, et al. Evaluation of the vacuum-assisted handpiece compared with the sapphire-cooled handpiece of the 800-nm diode laser system for the use of hair removal and reduction. J Cosmet Laser Ther 2010;12:264–8.

19. Melzack R, Wall PD. Pain mechanisms: A new theory. Science 1965;150:171–7.

20. Yeung CK, Shek SY, Chan HH. Hair removal with neodymium-doped yttrium aluminum garnet laser and pneumatic skin flattening in Asians. Dermatol Surg 2010;36:1664–70.

21. Allison KP, Kiernan MN, Waters RA, et al. Evaluation of the ruby 694 Chromos for hair removal in various skin sites. Lasers Med Sci 2003;18:165–70.

22. Nouri K, Chen H, Saghari S, et al. Comparing 18-versus 12-mm spot size in hair removal using a gentlease 755-nm alexandrite laser. Dermatol Surg 2004;30:494–7.

23. Fiskerstrand EJ, Svaasand LO, Nelson JS. Hair removal with long pulsed diode lasers: a comparison between two systems with different pulse structures. Lasers Surg Med 2003;32:399–404.

24. Handrick C, Alster TS. Comparison of long-pulsed diode and long-pulsed alexandrite lasers for hair removal: a long-term clinical and histologic study. Dermatol Surg 2001;27:622–6.

25. Clayton WJ, Lipton M, Elford J, et al. A randomized controlled trial of laser treatment among hirsute women with polycystic ovary syndrome. Br J Dermatol 2005;152:986–92.

26. Toosi P, Sadighha A, Sharifian A, et al. A comparison study of the efficacy and side effects of different light sources in hair removal. Lasers Med Sci 2006;21:1–4.

27. Smith SR, Piacquadio DJ, Beger B, et al. Eflornithine cream combined with laser therapy in the management of unwanted facial hair growth in women: a randomized trial. Dermatol Surg 2006;32:1237–43.

28. Hamzavi I, Tan E, Shapiro J, et al. A randomized bilateral vehicle-controlled study of eflornithine cream combined with laser treatment versus laser treatment alone for facial hirsutism in women. J Am Acad Dermatol 2007;57:54–9.

29. Sand M, Bechara FG, Sand D, et al. A randomized, controlled, double-blind study evaluating melanin-encapsulated liposomes as a chromophore for laser hair removal of blond, white, and gray hair. Ann Plast Surg 2007;58:551–4.

30. Davoudi SM, Behnia F, Gorouhi F, et al. Comparison of long-pulsed alexandrite and Nd: YAG lasers, individually and in combination, for leg hair reduction: an assessor-blinded, randomized trial with 18 months of follow-up. Arch Dermatol 2008;144:1323–7.

31. Rezvanian H, Adibi N, Siavash M, et al. Increased insulin sensitivity by metformin enhances intense-pulsed-light-assisted hair removal in patients with polycystic ovary syndrome. Dermatology 2009;218:231–6.

32. Braun M. Permanent laser hair removal with low fluence high repetition rate versus high fluence low repetition rate 810 nm diode laser–a split leg comparison study. J Drugs Dermatol 2009;8:s14–7.

33. Haak CS, Nymann P, Pedersen AT, et al. Hair removal in hirsute women with normal testosterone levels: a randomized controlled trial of long-pulsed diode laser vs. intense pulsed light. Br J Dermatol 2010;163:1007–13.

34. Bakus AD, Garden JM, Yaghmai D, et al. Long-term fine caliber hair removal with an electro-optic Q-switched Nd: YAG Laser. Lasers Surg Med 2010;42:706–11.

35. Braun M. Comparison of high-fluence, single-pass diode laser to low-fluence, multiple-pass diode laser for laser hair reduction with 18 months of follow up. J Drugs Dermatol 2011;10:62–5.

36. Pai GS, Bhat PS, Mallya H, et al. Safety and efficacy of low-fluence, high-repetition rate versus high-fluence, low-repetition rate 810-nm diode laser for

permanent hair removal – a split-face comparison study. J Cosmet Laser Ther 2011;13:134–7.

37. Haedersdal M, Beerwerth F, Nash JF. Laser and intense pulsed light hair removal technologies: from professional to home use. Br J Dermatol 2011;165(Suppl 3):31–6.

38. Richards RN, McKenzie MA, Meharg GE. Electroepilation (electrolysis) in hirsutism. 35,000 hours' experience on the face and neck. J Am Acad Dermatol 1986;15:693–7.

39. Görgü M, Aslan G, Aköz T, et al. Comparison of alexandrite laser and electrolysis for hair removal. Dermatol Surg 2000;26:37–41.

40. Shapiro J, Lui H. Treatments for unwanted facial hair. Skin Therapy Lett 2005;10:1–4.

41. Schulze R, Meehan KJ, Lopez A, et al. Low-fluence 1,064-nm laser hair reduction for pseudofolliculitis barbae in skin types IV, V, and VI. Dermatol Surg 2009;35:98–107.

42. Oram Y, Kahraman F, Karincaoglu Y, et al. Evaluation of 60 patients with pilonidal sinus treated with laser epilation after surgery. Dermatol Surg 2010;36:88–91.

43. Tierney E, Mahmoud BH, Hexsel C, et al. Randomized control trial for the treatment of hidradenitis suppurativa with a neodymium-doped yttrium aluminium garnet laser. Dermatol Surg 2009;35:1188–98.

44. Freedman BM, Earley RV. Comparing treatment outcomes between physician and nurse treated patients in laser hair removal. J Cutan Laser Ther 2000;2:137–40.

45. Wheeland RG. Simulated consumer use of a battery-powered, hand-held, portable diode laser (810 nm) for hair removal: a safety, efficacy and ease-of-use study. Lasers Surg Med 2007;39:476–93.

46. Adhoute H, Hamidou Z, Humbert P, et al. Randomized study of tolerance and efficacy of a home-use intense pulsed light (IPL) source compared to the hot-wax method. J Cosmet Dermatol 2010;9:287–90.

47. Spencer JM. Clinical evaluation of a handheld self-treatment device for hair removal. J Drugs Dermatol 2007;6:788–92.

48. Alster TS, Tanzi EL. Effect of a novel low-energy pulsed-light device for home-use hair removal. Dermatol Surg 2009;35:483–9.

49. Shulman S, Bichler I. Ocular complications of laser-assisted eyebrow epilation. Eye (Lond) 2009;23:982–3.

50. Alster TS, Khoury RR. Treatment of laser complications. Facial Plast Surg 2009;25:316–23.

51. Desai S, Mahmoud BH, Bhatia AC, et al. Paradoxical hypertrichosis after laser therapy: a review. Dermatol Surg 2010;36:291–8.

52. Alajlan A, Shapiro J, Rivers JK, et al. Paradoxical hypertrichosis after laser epilation. J Am Acad Dermatol 2005;53:85–8.

53. Moreno-Arias G, Castelo-Branco C, Ferrando J. Paradoxical effect after IPL photoepilation. Dermatol Surg 2002;28:1013–6 [discussion: 1016].

54. Landa N, Corrons N, Zabalza I, et al. Urticaria induced by laser epilation: a clinical and histopathological study with extended follow-up in 36 patients. Lasers Surg Med 2012;44:384–9.

55. Bernstein EF. Severe urticaria after laser treatment for hair reduction. Dermatol Surg 2010;36:147–51.

56. Tetzlaff MT, Evans K, DeHoratius DM, et al. Fox-Fordyce disease following axillary laser hair removal. Arch Dermatol 2011;147:573–6.

57. Hahn I, Hoffman RS, Nelson LS. EMLA-induced methemoglobinemia and systemic topical anesthetic toxicity. J Emerg Med 2004;26:85–8.

Utilizing Electromagnetic Radiation for Hair Growth
A Critical Review of Phototrichogenesis

Sunil Kalia, MD, MHSc, FRCPC*, Harvey Lui, MD, FRCPC

KEYWORDS

- Laser • Ultraviolet radiation • Hair stimulation • Photobiology • Alopecia areata
- Male and female pattern hair loss

KEY POINTS

- Although hair loss is a common medical problem with significant psychological consequences, satisfactory and effective treatment options are somewhat limited.
- Male pattern hair loss (MPHL), female pattern hair loss (FPHL), and alopecia areata (AA) represent the most prevalent disorders for which patients seek medical treatment of hair loss.
- MPHL/FPHL and AA represent the most common hair conditions for which patients consult dermatologists.

INTRODUCTION

Although hair loss is a common medical problem with significant psychological consequences, satisfactory and effective treatment options are somewhat limited. MPHL/FPHL and AA represent the most prevalent disorders for which patients seek medical treatment of hair loss.[1–3] Because conventional medical treatment has proved inadequate in many cases, a variety of novel treatment options have been investigated. Low-level laser therapy (LLLT) has recently been approved by the US Food and Drug Administration (FDA) for the treatment of MPHL/FPHL, and it is currently being studied for AA.[4,5] In this article, the evidence for using LLLT and other forms of light-based treatment for inducing hair growth (ie, phototrichogenesis) is critically reviewed and compared with conventional treatments.

PATTERN HAIR LOSS AND ITS DEPENDENCY ON ANDROGENS

MPHL/FPHL and AA represent the most common hair conditions for which patients consult dermatologists. The specific incidences of MPHL/FPHL vary according to the diagnostic criteria used, with clear trends toward higher prevalences with advancing age.[6] The white population tends to manifest MPHL/FPHL more commonly than Chinese, Japanese, or African American descendants.[7,8] Depending on the age group studied, prevalence estimates have ranged from 16% to 100%.[1,6,9,10] MPHL tends to affect the temporal and vertex areas and has been categorized into different stages with the Norwood-Hamilton classification,[1] whereas FPHL tends to have preservation of the frontal hair region and vertex and is evaluated using the Ludwig scale.[11]

Conflicts of Interest: The authors report no conflicts of interest that are relevant to this article.
Department of Dermatology and Skin Science, University of British Columbia, and Photomedicine Institute, Vancouver Coastal Health, Vancouver, BC
* Corresponding author. 835 West 10th Avenue, Vancouver, British Columbia, V5Z 4E8, Canada.
E-mail address: sunil.kalia@vch.ca

derm.theclinics.com

MPHL has been linked to the downstream effects of testosterone and develops in individuals who are genetically susceptible to the hair miniaturizing effects of androgens on hair follicles.[12] Because men with a genetic deficiency of the enzyme steroid 5α-reductase (5αR) type II do not develop MPHL, this enzyme was hypothesized as playing a pivotal role in the development of MPHL.[13] The enzyme, 5αR, converts testosterone to dihydrotestosterone, and this latter hormone binds 5 times more potently to androgen receptors.[14,15] Two isoforms are present for 5αR. Hair follicles on the scalp and the prostate gland contain mostly 5αR type II. The role of androgens in FPHL is less clear.[16] The duration of the anagen active growth phase is shortened in FPHL, but the detailed mechanism for this is poorly understood.[17] Growth factors have been proposed to play a role and their effects have been demonstrated in mice models, but consistent studies in humans are lacking.[18]

ALOPECIA AND THE IMMUNE SYSTEM

The prevalence of AA seems similar across different population groups, with a lifetime risk of approximately 1.5% to 2% in the general population.[3,19] In the United States, the incidence has been estimated at 0.1% to 0.2% per year and affects male and female patients equally.[20] Although AA most commonly presents with focal nonscarring isolated patches, patients may develop diffuse or refractory cases. Both MPHL/FPHL and AA are linked to severe psychosocial distress and social impairment, and, therefore, individuals with these conditions often seek therapy.[21]

The pathogenesis of AA is currently hypothesized to be an autoimmune mediated hair loss disorder because it is strongly associated with several other autoimmune-based disorders.[22] Furthermore, its relationship with autoimmunity is supported by its response to immunosuppressive agents. At the molecular level, HLA class II antigens are highly expressed in AA hair follicles and are responsible for up-regulating CD4+ T lymphocytes.[23] In addition, antigen-presenting cells, such as macrophages and Langerhans cells, are increased.[24] The hair cycle is also believed altered in AA, and the disruption depends on the stage of AA. In patients with early AA, the anagen phase predominates; however, increased numbers of dystrophic hair follicles are found.[25] With further progression of AA, there is increased follicular conversion to telogen, such that with chronic AA, hair follicles remain suspended in the telogen phase.

CONVENTIONAL MANAGEMENT OF MPHL/FPHL AND AA

Because androgenetic alopecia and extensive, refractory AA represent progressive and chronic conditions, patients seek therapy that is effective but with minimal long-term side effects. Available medical treatment options used to treat MPHL include minoxidil, finasteride, and dutasteride (although dutasteride is not currently FDA approved).[26] FPHL is more difficult to manage, because androgen effects do not seem to play as significant a role. Androgen receptor inhibitors are often not as effective and may be contraindicated, particularly in men.[27] Spironolactone is a viable option in some patients with FPHL. Patients who do not obtain satisfactory response from medical treatments may need to consider hair transplant surgery.[28]

AA is routinely managed with topical and intralesional corticosteroids.[29] Topical minoxidil or anthralin may be used in cases with inadequate response with corticosteroids. Refractory or severe cases may require additional treatment, such as contact therapy with diphenylcyclopropenone, dinitrochlorobenzene, or squaric acid dibutyl ester.[30] Short courses of systemic cyclosporine and corticosteroids are occasionally prescribed in widespread diseases of AA. Hairpieces, wigs, and toupees are other options for patients who find medical or surgical therapy unsatisfactory for extensive hair loss caused by MPHL/FPHL or AA. Despite all these readily available treatment options, there remains a need for more effective management options.

THE CLINICAL PHENOMENON OF LIGHT-INDUCED HAIR GROWTH

The putative effects of light, which is a form of electromagnetic radiation, on hair growth stimulation have been observed empirically by dermatologists, but there has been minimal insight into the responsible mechanisms. Hypertrichosis occurs on light-exposed skin sites in several types of porphyrias, including porphyria cutanea tarda, hepatoerythropoietic porphyria, variegate porphyria, and congenital erythropoietic porphyria.[31] Photoactivated porphyrins produce reactive single oxygen and free radicals that result in subsequent lipid peroxidation and protein cross-linking yielding alteration of cellular and tissue structures. Although it is well understood that porphyrins tend to accumulate with the pilosebaceous unit, the link between the photochemical activation of porphyrins and the induction of hair growth is essentially unknown.[32]

Hypertrichosis has also been reported to occur during psoralen–UV-A (PUVA) therapy. This phenomenon is also poorly understood, but it may be accounted for by the light-induced production growth factors and prostaglandins. There is one documented study where 15 of 23 female patients (65%) receiving systemic PUVA therapy developed moderate-severe hypertrichosis, compared with only 2 of 14 patients on UV-A therapy alone.[33,34] These observations led the author to evaluate 7 male patients receiving 8-methoxypsoralen with UV-A twice weekly. Hair lengthening was noted post-PUVA in all 7 patients after 8 weeks of therapy (range 17%–71%). Other studies, however, that evaluated PUVA patients retrospectively have shown hypertrichosis an uncommon occurrence at only in 4.4% of patients.[33]

Several reports have focused on the seemingly paradoxic development of hypertrichosis after laser epilation. In one retrospective study of 489 patients who were treated with long-pulsed alexandrite laser (755 nm), 3 patients (0.6%) reported increased hair growth after laser hair epilation.[35] This phenomenon tended to occur in darker skin phototypes (Fitzpatrick skin type >IV) and with black hair. The fluence settings used in these patients were 15 J/cm^2 to 40 J/cm^2 at pulse durations between 10 milliseconds and 40 milliseconds. Similar findings of paradoxic hair growth have been reported with the use of intense pulse light.[36] The mechanism for why hair growth is actually stimulated during the course of its attempted removal has not been studied in any detail, but one hypothesis is that the appearance of increased hair may simply reflect that laser treatments may serve to synchronize the hair growth cycles of all the follicles within the laser-exposed sites.[36] Once the hair follicles in a treatment site are synchronized they presumably enter anagen at the same time, such that the overall hair density seems to be increased relative to untreated areas where the hair cycling is typically asynchronous.

These unequivocal observations of increased hair growth in porphyria patients and those who have received PUVA or laser epilation have demonstrated that in principle the energy of electromagnetic radiation can be harnessed to treat hair loss.

LOW-LEVEL LASER THERAPY

LLLT has also been referred to red light therapy, cold laser, soft laser, biostimulation, and photobiomodulation. The characteristics of LLLT that distinguish it from other laser-based therapies, include the use of very low power densities and the requirement for continual maintenance treatment.[37] Most LLLT devices are within the red to near-infrared wavelength range (600–1000 nm) and use power densities much less than that required to heat tissue (10 mW/cm^2–5 W/cm^2).[38] The use of LLLT evolved after its first reported use in humans in the 1960s by the National Aeronautics and Space Administration to promote wound healing. Since then, LLLT devices have been used and promoted to treat patients with strokes, myocardial infarctions, major depression and anxiety, oral mucositis, arthritis, lateral epicondylitis, and carpal tunnel syndrome.[39–42] The hard clinical evidence, however, that LLLT is effective in these conditions is controversial because several studies have shown a lack of improvement.

PROPOSED MECHANISM OF ACTION OF LOW-LEVEL LASER THERAPY

The mechanism of action of LLLT continues to remain poorly understood. Several molecular theories regarding the biostimulatory effect with LLLT have been proposed. Studies have shown that the cellular respiratory chain of mitochondria absorbs LLLT energy. In particular, cytochrome C oxidase, a complex of the integral membrane protein of the inner mitochondria membrane, has an action spectrum ranging from 600 nm to 900 nm. Absorption of photons from LLLT oxidizes cytochrome C oxidase and increases electron transport, leading to increased ATP production. Both calcium ions and cAMP are upregulated via ATP, thus promoting cellular signaling and purportedly allowing for possible hair regrowth. Increased circulation caused by release of nitrogen oxide, promoting vasodilation, also allows for a metabolic boost. Endogenous growth factors, such as basic fibroblast growth factor and insulin-like growth factor, are also upregulated, allowing for cellular proliferation.[43]

A narrow-band red light-emitting diode, 638 nm (Mignon Belle LT-1, Crystalline, Mignon Belle, Osaka, Japan), studied mice in vivo and human dermal papilla in vitro at 1.0 J/cm^2 and 1.5 J/cm^2 respectively.[44] Six shaved BL-6 mice were irradiated with narrow-band red light-emitting diode and compared with placebo; statistically significant increased hair regrowth was detected. Evaluation of dermal papillae revealed agreement with previous observations, demonstrating (1) hair growth acceleration via human growth factor regulation and decreased number of hair follicles entering the catagen phase, (2) induction of anagen phase due to leptin expression, and (3) perifollicular angiogenesis due to vascular endothelial growth factor-A, resulting in increased hair follicle diameter size and accelerated hair regrowth.[44,45]

These theories need to be studied further, because confirmatory studies directly done on hair growth in vivo on humans are lacking. The majority of mechanistic studies are based on extrapolations on wound healing.

RECONCILING LOW-LEVEL LASER THERAPY WITH PHOTOBIOLOGIC PRINCIPLES

If LLLT leads to hair growth, then the mechanisms for this should be in accordance with other known photobiologic principles and reactions that are used therapeutically in dermatology. For all known uses of light in dermatology, the first law of photobiology requires the absorption of a photon by a putative chromophore to a higher energy state. The subsequent release of energy from this excited chromophore then results in either (1) the production of heat to drive photothermal effects or (2) the alteration of biomolecules through photochemical reactions. Because LLLT power densities are not expected to generate much tissue heat, any therapeutic effect on hair growth stimulation presumably arises from photochemistry. All of these photobiologic steps, including the role chromophores and the chemical/biomolecular mediators, are specific. Using the generic term, biostimulation, to describe how LLLT works implies a precision of understanding that has actually not yet been achieved.

Photobiologic effects should be predictable and relevant therapeutic parameters, such as wavelength, fluence, and exposure time, should thus be of critical importance to a large degree. The systematic evaluation of such parameters for LLLT hair growth is not well demonstrated in the literature, including the appropriate action spectrum and detailed dose-ranging studies.

CLINICAL STUDIES EVALUATING LOW-LEVEL LASER THERAPY USED TO TREAT HAIR LOSS

Notwithstanding the lack of a firmly established and well-understood mechanism of action for light-induced hair growth, the key clinical issue is whether LLLT can lead to visibly appreciable hair growth in controlled studies.

Male/Female Pattern Hair Loss

Different laser and light-emitting diodes have been studied to evaluate hair regrowth, including excimer (XeCl, 308 nm), helium-neon laser (HeNe, 632.8 nm), and fractional erbium-glass (1550 nm). The device that has been most thoroughly studied is the HairMax LaserComb (Lexington

International, Boca Raton, Florida), a handheld class 3R lower-level laser therapy device, which contains a single laser module that emulates 9 beams (total maximal output at 45 mW) at a wavelength of 655 nm.[46] Each of the teeth on the combs is aligned with a laser beam. The device is used by parting the user's hair with the comb that is attached to the device, which enhances delivery of the laser light. The study that led to this device's FDA approval was conducted at 4 sites and was a double-blinded, sham device–controlled, multicenter, 26-week trial[46]; 110 men completed the study and were aged 30 to 60 years with MPHL classified as Norwood-Hamilton classes IIa-V and Fitzpatrick skin types I to IV. Subjects were instructed to use the device 3 times per week for 15 minutes, on nonconsecutive days, for a total of 26 weeks. Sites were marked with a tattoo, and a circular area with a diameter of 2.96 cm was evaluated after hair clipping. Through computer-aided counts assessed by scalp macroimaging, the 655-nm laser comb demonstrated a hair density of 19.8 hairs per cm^2 compared with −7.6 hairs per cm^2 for the sham device treatment ($P<.0001$). No statistical improvement was noted on global investigator assessment. Independent prospective investigator studies have not been published to date, and case studies have shown a lack of effect for this particular device.[47]

To date, LLLT has not been compared in a clinical trial against current standard therapies for pattern hair loss, such as minoxidil and finasteride. Both of these treatments have been shown to stabilize pattern alopecia by preventing further hair loss in the long term (ie, at least 1 year). There have been no published studies on the use of LLLT for long-term hair stabilization. Thus, patients who use the laser comb should not necessarily expect that it will result in hair growth that is clinically or visibly apparent nor should they anticipate that it will reliably prevent their pattern hair loss from worsening with time.

Alopecia Areata

The use of the Lexington LaserComb has been studied for AA. Twelve C3H/HeJ mice induced with AA were randomized into 2 groups; 1 received the laser comb treatment (wavelength 655 nm, beam diameter <5 mm, divergence 57 mrad, 9 lasers) whereas the other group received sham-treatment.[48] The laser was given for 20 seconds for each session, 3 times per week for a total of 6 weeks. Hair regrowth was observed in all the mice in the treatment arm after 6 weeks, whereas no mice had regrowth in the sham-treatment group. Histologic evaluation demonstrated increased anagen hair follicles in those treated with the laser comb, whereas the control mice had hair follicles still present only in the telogen phase. Longer-term studies and evaluation need to be conducted in humans for this indication.

Currently, there are insufficient randomized, multicenter controlled trials to prove the efficacy of LLLT. Parameters, such as wavelength, fluence, pulse structure, power density, time, and number of treatment sessions, have not been fully defined for LLLT.[49] Proponents of LLLT claim that studies that demonstrate a lack of efficacy with LLLT are faulted due to inadequate parameter settings, yet there is a significant paucity of rigorous studies evaluating the optimal parameters for hair regrowth.

CLINICAL STUDIES EVALUATING OTHER FORMS OF RADIATION FOR HAIR LOSS

Ultraviolet phototherapy has also been studied for AA. For PUVA the published experience has yielded mixed results. The formation of monoadducts with pyrimidine bases and cross-links with opposite DNA strands inhibits DNA synthesis and culminates in the depletion of infiltrating T lymphocytes.[50] Furthermore, PUVA causes T-cell apoptosis. Studies of topical and oral PUVA differ widely in their results with 15% to 70% of patients experiencing improvement of AA lesions.[51–53] Two large retrospective studies showed no difference in the improvement of AA lesions treated with PUVA compared with control lesions.[52,54] Another device, the 308-nm excimer lamp, induces T-cell apoptosis and might, therefore, be capable of improving AA.[55] With this treatment device, the exposure field is more selective and targeted, which means that higher fluences can be more readily and safely used compared with fluorescent UV lamps. In a study evaluating 3 patients with AA, lesions were treated twice weekly (irradiance 150 mW/cm,^{2} spot size 18.9 cm^2).[56] Lesions were initially treated with a fluence of 150 mJ/cm,^{2} and irradiation doses were increased by 50 mJ/cm^2 until erythema was observed. After 10 treatment sessions, all 3 patients were noted to have hair regrowth. Also promising is 1 case report showing improvement with fractional erbium:glass photothermolysis therapy in a 35-year-old men who was refractory to conventional treatment.[57] Controlled trials are needed to properly assess the effectiveness of the 308-nm excimer lamp and fractional photothermolysis therapy for AA patients.

Topical photodynamic therapy with 5-aminolevulinic acid (ALA) has not been shown to induce hair growth in patients with extensive AA.[58] Six patients with extensive AA had different scalp areas exposed to topical ALA lotion at 5%, 10%, and 20% as well as vehicle lotion alone, followed 3 hours later by red light exposure at each treatment session. After 20 twice-weekly treatment sessions, no significant hair growth was seen between the vehicle and the 3 ALA-treated sites.

FUTURE STUDIES CONDUCTED EVALUATING RADIATION DEVICES FOR HAIR LOSS

Different radiation devices using LLLT are currently being evaluated for MPHL/FPHL, including the Hairmax LaserComb, LaserCap, TopHat 655 Rejuvenation System, and Erchonia ML Scanner devices. Similar to the trial done for MPHL, has been under way at multiple sites evaluating the Hairmax LaserComb in FPHL patients and is now reported as completed, although the results have not yet been disseminated.[59] This phase II study will also be a double-blind, sham-controlled trial evaluating changes in terminal hair count and global assessments and has enrolled 72 patients. The LaserCap (Transdermal Cap, Gates Mills, Ohio) contains 224 laser diodes (total maximum output of 1120 mW) affixed to a mesh framework under a cap. The LaserCap is currently being investigated in multicenter trial to gain FDA approval. A study sponsored by Apira Science is currently evaluating patients aged 18 to 48 years, with hair loss classified as Norwood-Hamilton IIa to V for men and Ludwig I or II for women.[60] This randomized, double-blinded study will evaluate the TopHat 655 Rejuvenation System (Apira Science, Newport Beach, California) in comparison with a sham device that will only contain red incandescent bulbs rather than laser beams at 655 nm. The study is expected to enroll 88 patients. The TopHat 655 system will be worn every other day for 16 weeks for a preprogrammed time period. Erchonia Corporation is currently evaluating their Erchonia ML Scanner (Erchonia Cooperation, McKinney, Texas), in 70 patients with FPHL.[61] Subjects will be randomly assigned to receive the scanner device or a sham device. The exact details of this device, including the laser beam, have not yet been released.

LLLT is also being evaluated for patients with telogen effluvium secondary to chemotherapy. A nonrandomized, open-label, safety/efficacy study is currently evaluating hair preservation with patients receiving chemotherapy for breast cancer.[62] A 670-nm LLLT device with laser beams affixed in a rotating helmet apparatus will be used by 15 subjects twice a week before receiving chemotherapy and once a week until 1 week after the last chemotherapy.

SUMMARY

Hair loss secondary to either MPHL/FPHL or AA is a common problem in the general population. Conventional management for MPHL/FPHL includes the use of minoxidil, finasteride, dutasteride, spironolactone, hair fillers, hairpieces, and wigs.[63] Most AA cases can be managed with intralesional steroids injections, but resistant cases can be treated with anthralin or diphenylcyclopropenone. Despite these available treatment options, LLLT and other forms of radiation have been investigated for both MPHL/FPHL and AA. Consistent results, however, showing beneficial improvement in clinical trials are lacking. Furthermore, LLLT has been criticized for several reasons, including (1) lack of independent peer-reviewed randomized trials showing efficacy, (2) inadequate explanation of LLLT's mechanism of action relating to the pathophysiology of MPHL/FPHL and AA, (3) failure to incorporate the fundamental laws of photochemistry in the mechanism of action for LLLT, and (4) lack of success with anecdotal experience of patients receiving treatment with LLLT. Further studies are being conducted to test the efficacy of LLLT for hair loss using different modes of light delivery.

REFERENCES

1. Hamilton J. Patterned loss of hair in man—types and incidence. Ann N Y Acad Sci 1951;53(3):708–28.
2. Guzman-Sanchez DA, Villanueva-Quintero GD, Alfaro NA, et al. A clinical study of alopecia areata in mexico. Int J Dermatol 2007;46(12):1308–10.
3. Chu S, Chen Y, Tseng W, et al. Comorbidity profiles among patients with alopecia areata: the importance of onset age, a nationwide population-based study. J Am Acad Dermatol 2011;65(5):949–56.
4. Stillman L. Reply to: the use of low-level light for hair growth: part I. J Cosmet Laser Ther 2010;12(2):116.
5. Avram MR, Rogers NE. The use of low-level light for hair growth: part I. J Cosmet Laser Ther 2009;11(2):110–7.
6. Gan DC, Sinclair RD. Prevalence of male and female pattern hair loss in Maryborough. J Investig Dermatol Symp Proc 2005;10(3):184–9.
7. Goh CL. A retrospective study on the characteristics of androgenetic alopecia among asian races in the national skin centre, a tertiary dermatological referral centre in singapore. Ann Acad Med Singap 2002; 31(6):751–5.
8. Severi G, Sinclair R, Hopper JL, et al. Androgenetic alopecia in men aged 40–69 years: prevalence and risk factors. Br J Dermatol 2003;149(6):1207–13.
9. DeMuro-Mercon C, Rhodes T, Girman CJ, et al. Male-pattern hair loss in norwegian men: a community-based study. Dermatology 2000;200(3):219–22.
10. Wang TL, Zhou C, Shen YW, et al. Prevalence of androgenetic alopecia in china: a community-based study in six cities. Br J Dermatol 2010; 162(4):843–7.
11. Norwood O. Incidence of female androgenetic alopecia (female pattern alopecia). Dermatol Surg 2001;27(1):53–4.
12. Carmina E, Rosato F, Janni A, et al. Extensive clinical experience: relative prevalence of different androgen excess disorders in 950 women referred because of clinical hyperandrogenism. J Clin Endocrinol Metab 2006;91(1):2–6.
13. Schweiger ES, Boychenko O, Bernstein RM. Update on the pathogenesis, genetics and medical treatment of patterned hair loss. J Drugs Dermatol 2010;9(11):1412–9.
14. Alsantali A, Shapiro J. Androgens and hair loss. Curr Opin Endocrinol Diabetes Obes 2009;16(3):246–53.
15. Kwack MH, Ahn JS, Kim MK, et al. Dihydrotestosterone-inducible IL-6 inhibits elongation of human hair shafts by suppressing matrix cell proliferation and promotes regression of hair follicles in mice. J Invest Dermatol 2012;132(1):43–9.
16. Messenger AG. Hair through the female life cycle. Br J Dermatol 2011;165(Suppl 3):2–6.
17. Camacho-Martinez FM. Hair loss in women. Semin Cutan Med Surg 2009;28(1):19–32.
18. Hamada K, Randall VA. Inhibitory autocrine factors produced by the mesenchyme-derived hair follicle dermal papilla may be a key to male pattern baldness. Br J Dermatol 2006;154(4):609–18.
19. Roselino A, Almeida A, Hippolito M, et al. Clinical-epidemiologic study of alopecia areata RID F-7487-2010. Int J Dermatol 1996;35(3):181–4.
20. Safavi K, Muller S, Suman V, et al. Incidence of alopecia-areata in olmsted county, minnesota, 1975 through 1989. Mayo Clin Proc 1995;70(7):628–33.
21. Cash TF. Attitudes and practices of dermatologists and primary care physicians who treat patients for MPHL: results of a survey. Curr Med Res Opin 2010;26(2):345–54.
22. Sundberg JP, McElwee KJ, Carroll JM, et al. Hypothesis testing: CTLA4 co-stimulatory pathways critical in the pathogenesis of human and mouse alopecia areata. J Invest Dermatol 2011;131(11):2323–4.
23. Zoller M, McElwee KJ, Engel P, et al. Transient CD44 variant isoform expression and reduction in CD4(+)/ CD25(+) regulatory T cells in C3H/HeJ mice with alopecia areata. J Invest Dermatol 2002;118(6):983–92.
24. Freyschmidt-Paul P, Zoller M, McElwee KJ, et al. The functional relevance of the type 1 cytokines IFN-gamma and IL-2 in alopecia areata of C3H/HeJ mice. J Investig Dermatol Symp Proc 2005;10(3):282–3.
25. Tang L, Cao L, Bernardo O, et al. Topical mechlorethamine restores autoimmune-arrested follicular

activity in mice with an alopecia areata-like disease by targeting infiltrated lymphocytes. J Invest Dermatol 2003;120(3):400–6.

26. Shapiro J, Kaufman KD. Use of finasteride in the treatment of men with androgenetic alopecia (male pattern hair loss). J Investig Dermatol Symp Proc 2003;8(1):20–3.

27. Shapiro J. Clinical practice. Hair loss in women. N Engl J Med 2007;357(16):1620–30.

28. van Zuuren EJ, Fedorowicz Z, Carter B, et al. Interventions for female pattern hair loss. Cochrane Database Syst Rev 2012;(5):CD007628.

29. Alkhalifah A. Topical and intralesional therapies for alopecia areata. Dermatol Ther 2011;24(3):355–63.

30. Gilhar A, Etzioni A, Paus R. Alopecia areata. N Engl J Med 2012;366(16):1515–25.

31. Elder GH. The cutaneous porphyrias. Semin Dermatol 1990;9(1):63–9.

32. Grossman ME, Bickers DR, Poh-Fitzpatrick MB, et al. Porphyria cutanea tarda. Clinical features and laboratory findings in 40 patients. Am J Med 1979;67(2):277–86.

33. Rampen FH. Hypertrichosis in PUVA-treated patients. Br J Dermatol 1983;109(6):657–60.

34. Rampen FH. Hypertrichosis: a side-effect of PUVA therapy. Arch Dermatol Res 1985;278(1):82–3.

35. Alajlan A, Shapiro J, Rivers JK, et al. Paradoxical hypertrichosis after laser epilation. J Am Acad Dermatol 2005;53(1):85–8.

36. Desai S, Mahmoud BH, Bhatia AC, et al. Paradoxical hypertrichosis after laser therapy: a review. Dermatol Surg 2010;36(3):291–8.

37. Chung H, Dai T, Sharma SK, et al. The nuts and bolts of low-level laser (light) therapy. Ann Biomed Eng 2012;40(2):516–33.

38. Bjordal JM. Low level laser therapy (LLLT) and world association for laser therapy (WALT) dosage recommendations. Photomed Laser Surg 2012; 30(2):61–2.

39. Dakowicz A, Kuryliszyn-Moskal A, Kosztyla-Hojna B, et al. Comparison of the long-term effectiveness of physiotherapy programs with low-level laser therapy and pulsed magnetic field in patients with carpal tunnel syndrome. Adv Med Sci 2011;56(2):270–4.

40. Martu S, Amalinei C, Tatarciuc M, et al. Healing process and laser therapy in the superficial periodontium: a histological study. Rom J Morphol Embryol 2012;53(1):111–6.

41. Tumilty S, McDonough S, Hurley DA, et al. Clinical effectiveness of low-level laser therapy as an adjunct to eccentric exercise for the treatment of achilles' tendinopathy: a randomized controlled trial. Arch Phys Med Rehabil 2012;93(5):733–9.

42. Wu Q, Xuan W, Ando T, et al. Low-level laser therapy for closed-head traumatic brain injury in mice: effect of different wavelengths. Lasers Surg Med 2012; 44(3):218–26.

43. Saygun I, Nizam N, Ural AU, et al. Low-level laser irradiation affects the release of basic fibroblast growth factor (bFGF), insulin-like growth factor-I (IGF-I), and receptor of IGF-I (IGFBP3) from osteoblasts. Photomed Laser Surg 2012;30(3):149–54.

44. Fushimi T, Inui S, Ogasawara M, et al. Narrow-band red LED light promotes mouse hair growth through paracrine growth factors from dermal papilla. J Dermatol Sci 2011;64(3):246–8.

45. Feng J, Zhang Y, Xing D. Low-power laser irradiation (LPLI) promotes VEGF expression and vascular endothelial cell proliferation through the activation of ERK/Sp1 pathway. Cell Signal 2012; 24(6):1116–25.

46. Leavitt M, Charles G, Heyman E, et al. HairMax LaserComb laser phototherapy device in the treatment of male androgenetic alopecia: a randomized, double-blind, sham device-controlled, multicentre trial. Clin Drug Investig 2009;29(5):283–92.

47. Rushton DH, Gilkes JJ, Van Neste DJ. No improvement in male-pattern hair loss using laser hair-comb therapy: a 6-month, half-head, assessor-blinded investigation in two men. Clin Exp Dermatol 2012; 37(3):313–5.

48. Wikramanayake TC, Rodriguez R, Choudhary S, et al. Effects of the lexington LaserComb on hair regrowth in the C3H/HeJ mouse model of alopecia areata. Lasers Med Sci 2012;27(2):431–6.

49. Avram MR, Leonard RT Jr, Epstein ES, et al. The current role of laser/light sources in the treatment of male and female pattern hair loss. J Cosmet Laser Ther 2007;9(1):27–8.

50. Healy E, Rogers S. PUVA treatment for alopecia areata—does it work? A retrospective review of 102 cases. Br J Dermatol 1993;129(1):42–4.

51. Sahin S, Yalcin B, Karaduman A. PUVA treatment for alopecia areata. Experience in a turkish population. Dermatology 1998;197(3):245–7.

52. Taylor CR, Hawk JL. PUVA treatment of alopecia areata partialis, totalis and universalis: audit of 10 years' experience at st john's institute of dermatology. Br J Dermatol 1995;133(6):914–8.

53. Weissmann I, Hofmann C, Wagner G, et al. PUVA-therapy for alopecia areata. An investigative study. Arch Dermatol Res 1978;262(3):333–6.

54. Whitmont KJ, Cooper AJ. PUVA treatment of alopecia areata totalis and universalis: a retrospective study. Australas J Dermatol 2003;44(2):106–9.

55. Al-Mutairi N. 308-nm excimer laser for the treatment of alopecia areata in children. Pediatr Dermatol 2009;26(5):547–50.

56. Al-Mutairi N. 308-nm excimer laser for the treatment of alopecia areata. Dermatol Surg 2007;33(12): 1483–7.

57. Yoo KH, Kim MN, Kim BJ, et al. Treatment of alopecia areata with fractional photothermolysis laser. Int J Dermatol 2010;49(7):845–7.

58. Bissonnette R, Shapiro J, Zeng H, et al. Topical photodynamic therapy with 5-aminolaevulinic acid does not induce hair regrowth in patients with extensive alopecia areata. Br J Dermatol 2000;143(5): 1032–5.

59. National Institutes of Health. Treatment of androgenetic alopecia in females, 9 beam. Available at: http://clinicaltrials.gov/ct2/show/NCT00981461?term=lasercomb&rank=4. Accessed on August 1, 15, 2012. Last updated August 7, 2012.

60. National Institutes of Health. Treatment of androgenetic alopecia in males and females (LLLT). Treatment of Androgenetic Alopecia in Males and Females (LLLT), accessed on August 15, 2012. Last updated July 2012.

61. National Institutes of Health. Study of the effect of low level laser light on hair growth on the female human scalp. Available at: http://clinicaltrials.gov/ct2/show/NCT01292746?term=laser+hair&rank=11. Accessed on August 15, 2012. Last updated February 8, 2011.

62. National Institutes of Health. Low level laser therapy for hair preservation with chemotherapy for breast cancer. Available at: http://clinicaltrials.gov/ct2/show/NCT01081106?term=laser+hair&rank=9. Accessed on August 15, 2012. Last updated August 1, 2012.

63. Otberg N, Finner AM, Shapiro J. Androgenetic alopecia. Endocrinol Metab Clin North Am 2007; 36(2):379–98.

Index

A

AA. See Alopecia areata (AA)
Acne keloidalis, 164
  histopathology of, 48
AGA. See Androgenetic alopecia (AGA)
Alexandrite laser
  for hair removal, 182
Alopecia. See also specific types and Hair loss
  androgenetic. See Androgenetic alopecia (AGA)
  cicatricial. See Cicatricial alopecia
  drugs effects on, 68
  frontal fibrosing
    histopathology of, 49
    trichoscopy features of, 36
  immune system and, 194
  noncicatricial. See Noncicatricial alopecia
  nonscarring
    differential diagnosis of, 31–35
    histopathology of, **43–56**
    in SLE, 75–77
  postoperative, pressure-induced
    histopathology of, 52
  psoriatic. See Psoriatic alopecia
    histopathology of, 53–54
    TNF-α–induced
      histopathology of, 54
  scarring
    histopathology of, **43–56**
    in SLE, 77–80
  syphilitic
    histopathology of, 54–55
  in systemic autoimmune diseases, 75–80
  temporal triangular
    histopathology of, 52
  traction
    histopathology of, 51–52
Alopecia areata (AA), 7–9, **93–108**
  abnormalities associated with, 94
  autoimmune diseases and, 113–114
  causes of, 109–110
  clinical picture of, 93–94, 109–110
  differential diagnosis of, 94
  environment and, 8–9
  epidemiology of, 93, 109
  etiopathogenesis of, 95
  genetic basis of, 8, **109–117**
    candidate gene and linkage studies in, 110
    genome-wide association studies in, 111
    hair follicle–specific genes, 113

  immune genes in, 111–113
  histopathology of, 52–53, 96
  hormones and, 8–9
  investigations in, 96
  prognosis of, 95
  treatment of, 96–103
    anthralin in, 98
    azathioprine in, 102
    conventional, 194
    corticosteroids in, 101
      intralesional, 96–97
      topical, 97
    cyclosporine in, 101
    failures, 102
    immunotherapy in
      topical, 98–99
    LLLT in
      evaluation of
        clinical studies in, 196–197
    localized, 96–101
      potential, 100–101
    management plan in, 102–103
    methotrexate in, 101–102
    minoxidil in, 97–98
    phototherapy in, 100
    preventive
      lack of, 110
    prostaglandin analogs in, 99–100
    psychosocial support in, 102
    sulfasalazine in, 101
    systemic, 101–102
  trichoscopy features of, 33–34
Alopecia mucinosa, 160–161
Anagen effluvium
  drug effects on, 68–69
Anagen growth phase
  of hair follicle, 4–5
Anagen hair
  anatomy of, 45
Androgen(s)
  in FPHL, 193–194
  hair growth related to, 11–12
  in MPHL, 193–194
Androgen hormones
  TE related to, 70–71
Androgenetic alopecia (AGA)
  genetics and, 12–13
  histopathology of, 49–50
  hormones and, 12

Dermatol Clin 31 (2013) 201–209
http://dx.doi.org/10.1016/S0733-8635(12)00146-5
0733-8635/13/$ – see front matter © 2013 Elsevier Inc. All rights reserved.

Androgenetic (*continued*)
   molecular mechanism of, 12
   trichoscopy features of, 31–33
Anthralin
   for AA, 98
Antiandrogen(s)
   for FPHL, 121–123
   for hirsutism, 59–61
Anticoagulant(s)
   TE related to, 70
Antimicrobial agents
   TE related to, 70
Autoimmune disease(s)
   hair loss in, **75–91**
      AA, 113–114
      dermatomyositis, 80, 83–85
      fibromyalgia, 86, 88
      scleroderma, 85–86
      SLE, 75–80
     systemic
      alopecia in, 75–80
Azathioprine
   for AA, 102

B

Beard
   hair transplantation for, 150
Bicalutamide
   for hirsutism, 61
Biotin
   hair effects of, 168
Blood vessels
   evaluation of
     in scalp diseases, 31

C

Camouflage
   for FPHL, 123
   hair-styling product techniques in, 177
   for MPHL, 137
Candidate gene studies
   in AA, 110
Cardiovascular drugs
   TE related to, 70
Catagen hair
   anatomy of, 45
CCCA. *See* Central centrifugal cicatricial alopecia
   (CCCA)
CCLE. *See* Chronic cutaneous (discoid) lupus
   erythematosus (CCLE)
Cell therapy/follicular cell implantation
   for MPHL, 137–138
Cellulitis
   dissecting
     histopathology of, 48
     trichoscopy features of, 36–37

Central centrifugal cicatricial alopecia (CCCA), 160
   histopathology of, 46
Chlormadione acetate
   for hirsutism, 60
Chronic cutaneous (discoid) lupus erythematosus
   (CCLE), 157–158
   histopathology of, 47–48
Cicatricial alopecia
   central centrifugal, 160
     histopathology of, 46
   differential diagnosis of, 35–37
   drug effects on, 71
   hair transplantation for, 150–151
   histopathology of, 46–49
   inflammation and, 9
   neutrophilic, 161–163
   primary, **155–166**. *See also* Primary cicatricial
     alopecias
Classic lichen planopilaris
   trichoscopy features of, 36
CLEC16A on chromosome 16p13.13
   in AA, 112–113
Conditioners
   formulation of, 176–177
   for hair loss, **176–177**
Contraceptives
   oral
     TE related to, 70
Copper
   hair effects of, 170
Corticosteroid(s)
   for AA, 101
   intralesional
     for AA, 96–97
   topical
     for AA, 97
CTLA4 on chromosome 2q33.2
   in AA, 111
Cyclosporine
   for AA, 101
Cyproterone acetate
   for FPHL, 122
   for hirsutism, 60

D

Dermatomyositis
   hair loss in, 80, 83–85
Dermatoscopy
   in MPHL diagnosis, 133
Dienogest
   for hirsutism, 60
Diet(s)
   weight loss
     hair effects of, 168
Diode laser
   for hair removal, 182

Discoid lupus erythematosus (DLE), 157–158
  chronic
    histopathology of, 47–48
  trichoscopy features of, 35–36
Dissecting cellulitis
  histopathology of, 48
  trichoscopy features of, 36–37
Dissecting folliculitis, 163–164
DLE. *See* Discoid lupus erythematosus (DLE)
Drospirenone
  for hirsutism, 61
Drug(s)
  hair loss related to, **67–73**. *See also specific
    disorders and drugs*
    alopecia, 68
    anagen effluvium, 68–69
    cicatricial alopecia, 71
    systemic autoimmune disease treatment–
      related, 88
    TE, 69–71
Dutasteride
  for FPHL, 122
  for MPHL, 136
Dystrophic anagen growth phase
  of hair follicle, 6

E

E-One
  for hair removal, 188
Eflornithine
  for hirsutism, 62
Electrolysis
  for hirsutism, 63
Electromagnetic radiation
  for hair growth, **193–200**
Environment
  AA related to, 8–9
  hair disorders associated with, 10–11
Enzyme inhibitors
  for hirsutism, 61–62
EOS/ERBB3 on chromosome 12q13
  in AA, 112
Epidermis
  perifollicular
    evaluation of, 31
Epilation
  physical and chemical
    for hirsutism, 62–63
Essential fatty acids
  hair effects of, 169
Excessive hair
  described, 180–181
  women with, **57–65**. *See also* Women, excessive
    hair growth in
Eyebrow
  hair transplantation for, 149–150

Eyelash(es)
  hair transplantation for, 150

F

Fatty acids
  essential
    hair effects of, 169
Female pattern hair loss (FPHL), **119–127**
  androgens in, 193–194
  defined, 119
  diagnosis of, 119–120
  genetic studies in, 120
  hair transplantation for, 148–149
  pathogenesis of, 120
  treatment of, 120–125
    adjunctive therapies in, 123–124
    androgen-independent agents in, 123
    antiandrogen therapies in, 121–123
    camouflage in, 123
    conventional, 194
    cyproterone acetate in, 122
    dutasteride in, 122
    5-α reductase inhibitors in, 122
    fluridil in, 122
    flutamide in, 122
    fulvestrant in, 122–123
    future directions in, 124–125
    goal of, 120–121
    ketoconazole in, 123
    light therapy in, 123–124
    LLLT in
      evaluation of
        clinical studies in, 196
    minoxidil in, 123
    spironolactone in, 121–122
FFA. *See* Frontal fibrosing alopecia (FFA)
Fibromyalgia
  hair loss in, 86, 88
Fibrosing alopecia
  in patterned distribution
    histopathology of, 49
Finasteride
  for hirsutism, 61–62
  for MPHL, 135–136
5-α reductase inhibitors
  for FPHL, 122
Fluridil
  for FPHL, 122
  for MPHL, 137
Flutamide
  for FPHL, 122
  for hirsutism, 61
Folliculitis
  dissecting, 163–164
Folliculitis decalvans, 161–162
  trichoscopy features of, 37

Folliculitis keloidalis
    histopathology of, 48
Folliscope
    in MPHL diagnosis, 133
FPHL. *See* Female pattern hair loss (FPHL)
Frontal fibrosing alopecia (FFA)
    histopathology of, 49
    trichoscopy features of, 36
Fulvestrant
    for FPHL, 122–123

G

Genetic(s)
    AA and, 8, **109–117**. *See also* Alopecia areata (AA),
        genetic basis of
    AGA and, 12–13
    in FPHL, 120
    hair disorders and, 9–10
    in MPHL, 130
Genome-wide association studies
    in AA, 111

H

Hair
    anagen
        anatomy of, 45
    basic structures of
        evaluation of, 29–31
    catagen
        anatomy of, 45
    excessive
        described, 180–181
        in women, **57–65**. *See also* Women, excessive
            hair growth in
        nutrition effects on, **167–172**. *See also* Nutrition,
            hair effects of
        shampoo effects on, **173–176**. *See also*
            Shampoos
    telogen
        anatomy of, 45
Hair analysis, 167
Hair biology
    basic science of, **1–19**
    contribution to hair disorders, 2–4
        dermatologist's point of view, 2
        hair follicle density, 3
        hair follicle embryogenesis, 2–3
        hair follicle growth rate, 3–4
        hair follicle size, 3
        patient's point of view, 2
Hair breakage
    in hair loss diagnosis, 23
Hair coming out by roots
    in hair loss diagnosis, 22–23
Hair conditioners
    formulation of, 176–177
    in hair loss management, **176–177**
Hair cycle
    contribution to hair disorders, 4–6
    normal, 68
Hair cycle clock, 6
Hair disorders. *See also specific types*
    causes of, 6–13
        environment, 10–11
        genetics, 9–10
        hair biology–related, 2–4
        hair cycle–related, 4–6
        hormones, 11–13
        inflammation, 7–9
    treatment of
        development of, 13–14
Hair follicle(s)
    anagen growth phase, 4–5
    density of, 3
        genetics and, 9
    dystrophic anagen growth phase, 6
    embryogenesis of, 2–3
    exogen event, 6
    growth cycle of
        genetics and, 10
    growth rate of, 3–4
    immune privilege and, 7
    kenogen event, 6
    size of, 3
        genetics and, 10
    telogen phase of, 5–6
    turnover of, 167
Hair follicle cycle, 21
Hair follicle disorder. *See also* Hair disorders
    described, 1–2
Hair follicle openings
    evaluation of, 30–31
Hair follicle–specific genes
    in AA, 113
Hair growth
    androgens and, 11–12
    electromagnetic radiation for, **193–200**
    light-induced
        clinical phenomenon of, 194–195
    LLLT for, 195. *See also* Low-level laser therapy
        (LLLT)
    normal
        defined, 1
Hair loss. *See also specific types and* Alopecia
    autoimmune disease and, **75–91**. *See also*
        Autoimmune disease(s), hair loss in
    conditioners for, **176–177**
    described, 67–68
    diagnosis of, **21–28**
        clinical examination in, 23–27
        laboratory tests in, 27
        patient evaluation in, 21–27

patient history in, 21–23
    scalp biopsy in, 27
drugs effects on, **67–73**. *See also* Drug(s), hair loss
    related to
environment and, 10–11
female pattern, **119–127**. *See also* Female pattern
    hair loss (FPHL)
genetics and, 9
hair grooming for patient with, 177
hormones and, 11
inflammation and, 7
male pattern, **129–140**. *See also* Male pattern hair
    loss (MPHL)
nonscalp
    hair transplantation for, 149–150
nonscarring
    histopathology of, **43–56**. *See also* Hair loss,
        scarring and nonscarring, histopathology of
radiation for
    evaluation of
        clinical studies in, 197
        future studies in, 197
scarring and nonscarring
    histopathology of, **43–56**
        biopsy and processing technique, 44
        cicatricial alopecia, 46–49
        described, 43
        expected findings in transverse sections,
            45–46
        noncicatricial, inflammatory forms of
            alopecia, 52–55
        noncicatricial, noninflammatory forms of
            alopecia, 49–52
    shampoos and, **173–176**. *See also* Shampoos
Hair mount
    in hair loss diagnosis, 25–27
Hair removal
    long-term
        using light, **179–191**
            complications of, 189
            described, 179–180
            efficacy of, 184, 188
            laser and light biophysics, 181
            nonlaser devices, 182
            photoepilation devices, 181–182
            photoepilation techniques, 182–184
            radiofrequency with IPL, 182
            safety of, 189
        skin cooling in, 181
Hair shafts
    abnormalities of
        differential diagnosis of, 38
    evaluation of, 29–30
Hair shedding, 68
Hair transplantation, **141–153**
    for cicatricial alopecia, 150–151
    complications of, 148

described, 141
    donor harvesting for, 142–145
        closure techniques in, 143
        follicular unit extraction in, 143–144
        hair regeneration from bisected follicles
            in, 145
        manual punches in, 144
        motorized and automated punches in, 144
        nonscalp donor area in, 144–145
        robotics in, 144
        strip method in, 142
        trichophytic closure in, 143
    for FPHL, 123
    graft dissection and handling in, 145–147
    indications for, 148–151
        FPHL, 148–149
        MPHL, 148–149
        nonscalp hair loss, 149–150
    postoperative considerations in, 148
    procedural techniques, 141–142
    recipient graft creation and placement in, 147–148
HairDX test
    in MPHL diagnosis, 134
Hirsutism, 181
    diagnosis of, 57–59
    treatment of
        antiandrogens in, 59–61
        electrolysis in, 63
        enzyme inhibitors in, 61–62
        holistic, 63
        laser epilation/photoepilation in, 63
        medical, 59–62
        physical and chemical epilation in, 62–63
HLA on chromosome 6p21.32
    in AA, 111
Holistic treatment
    for hirsutism, 63
Hormone(s)
    AA related to, 8–9
    androgen
        TE related to, 70–71
    hair disorders associated with, 11–13
Hypertrichosis, 181
    diagnosis of, 59–62

I

IL2/IL21 on chromosome 4q27
    in AA, 111
IL13 on chromosome 5q31
    in AA, 112–113
IL2RA on chromosome 10p15.1
    in AA, 112
Immune genes
    AA and, 111–113
Immune system
    alopecia and, 194

Immunotherapy
   topical
      for AA, 98–99
Inflammation
   hair disorders associated with, 7–9
Insulin-sensitizing agents
   for hirsutism, 62
Iron
   hair effects of, 169–170

K

Keratosis follicularis spinulosa decalvans (KFSD), 161
Ketoconazole
   for FPHL, 123
KFSD. See Keratosis follicularis spinulosa decalvans
   (KFSD)

L

Laser epilation
   complications of, 189
   for hirsutism, 63
   safety of, 189
Laser therapy. See also specific types
   for hair removal, 181–182
   low-level
      for hair growth, 195–197. See also Low-level
        laser therapy (LLLT)
   for MPHL, 137
Lichen planopilaris (LPP), 158–159
   classic
      trichoscopy features of, 36
   drug effects on, 71
   histopathology of, 46–47
Light-induced hair growth
   clinical phenomenon of, 194–195
Light therapy
   for FPHL, 123–124
   in hair removal, **179–191**. See also Hair removal
Linkage studies
   in AA, 110
LLLT. See Low-level laser therapy (LLLT)
Low-level laser therapy (LLLT)
   for hair growth, 195–197
      evaluation of
        clinical studies in, 196–197
      with photobiologic principles, 196
      proposed mechanism of action of, 195–196
LPP. See Lichen planopilaris (LPP)

M

Male pattern hair loss (MPHL), **129–140**
   androgens in, 129–130, 193–194
   clinical features of, 131–132
   described, 129

diagnosis of, 132–134
diseases associated with, 134
genetics in, 130
hair-cycle dynamics in, 130–131
hair transplantation for, 148–149
histopathology of, 131
monitoring of
   global photograph in, 136
pathophysiology of, 129–131
treatment of, 134–138
   cell therapy/follicular cell implantation in,
      137–138
   combination therapy in, 136–137
   conventional, 194
   cosmetic camouflage in, 137
   dutasteride in, 136
   emerging, 137–138
   finasteride in, 135–136
   fluridil in, 137
   laser therapy in, 137
   LLLT in
      evaluation of
        clinical studies in, 196
   minoxidil in, 134–135
      vs. finasteride, 136
   prostaglandin analogues in, 137
   surgical, 136
Malnutrition
   hair effects of, 168
Men
   pattern hair loss in, **129–140**. See also Male
      pattern hair loss (MPHL)
Methotrexate
   for AA, 101–102
Minoxidil
   for AA, 97–98
   for FPHL, 123
   for MPHL, 134–135
Moustache
   hair transplantation for, 150
MPHL. See Male pattern hair loss (MPHL)

N

ND:YAG laser
   for hair removal, 181–182
Neodymium:yttrium-aluminum-garnet (Nd:YAG) laser
   for hair removal, 181–182
Neutrophilic cicatricial alopecias, 161–163
Niacin
   hair effects of, 169
No! No!
   for hair removal, 188
Noncicatricial alopecia
   inflammatory forms of
      histopathology of, 52–55
   noninflammatory forms of

histopathology of, 49–52
SLE and, 55
Nonscalp hair loss
hair transplantation for, 149–150
Nutrition
hair effects of, **167–172**
biotin, 168
copper, 170
essential fatty acids, 169
iron, 169–170
malnutrition, 168
niacin, 169
nutritional supplements, 170
proteins, 168
selenium, 170
toxins, 170
vitamins
A, 170
B12, 168
C, 168
D, 170
weight loss diets, 168
zinc, 168–169
Nutritional supplements
hair effects of, 170

O

Oral contraceptives
TE related to, 70

P

Perifollicular epidermis
evaluation of, 31
pH
shampoos and, 176
Photoepilation
for hair removal
anesthesia for, 183
complications of, 189
devices, 181–182
frequency and number of treatments, 184
in home, 188
laser and light treatment parameters in,
183–184
location of sites for, 188
pain control in, 183
patient preparation and selection, 182–183
safety of, 189
scanners in, 184
skin cooling in, 184
techniques, 182–184
vaccuum-assisted treatment in, 184
for hirsutism, 63
home, 188
Phototherapy
for AA, 100

Phototrichogram
in MPHL diagnosis, 133–134
Pluck test
in MPHL diagnosis, 133
PRDX5 on chromosome 11q13
in AA, 113
Primary cicatricial alopecias, **155–166**
acne keloidalis, 164
alopecia mucinosa, 160–161
CCCA, 160
CCLE, 157–158
classification of, 155
clinical findings in, 156
described, 155
diagnosis of, 156
DLE, 157–158
epidemiology of, 155–156
KFSD, 161
LPP, 158–159
lymphocytic, 157–161
management of, 156–157
mixed, 164
neutrophilic, 161–163
pathogenesis of, 155–156
pseudopelade of Brocq, 159–160
Prostaglandin analogues
for AA, 99–100
for MPHL, 137
Protein(s)
hair effects of, 168
Pseudopelade of Brocq, 159–160
trichoscopy features of, 37
Psoriatic alopecia
histopathology of, 53–54
TNF-α–induced
histopathology of, 54
Psychosocial support
for AA, 102
Psychotropic drugs
TE related to, 69–70
Pubic hair
hair transplantation for, 150
Pull test
in hair loss diagnosis, 24–25
in MPHL diagnosis, 132–133

R

Radiation
electromagnetic
for hair growth, **193–200**
for hair loss
evaluation of
clinical studies in, 197
future studies in, 197
Retinoids
TE related to, 70

Robotics
    in hair transplantation, 144
Ruby lasers
    for hair removal, 181

S

Scalp
    normal
        described, 44–45
Scalp biopsy
    in hair loss diagnosis, 27
    in MPHL diagnosis, 134
Scalp diseases
    blood vessel evaluation in, 31
Scanners
    in photoepilation, 184
Scleroderma
    hair loss in, 85–86
Selenium
    hair effects of, 170
Shampoos
    conditioning, 175
    described, 173–174
    hair loss and, **173–176**
        described, 173–174
    pH and, 176
Silk'n
    for hair removal, 188
Skin cooling
    in hair removal, 181
    in photoepilation, 184
SLE. See Systemic lupus erythematosus (SLE)
Spironolactone
    for FPHL, 121–122
    for hirsutism, 60–61
STX17 on chromosome 9q31.1
    in AA, 113
Sulfasalazine
    for AA, 101
Syphilitic alopecia
    histopathology of, 54–55
Systemic lupus erythematosus (SLE)
    hair loss in, 75–80
        noncicatricial alopecia
            histopathology of, 55
        nonscarring alopecia, 75–77
        scarring alopecia, 77–80

T

TE. See Telogen effluvium (TE)
Telogen effluvium (TE)
    drug effects on, 69–71
        androgen hormones, 70–71
        anticoagulants, 70
        antimicrobial agents, 70

        cardiovascular drugs, 70
        oral contraceptives, 70
        psychotropic drugs, 69–70
        retinoids, 70
    environment and, 10–11
    histopathology of, 50–51
    trichoscopy features of, 31
Telogen hair
    anatomy of, 45
Telogen phase of hair follicle, 5–6
Temporal triangular alopecia
    histopathology of, 52
Tinea capitis
    histopathology of, 49
TNF-α. See Tumor necrosis factor–α (TNF-α)
Toxin(s)
    hair effects of, 170
Traction alopecia
    histopathology of, 51–52
Transplantation
    hair, **141–153**. See also Hair transplantation
Tria laser
    for hair removal, 188
Trichogram/pluck test
    in MPHL diagnosis, 133
TrichoScan
    in MPHL diagnosis, 134
Trichoscopy, **29–41**
    in basic hair structures evaluation, 29–31
    in differential diagnoses, 31–38
        AA, 33–34
        AGA, 31–33
        cicatricial alopecia, 35–37
        classic LPP, 36
        dissecting cellulitis, 36–37
        DLE, 35–36
        FFA, 36
        folliculitis decalvans, 37
        hair shaft abnormalities, 38
        pseudopelade of Brocq, 37
        TE, 31
        trichotillomania, 34–35
    UV-enhanced, 38–39
Trichotillomania
    histopathology of, 51
    trichoscopy features of, 34–35
Tug test
    in hair loss diagnosis, 25
Tumor necrosis factor–α (TNF-α)–induced psoriatic
        alopecia
    histopathology of, 54

U

ULBP3/ULBP6 on chromosome 6q25.1
    in AA, 112
Ultraviolet (UV)-enhanced trichoscopy, 38–39

V

Vaccuum-assisted treatment
in photoepilation, 184
Videodermoscope/folliscope
in MPHL diagnosis, 133
Vitamin(s)
hair effects of
A, 170
B12, 168
C, 168
D, 170

W

Weight loss diets
hair effects of, 168

Women
excessive hair growth in, **57–65**. *See also*
Hirsutism
diagnosis of, 57–59
prevalence of, 57
treatment of
medical, 59–62
pattern hair loss in, **119–127**.
See also Female pattern
hair loss (FPHL)

Z

Zinc
hair effects of, 168–169

Printed and bound by CPI Group (UK) Ltd, Croydon, CR0 4YY

03/10/2024

01040346-0003